missing Voices
The Experience of Motherhood

ALS? ✓ CRW PIC

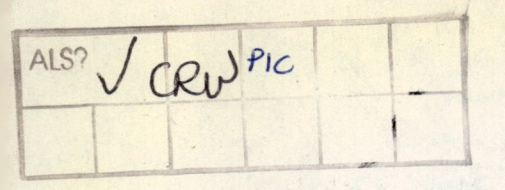

missing Voices
The Experience of Motherhood

STEPHANIE BROWN

JUDITH LUMLEY

RHONDA SMALL

JILL ASTBURY

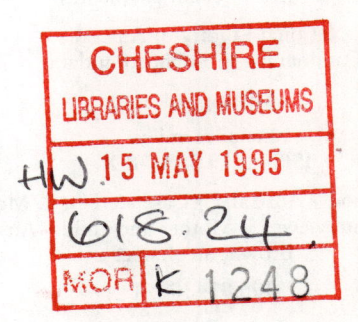

Melbourne
OXFORD UNIVERSITY PRESS
Oxford Auckland New York

OXFORD UNIVERSITY PRESS AUSTRALIA
Oxford New York
Athens Auckland Bangkok Bombay
Calcutta Cape Town Dar es Salaam Delhi
Florence Hong Kong Istanbul Karachi
Kuala Lumpur Madras Madrid Melbourne
Mexico City Nairobi Paris Singapore
Taipei Tokyo Toronto
and associated companies in
Berlin Ibadan

OXFORD is a trade mark of Oxford University Press

© Stephanie Brown, Judith Lumley, Rhonda Small, Jill Astbury 1994
First published 1994

This book is copyright. Apart from any fair
dealing for the purposes of private study,
research, criticism or review as permitted under
the Copyright Act, no part may be reproduced,
stored in a retrieval system, or transmitted, in
any form or by any means, electronic, mechanical,
photocopying, recording or otherwise without
prior written permission. Enquiries to be made to
Oxford University Press.

Copying for educational purposes
Where copies of part or the whole of the book are
made under Section 53B or Section 53D of the Act,
the law requires that records of such copying be
kept. In such cases the copyright owner is
entitled to claim payment.

National Library of Australia
Cataloguing-in-Publication data:

Missing voices.

Includes index.
ISBN 0 19 553378 X.

1. Motherhood – Australia – Case studies. 2. Mothers –
Australia – Interviews. 3. Mother and child – Australia. I.
Brown, Stephanie.

306.87430994

Edited by Jo McMillan
Cover design and illustration by Guy Mirabella
Designed by Guy Mirabella
Typeset by Mackenzies, Victoria
Printed by Australian Print Group, Victoria
Published by Oxford University Press
253 Normanby Road, South Melbourne, Australia

CONTENTS

ACKNOWLEDGEMENTS		vii
PREFACE On Believing Women		1
1	Researching Pregnancy, Birth, Motherhood and Depression	9

The Survey of Recent Mothers

2	Care in Pregnancy	31
3	Thoughts About the Birth Eight Months Later	50
4	Childbirth Classes: Making a Difference?	84
5	Thrown into a New Job	100
6	One in Seven: Depression after Birth	120

The Follow-Up Study

	Introduction	136
7	Troubled Thoughts on Being a 'Good' Mother	139
8	The Experience of Motherhood	161
9	Depression: Women's Voices	173
10	The Social Context of Motherhood	190
11	Balancing Acts: Work and Family	202
12	Three Women's Accounts of Motherhood	227
13	What Women Do About Depression	249
	AN AFTERWORD	263
	APPENDIX 1 Other Research Issues	264
	APPENDIX 2 Glossary of Statistical Terms	271
	APPENDIX 3 Standardised Questionnaires and Obstetric Procedure Score	274
	NOTES	278
	INDEX	295

ACKNOWLEDGEMENTS

First and most we want to thank all the women who took part in the two research projects: the 790 women who filled in a questionnaire, which arrived out of the blue when their babies were eight to nine months old, and the 90 women who allowed us into their homes and talked so candidly and with such feeling about the experience of becoming and being a mother.

Both pieces of research were awarded public health project grants by the Victorian Health Promotion Foundation, with some additional support coming in 1993 from the Foundation's program grant to the Centre for the Study of Mothers' and Children's Health. It would have been impossible to carry out the research without the Foundation's support, and we are grateful for the recognition that this is an important area of public health.

Many other people and institutions played a part. We thank Ann Cartwright and the Institute for Social Studies in Medical Care for permission to adapt the Institute's national postal questionnaire on satisfaction with maternity care for use in an Australian context; the Health Department of Western Australia for permission to use questions contained in their Consumer Survey of Recent Mothers; the women attending Sunbury and Mill Park Maternal and Child Health Centres, and the members of the Post and Ante Natal Depression Association (PaNDA), who took part in the final piloting of the questionnaires and the home interview schedule; the Victorian hospitals and home-birth practitioners who assisted in the distribution of the original survey; the Social Biology Resources Centre, which acted as a financial auspice for the first project; and the members of the Reference Group for the follow-up study (Marion Allen, Dorothy Scott and Ros Stevens).

We thank the editors of the following journals (the Public Health Association and Oxford University Press) for permission to use material that has appeared in the *Australian Journal of Public Health*[1] (Chapters 2 and 6), *Birth*[2] (Chapters 3 and 4), the *Journal of Reproductive and Infant Psychology*[3] (Chapters 8, 9, 10 and 13), the *Medical Journal of Australia*[4] (Chapter 10), *Midwifery*[5] (Chapter 5), *Choice and Change: Ethics, Politics and Economics of Public Health*[6] (Chapters 1 and 3) and *A Dictionary of Epidemiology*[7] (Appendix 2).

We are very grateful to Jen Lunt and Bonnie Simons for their thoughtful transcriptions and to other staff from the Centre for the Study of Mothers' and Children's Health — Anne Potter, Anne Unger, Alison Venn, Lyn Watson, Judith Yates, Jane Yelland — who provided help ranging from advice and feedback on questionnaire design to statistics, computing and financial administration.

We thank Russell Wright, Hans Löfgren and Peter Lumley whose sharing of the responsibility for domestic labour and the care of children made it all possible.

We wish to make it clear that this book is a collaborative effort and we thus share the responsibility for it. What we have done is to give priority in the linear listing of authors to the Centre for the Study of Mothers' and Children's Health, which was the auspice for the research projects. However, the end of each chapter is annotated to show our relative contributions to its production.

PREFACE

On Believing Women

John Stuart Mill, the 19th-century British philosopher, in one of the earliest formulations of the need for women-centred research, wrote 'respecting the mental characteristics of women': 'It is a subject on which nothing final can be known, so long as those who alone can really know it, women themselves, have given but little testimony, and that little, mostly suborned.'[1] Unusually for his time, Mill believed that women possessed crucial knowledge about themselves. Even today, as we shall see, such a view is still far from being unequivocally endorsed by those carrying out research and deciding what should be published in the journals concerned with professional practice, especially where childbearing women are concerned.

Ann Oakley in *Women Confined* documented a number of telling exchanges between childbearing women and their doctors.[2] The following interchange witnessed by Oakley illustrates just how little women can be thought to know by their medical attendants.

Doctor (reading case notes): Ah, I see you've got a boy and a girl.
Patient: No, two girls.
Doctor: Really, are you sure? I thought it said ... (checks in case notes) oh no, you're quite right, two girls.

Significantly, the generous admission by the doctor that the woman is right about the sex of her children, does not come about because he realises he is being ludicrous in asking if she is sure, but from his own checking of the medical case notes, reinforcing the idea that a source of knowledge outside the woman has a higher level of credibility than anything she might say.

In the research that forms the basis of this book we started from a different vantage point and an opposite set of assumptions. The focus of our study was deliberately on women's own views of their childbearing experiences from pregnancy to the postpartum period. We asked women to tell us what they knew, how satisfied they were with the birthing services they received, and what they liked and disliked about their medical and nursing care. We asked them to describe what happened to them in the course of their childbearing and we proceeded on the assumption that we could believe what they said — that they did know what they were talking about. For this reason, we have made extensive use both of the written comments about childbirth that women made on the survey forms, and of quotations from the interview transcripts. The questions we asked were also informed by our knowledge of the issues that are of concern to women. For example, the questionnaire used in the eight-month survey included several questions seeking women's views about issues that women attending public meetings during the Ministerial Review of Birthing Services in Victoria had raised as problematic for them. Further, in our interviews with women two years after the birth of their babies, one of the questionnaires we used, on the experience of motherhood, was based on the many years of clinical experience of one of the authors concerning the life changes and emotional issues women themselves brought up in interviews that formed part of a longitudinal follow-up study of pre-term infants.[3] Indeed, the follow-up study was built around exploration of issues that we were aware women saw as pertinent to their experiences after having a child.

We were also ourselves 'subjects' in the research process. Each of us is a mother. When we began this project we had children ranging in age from three to 21 years, and two of us each had another child during the course of the project. Our own interest in, and enjoyment and awareness of, the emotional strain involved in caring for young children was vividly relived as we sat in women's kitchens and shared their experiences. We were not passive observers in women's homes recording their lives as hard-and-fast, objective data — nor did we seek to be. Sandra Harding argues that 'the class, race, culture and gender assumptions, beliefs and behaviours of the researcher her/himself must be placed within the frame of the picture that she/he attempts to paint'.[4] In this way the researcher is not, according to Harding, 'an invisible, anonymous voice of authority', but an active participant in the research process. Most 'scientific' research proceeds on the assumption that correct method renders 'good' research entirely objective. This is an assumption we would dispute, and for this reason we have tried to make our own constitutive role in designing and conducting the two studies apparent.

Our assumption that women can be believed when they report on their lives — that their reports have indisputable authenticity — is still seen as extremely dubious. This is illustrated by the letters we received from professional journals rejecting a paper — subsequently published elsewhere — about the links between postnatal depression and women's obstetric experiences (see Chapter 6). A fundamental objection to the paper was that we relied on and believed what women told us. The assistant editor of the *British*

Medical Journal wrote expressing concern that the 'data depend very much on recall of events during labour and pregnancy and no attempt is made *to validate the mothers' recall with what actually happened*' [emphasis added].

This view closely recalls the attitudes towards women's words expressed by clinicians in Ann Oakley's book. From both a scientific and a clinical perspective, it is clear that women are seen as unreliable informants who do not know what has happened to them and who cannot and should not be believed without corroborating evidence from a superior source. From this perspective, it does not seem at all odd to question whether women can be relied upon to recall if their labour was induced, or if they had a caesarean section, a birth assisted by forceps or an epidural anaesthetic.

A reviewer for the *British Journal of Psychiatry* saw the key problem as distortion and contamination rather than mere recall: he or she believed that if women were depressed eight months after giving birth then nothing they had to say about their experience of pregnancy, labour, birth or the postpartum period was relevant because it would be 'contaminated with a depressive memory distortion'. In this view, depression is seen as the cause of expressed dissatisfaction about antenatal care or adverse events of labour, rather than as a possible effect of these stressful events. Apart from anything else, such a view precludes an examination of, or changes to, maternity services so as to meet the criticisms of depressed women — if anything they say can be dismissed as 'unreliable' and 'distorted', then the status quo can be maintained unquestioningly.

'There is no need to write about satisfaction, dissatisfaction of maternity services and so forth.' The reviewer expressed the belief that depressed women 'will talk about everything in an ill light ... and many of them must have been complaining and feeling angry about labour when in fact this must represent the depressive distortion rather than the statements made at the time of labour.'

The strength of the belief in the primacy of 'depressive distortion' over the credibility of women's anger and grievances is illustrated by the use of the word 'must' on two occasions. In the absence of any supporting evidence, the only reason that women's anger and dissatisfaction 'must' be due to depressive memory distortion is if one holds to a theory of depression that deems this to be so. Two unpleasant intellectual and emotional operations are avoided; one relates to examining and paying attention to the quality of maternity services about which women express discontent. The other concerns questioning a model of depression that holds that women's opinions of why they are depressed is of little or no account, either theoretically or in deciding on appropriate intervention. The reviewer seems to believe that if a woman is depressed and complains and expresses anger about her obstetric care, then both her anger and criticisms should be disregarded as unrealistic and distorted.

To what extent women's opinions about the causes of their depression should be given credence over the opinions of others, including health-care professionals, may perhaps be questioned. What has been unequivocally established is that women's recall of being depressed is highly reliable.

John Cox and his colleagues, who have done extensive research into postnatal depression, found that women's recall of depression was accurate. 'Furthermore, the results of a follow-up study showed that postnatal depression was usually accurately recalled by the mothers *3 years later*'[5] [emphasis added]. This research shows that women did not suffer from memory distortion and, in fact, were able to remember and describe their feelings of depression three years after the event.

The assertion that women who are depressed see everything in a pervasively bleak light was also not borne out by the findings of our own study. Neither was the argument that because we asked women about their experiences of pregnancy and childbirth some eight months after birth, the findings would be unreliable. When we undertook the second part of our study, some two years after the births, we were able to check how accurately the same women remembered how they were feeling eight to nine months after the birth of their infants. We found the overwhelming majority of women could clearly remember if they had been depressed at the earlier time and why.

The way in which the salience or significance of an event might affect one's recollection of it,[6] does not seem to occur to the proponents of the 'women never know' school. Thus, having a caesarean section is apparently placed on a flat plane of memorability where no event is intrinsically more (or less) memorable than any other. Birth events, from this perspective, have no greater likelihood of being accurately recalled by women than when a bill was paid or what they ate for dinner three weeks ago. A forceps delivery or caesarean birth might be something one forgets, imagines, or remembers only hazily, and it therefore becomes imperative to check women's recall against 'what actually happened'.

It is not immediately obvious why medical records should be seen as a more accurate source of the 'facts', of 'what actually happened', than the woman herself. Indeed, several studies have been carried out on the congruity between mothers' reports and their obstetric records. Two important findings emerge from this research; first, maternal recall is highly accurate, and second, obstetric records can fall far short of constituting a faultless gold standard against which all other forms of evidence can be validly measured.[7]

In 'woman-centred' research, women are acknowledged as active, conscious, intentional authors of their own lives. As an ideal, this notion of 'woman-centred' research is appealing. As a description of reality, however, the term 'woman-centred' is not entirely satisfactory because it seems to suggest that women can occupy a powerful, authoritative and controlling position in their lives; lives often hemmed in by social arrangements and structural inequalities not of their own making.

Harding,[8] in a discussion of the influence of gender in the construction of theories of knowledge, notes how any epistemology, even if this is done implicitly, offers answers to questions about who can be a 'knower'. She then asks 'can women?'. This is the question that John Stuart Mill answered affirmatively, but which still generates doubt, as the above examples demonstrate. Woman-centred research proceeds on the assumption that women can indeed be knowers. This is a deliberately self-conscious assumption, which in part serves to highlight the structural inequalities of a research tradition in which women have not been thought of as capable of constructing knowledge, have not carried out most of the research or defined the problems worth researching, and have mainly occupied the role of research 'subjects' or research assistants; the researched rather than the researchers.

Traditional philosophy of science holds that the origin of scientific problems, the 'context of discovery', is inconsequential; what is important is the 'context of justification', or the process by which hypotheses are tested. But as Harding argues, 'the questions that are asked — and, even more significantly, those that are not asked — are at least as determinative of the adequacy of our total picture as are any answers that we can discover.' She goes on to say that 'defining what is in need of scientific explanation only from the perspective of bourgeois, white men's experiences leads to partial and even perverse understandings of social life. One distinctive feature of feminist research is that it generates its problematic from the perspective of women's experiences. It also uses these experiences as a significant indicator of the "reality" against which hypotheses are tested.'

Typically, within the framework of positivistic science women have been primarily positioned as passive, unreflective and uninformed sources of 'raw data'. This data is considered to belong to the researcher, on the grounds that only he (more rarely, she) has the proper qualifications to analyse it and extract its meaning. In the past there has been no ethical requirement that research findings should be taken back to the people researched. The researcher uses the results to construct a plausible scientific account structured by the hypotheses that the results are thought to confirm or refute. However, the notion that the data 'speak for themselves' in a completely impartial, archetypally 'scientific' way overlooks the part that can be played by interpreter bias. The interpretation of data has been found to vary widely between different groups of scientists and is influenced by such things as culture, commitment to a particular school of thought, and contextual factors.[9] Further, when there is the same amount of evidence *for* a preferred theory as *against* it, scientific researchers will judge the evidence that supports their preferred theory as significantly 'more convincing' and 'better conducted' than evidence that opposes it.[10]

From the outset, the way in which a problem is selected, defined and formulated will be affected by the value structure, interests, goals and motives of the researcher, not on purely logical or impartial grounds.[11] For this reason we have attempted to state our own roles and interests in the research that forms the basis of this book.

Despite some reservations about the term 'woman-centred' research, a strength of this model as a way of approaching research is that it relies on, and considers valid, women's own words and interpretations of events. It is research in which the 'subjects' actually remain as subjects, rather than being transformed into objects. Women's judgements, evaluations, and the meanings they make of their experiences are a central rather than a peripheral feature of such research, and these considerations powerfully inform our work on the experience of motherhood.

Although much research effort has been dedicated to establishing a causal connection between women's reproductive processes and their mental health and well-being, there seems to be an inverse relationship between the effort expended in trying to prove this link and the actual knowledge that has resulted. Thus, a recent comprehensive review of the evidence linking women's reproductive functioning to four supposed psychiatric syndromes (postpartum depression, pre-menstrual syndrome, post-hysterectomy depression and involutional melancholia) found little in the way of well-designed, properly executed studies, or reliable research evidence to support commonly held beliefs.[12] The review concluded that postpartum depression actually comprised three separate syndromes, that the effective study of pre-menstrual syndrome was awaiting the development of improved methodologies, and that there was no evidence for either post-hysterectomy depression or involutional melancholia.

The researchers argued that the current poor level of understanding of the relationship between reproductive functioning and women's emotional states arises because past research has been characterised by unwarranted assumptions and untenable conclusions. Many flawed studies were directed by myths and culturally biased attitudes towards women. As a result, research to date has been far from objective or impartial. These researchers assert that supposed observations of women actually tell us more about the psychology of the observer, usually male, than anything worthwhile about the psychology of the observed.

Much of the research on reproduction and mental well-being attempts to find the cause or causes of a positive or negative childbearing experience within the woman herself. It is as if childbearing occurs within a social and cultural vacuum, that nothing happens to the parturient woman and that no one else, least of all medical or nursing personnel, contribute anything to the quality of her experience by determining whether it is positive or negative. This emphasis on 'within person' variables has also been found in research undertaken on such problems as alcohol and drug abuse, delinquency, rape, and race relations: the majority of studies reviewed from the years 1936, 1956 and 1976 relied upon theories that attributed these problems to personality variables.[13]

The bulk of existing research is reminiscent of two people in a darkened room. One, the researcher, has a torch, which is turned on and shone at the other person, the parturient woman, who seems to be the only one there. The person holding the torch remains hidden in darkness, as does the rest of the room. We wanted in this study to look at the whole room and at the practices that occurred there, including the tests, interventions and obstetric procedures used.

We were interested in what childbearing women thought of the people who provided the care and administered the tests, interventions and procedures, and how these affected the childbearing experience and women's emotional well-being. Unlike most previous researchers, we were more interested in what women thought of their care-providers than in what care-providers thought of women. We also wanted to discover what role women felt they were able to play in decision making and how far this depended on whether their care-giver was a doctor or a midwife, or whether they gave birth in a labour ward or a birth centre. We were also vitally interested in how the social context in which women experienced motherhood itself impacted upon and shaped this experience.

In this way, our research is an example of 'researching up' rather than 'researching down', in that it did not set out with the preconception that the problem resides within the woman and her psyche or endocrine system, nor that these factors will ultimately yield 'the answer' to the problem if they are searched thoroughly enough.[14] Conversely, care-providers and their practices are not assumed to be unproblematic and outside the arena for exploration. Rather, care-givers are viewed as active and influential contributors to the way in which a woman constructs her pregnancy, birth and postpartum experience.

Our research attempts to provide a fuller picture of the experience of motherhood. It departs from previous research that has sought to find 'the cause' of postnatal depression in intrapsychic pathology and/or hormonal factors. Our study does not attempt to measure changes in hormones; there are many others available to carry out that research. We believe that because potentially significant factors outside this sphere, especially women's own views, have often been ignored in much existing research, our current understanding of what contributes to mothers' emotional well-being on the one hand, and emotional distress on the other, remains incomplete and distorted. We hope that our research will go some way towards redressing this situation.

Jill Astbury, Stephanie Brown, Judith Lumley

ONE

Researching Pregnancy, Birth, Motherhood and Depression

INTRODUCTION
The reasons for beginning this book with a description of the research methods are two-fold. The first and most important was to give a sense of what research involves and to demystify the process for those unfamiliar with it. The second was to bridge the divide that often separates those interested in different ways of doing research by describing the variety of research approaches we took to explore what happens to women in becoming and being mothers.

BACKGROUND
In the late 1980s health ministers in three Australian States (New South Wales, Western Australia and Victoria) commissioned reviews of the health services involved in the care of women during pregnancy and birth.[1] These reviews involved consultation with those who used the services and those who provided the services: calling for written submissions; holding public meetings; meeting with consumer and professional organisations; and meeting with hospitals. One of the most controversial questions to arise during the Ministerial Review of Birthing Services in Victoria was how representative the consumer perspectives gleaned through consultations and submissions were. It was often said that it was mainly middle-class women with 'unrealistic' expectations who complained about their experiences of maternity care. An application was made for a research grant to conduct a postal survey of recent mothers in order to obtain a representative picture of what Victorian women thought about maternity care. The two resulting projects are the basis for this book.

SURVEY OF RECENT MOTHERS
We originally planned to base the survey on a single sample comprising all women who gave birth in Victoria in a one-week period (6–12 February) in 1989. We intended to send questionnaires to women about six months after the births of their babies. All

Victorian maternity hospitals and home-birth practitioners were contacted in June or July 1989 and asked to assist the project, either by agreeing to post questionnaires to women listed in their records as having given birth during the chosen period or by providing a mailing list on a confidential basis to the project's research officer.

As the study called for participation by almost 150 maternity hospitals we sought initial approval from the Ethics Committee of the Health Department of Victoria, a process that took more than six months. Although this committee was established to circumvent problems associated with multiple applications to separate hospital ethics committees, each requiring a project summary and specific forms, many hospitals still wanted their own committees to review the project before agreeing to participate. This delayed the project considerably, and even jeopardised the original aim of providing information to the Review of Birthing Services.

Eventually, all but one country-based private hospital, which had twelve births in the chosen week, agreed to participate. One major hospital did not respond until March 1990 and as the mailing of the questionnaires could not be delayed if we were to make a submission to the review group, this hospital was omitted from the February survey period. Instead, the survey period for this hospital was the second week in September 1989. Due to the delay in obtaining permission for the study, women were sent the questionnaires eight to nine months after the birth of their babies, not six months as originally intended.

Research into women's views of maternity care has found that women are less likely to be critical of their care immediately after birth. This suggests that there is a 'halo' around the birth following the arrival of a healthy baby.[2] With time, this effect wears off. A more critical account is given in the second half of the year after birth as women reflect on the experience.[3]

Most hospitals sent the questionnaires directly to women, sometimes adding their own covering letter. A few, mostly smaller hospitals, gave us a mailing list. We requested that any mother whose baby had been stillborn or whose baby had died since birth be excluded (an estimated number of 10 to 20 babies in Victoria in any one week). In all, 1193 women were sent questionnaires.

Three mailings took place at two-weekly intervals. Each time women were sent a covering letter, the questionnaire, and a freepost envelope for its return. The covering letter was addressed by the researchers and printed on Melbourne's Social Biology Resources Centre letterhead, which was the auspice body for the project. This letter made it clear that the study was being undertaken across the State, that it was independent of individual hospitals or service providers, and that all information provided would be regarded as completely confidential. As no identifying information was sought, women were reassured that their replies were truly anonymous. The letter also stated clearly that any woman who did not wish to participate should feel free not to.

A brief explanation of the study, translated into six languages (Arabic, Cambodian, Chinese, Spanish, Turkish and Vietnamese), was included with all covering letters. The six languages were chosen in consultation with the Ethnic Affairs Commission and major public hospitals after checking the pattern of mothers' countries of birth across Victoria.

Considerable thought was given to ways of facilitating the involvement of women of non-English speaking backgrounds (NESB) in the study. Work in other countries[4] had demonstrated that women of NESB tend to be under-represented in postal surveys of this kind. We considered two options. The first was translating the questionnaire into all community languages. The second was offering the option of a telephone interview with a trained bilingual interviewer. Both options involved substantial costs not covered in the grant. We were wary of the second option because the comparison of structured telephone interviews with postal questionnaires in the United Kingdom had shown that the higher response rate by Asian mothers gave limited information: four-fifths of the responses were categorised as not satisfactory by the interviewer.[5] In addition, when we discussed this option with people working with ethnic communities, it seemed that a home-based interview would be preferable, given the breadth of topics covered by the questionnaire. Not only were there insurmountable cost factors, but we would have ended up comparing two groups of women studied in different ways.

The other option, translating the questionnaire into community languages, was also not satisfactory. Once again, people working with ethnic communities suggested that we were likely to encounter difficulties, particularly among ethnic groups in which literacy levels, even in their own language, were not high or for whom the technical language involved might prove difficult even in translation. A further practical problem was that we were unable to mail questionnaires in the appropriate language directly to each woman because of the emphasis on confidentiality in the research design. Hence we would have had to rely on women responding to our brief account of the study in their own language by telephoning us to ask for a copy of the translated questionnaire, an added hurdle that we anticipated would dissuade many women from participating.

Despite these concerns we decided to translate the questionnaire into two community languages, Vietnamese and Arabic, and included an invitation to women speaking these languages to contact the research officer for a translation. Our funds would cover the costs of only two translations.

The reason for sending out three copies of everything was also linked to the research design. Usually, when a questionnaire is sent out, those who have not replied after two weeks are sent a reminder letter or perhaps telephoned. If this is unsuccessful they get a second reminder, sometimes with a new copy of the questionnaire. The anonymity of our survey, the fact that hospitals sent it out, and that women were not asked to supply their names, meant that we could not use the usual reminder system. Instead we asked hospitals to send out all the material three times, as this is necessary to get a good response rate. We then had to make sure that no one had sent us more than one reply!

The questionnaire consisted of an A5-size booklet containing 66 pre-coded questions and a blank page for comments. Questions covered information about the baby and any previous pregnancies; antenatal care; labour and delivery; postnatal care; socio-demographic information such as the mother's age, country of birth, income, education, marital status and health insurance status. They were designed to find out what had actually happened — what procedures were used, who provided care, what pain relief was used, whether the woman breastfed, etc. — and also how satisfied women were with the care they received, about their preferences for future births, and about their emotional well-being at the time they received the questionnaire.

Developing the Questionnaire

In the development of any questionnaire there is a great deal of what could be called 'informal pilot testing'. Friends and colleagues are asked to examine a draft version and criticise the questions, the format, the language, the sequence of the questions, and to draw attention to any omissions. This developmental work was made easier in the case of our questionnaire since the survey was modelled on national population-based surveys of satisfaction with maternity care developed at the Institute for Social Studies in Medical Care in England.[6]

We made slight modifications to the institute's longer survey instrument to fit the Australian context. Our questionnaire also incorporated questions from a similar survey being conducted concurrently for the Western Australian Ministerial Task Force to Review Obstetric, Neonatal and Gynaecological Services.[7] New questions were added to deal with issues specific to the terms of reference of the Ministerial Review of Birthing Services in Victoria, including some arising from the submissions and public meetings that were part of the community consultation.[8] The questions relating to length of stay in hospital after birth, for example, were added for this reason. Another addition, which turned out to be very significant, was the inclusion of the Edinburgh Postnatal Depression Scale (EPDS).

Many of the hospital ethics committees wondered whether women would understand the questions we asked. We tried to make the language as clear as possible, and where technical language *was* used we provided a brief explanation in brackets. For example, 'induction of labour' was also described as 'a drip or breaking your waters/membranes to start off contractions'. The option of 'don't know' was also given where women might have been unfamiliar with particular procedures or with the terminology used to describe them.

Another issue was the possible need to compare women's recollections with 'what really happened' according to hospital records. Given the confidentiality and anonymity requirements of the study, we could not have sought permission for access to medical records across the State. Even if it had been possible it would have added very little to the study. Comparisons of women's reports about the events of pregnancy and labour with their hospital notes have been studied extensively, the conclusion being that women do know and can tell.

There are a few exceptions to this general rule, notably the distinction between induction of labour (starting labour off) and augmentation of labour (speeding up a labour which started spontaneously). Since these distinctions are known to be prone to error, even in official information systems,[9] it is not surprising that they are also problematic in surveys.

The issue of the acceptability of the questionnaire to women receiving it was also raised by some ethics committees, particularly the questions about past contraception, whether the pregnancy had been planned, and whether women planned to have more children. Two hospitals objected to one or two of these questions, which were subsequently deleted. The acceptability of the questionnaire was examined in the piloting phase, with no one indicating that any question was intrusive or unacceptable.

The questionnaire was pre-tested in Maternal and Child Health Centres in Sunbury and Mill Park. These two locations were chosen to ensure that twenty women from a range of social backgrounds were involved. Women attending the centres for routine appointments, mostly women with babies under twelve months old, were asked to complete a questionnaire with one of the authors there to answer any questions, to check whether any of the questions were unacceptable to recent mothers, and to identify any questions or terms that were not readily understood. As a result of this process some minor modifications were made to the wording and layout of the questionnaire.

Sample Size
A one-week period, yielding a potential sample of 1193 women, was selected for three reasons: to minimise confusion about the study dates for hospital staff mailing the questionnaire; to satisfy service-providers and professionals that at least 1 per cent of all births in Victoria in 1989 would be included; and to ensure that the study would include large enough numbers of certain groups of women to allow comparison of their satisfaction with care with that of the whole sample. Examples of these groups were women living outside the metropolitan area (perhaps 175 to 200 responding) and those who had a caesarean birth (perhaps 100 to 120 responding). Another group of special interest was women of NESB, where the potential sample was 150 to 175 women giving birth in a week, but in their case we were much less confident about what the response rate would be. Since very few women in Victoria give birth at home (two to four a week) or in a birth centre (1 to 2 per cent of births), we knew in advance that the sample would not be large enough to assess differences in these women's experiences.

Who Replied to the Questionnaire?
In Victoria, as in other Australian States, the Health Department collects detailed information on all births that occur within State boundaries.[10] This includes information about the mother herself — unfortunately there is nothing about fathers — about her pregnancy, labour, birth and immediate hospital stay, and about the baby's size and condition at birth and immediately afterwards. We were able to use this information to describe the characteristics of all the women who gave birth in the chosen weeks and to compare these characteristics with those of the women who sent back the questionnaires. We were able to assess the extent to which the mother's age, marital status or country of birth affected the likelihood of her participation in the study.

Responders and Non-Responders
A total of 799 completed questionnaires were returned. Nine had to be excluded because the baby's date of birth fell outside the study weeks or because they duplicated a form already sent in by the same woman. This left 790 replies. Another 77 questionnaires were returned undelivered, the majority because the woman had moved house since the birth or was not known at that address. The final response rate was 790/1107 (71.4 per cent). This is likely to be an under-estimate since households who did not return the envelope when the addressee was unknown would not have been identified as such. Some other women who received the survey booklet would have been unable to read English and, as discussed

above, our strategies for assisting them to respond were very limited. Given that every woman who received the questionnaire had an eight to nine month old baby, the response rate was highly satisfactory and strong evidence of the acceptability of this method of finding out women's views. Several women wrote comments on the form or rang the research officer to say how much they had enjoyed filling in the questionnaire and how glad they were that a study like this was being done. The response rate was within the range of similar studies elsewhere,[11] including the survey carried out in Western Australia in the same year for its review of maternity services.[12]

When we compared women who responded with all the women who should have received questionnaires we found that the groups were very similar in several important ways. Women living in the city and those living in the country were equally likely to respond. Those who responded were also representative in terms of their method of birth (spontaneous vaginal, caesarean, forceps, vacuum), the birthweight of their babies, the number of previous children, and the length of their hospital stay after birth.

There were, however, some important differences between those who responded and those who did not. Women born overseas in countries where English is not the first language were less likely to respond. There were 181 births to women in this category in the survey week, with 92 returning a completed form (50.8 per cent). The strategies of providing brief information about the study in six community languages and of making the questionnaire available in two of them did not work. Only one request for a copy of the questionnaire in Arabic was received and none was received for a Vietnamese translation.

Young women were another group with a low response rate. Only eleven of the 53 women under 20 years (20.8 per cent) and 78 of the 201 women aged 20 to 24 years (38.8 per cent) responded. These two groups overlap substantially with the other group of women who had a low response: among single women, two-thirds of whom would have been under 25 years, only 26 of 89 responded (29.2 per cent). The extra pressures of being young or single or both while also dealing with a new baby probably explain the low response rate. It is also likely that more of these young women had moved since the birth. This low participation rate by young women and women of NESB has been found consistently in community surveys[13] and it must be recognised as one of the limitations of the postal method. It always has to be borne in mind in the interpretation of the questionnaire findings. By contrast, women in another age group, those who were 30 to 34 years old at the time of birth, had an extremely high response rate: 304 of 332 (91.6 per cent) replied. A brief summary of some social and demographic characteristics of women who replied to the questionnaire is given in tables 1.1 and 1.2.

Table 1.1 Characteristics of the survey sample and of all Victorian births, 1989

		1989 Survey (%)	Victoria (%)
Maternal age	Under 20	1.4	4.3
	20–24	10.1	18.8
	25–29	38.6	38.7
	30–34	39.1	27.9
	35–39	9.1	9.0
	40 and over	1.8	1.3
Marital status	Married	88.7	84.7
	De Facto	6.3	5.1
	Single	3.3	8.9
	Other	1.7	1.3
Place of birth	Australia	78.7	75.4
	ESB*	9.5	9.2
	NESB**	11.8	15.4
Residence	Melbourne	71.7	71.5
	Other	28.3	28.5
Previous births	None	38.5	40.0
	One	35.2	33.4
	Two	18.4	17.4
	Three	6.1	6.2
	Four or more	1.8	3.0
Multiple birth		1.0	1.2

Missing values excluded
*ESB born overseas in a country where English is the first language
**NESB born overseas in a country where English is not the first language

Almost one-third of women who responded (31 per cent) added comments on the blank pages at the end of the questionnaire, giving 261 contributions ranging from a single sentence to several pages. Over half responded positively to a question asking whether they would be willing to take part in other research in the future, providing us with a contact phone number or an address.

Research Methods
The research methods used in this study and the follow-up study were quite diverse and incorporated both quantitative and qualitative approaches. Each of these approaches has distinctive advan-

tages and strengths along with characteristic limitations. Some of these strengths and weaknesses have already come up in the description of the Survey of Recent Mothers, but others are also relevant.

Table 1.2   Other characteristics of the women in the study

Characteristic	%
Socio-demographic	
Family income < $20 000 a year	18.0
Family income < $30 000 a year	47.2
Secondary school less than Yr 12	56.1
Completed an apprenticeship	13.8
Held a diploma or degree	33.2
Had private health insurance	61.9
Antenatal care	
Specialist obstetrician	52.4
General practitioner	28.9
Public hospital clinic	16.7
Midwife/birth centre	<1.0
Birth	
Hospital labour ward	97.2
Birth centre	2.4
Home	(1 woman)

There are no comparative data available for all women giving birth in Victoria.

The advantage of postal questionnaires is that they are relatively inexpensive. It is possible to include a large sample in the research; much larger than would be possible if everyone had to be interviewed, whether face-to-face or by telephone. With a postal questionnaire, unlike the other two approaches, distance makes no difference to the cost of contact. The whole population, city and country, can be sampled.

Having a large sample is important in two ways. First, any estimates of how common an event or experience was in the study group can be reasonably precise. In the Survey of Recent Mothers, 15.4 per cent of women were probably depressed at the time they filled in the EPDS and, given the numbers of women in the study, we can be confident, from a statistical standpoint, that if we repeated the study on several occasions the proportion depressed would lie between 12.8 and 18.0 per cent. If the whole study had included only 77 women then with the same finding of 15.4 per cent probably depressed we could only be confident that the 'true' proportion could lie anywhere from 7.3 to 23.5 per cent.

Second, a large sample allowed us to compare the experiences of important sub-groups: rural and city women, women who attended or did not attend childbirth preparation classes, women who went to public hospitals and women who went to private obstetricians. The study had sufficient power to detect small differences between these sub-groups of real and practical importance. Conversely, there were sub-groups that even in this large sample were too small to be compared with other groups, for example, women giving birth at home, and mothers of twins.

The anonymity and confidentiality aspects of the study are not intrinsic to postal questionnaires, but they were features of this one. It was an advantage that women knew they could not be identified and that the survey forms were returned to an independent auspice, rather than to the hospital where they had given birth. Feedback to hospitals about their own clients was limited to tables and the unattributed quotations of their clients and even this was available only if they had at least five or more responses. Women were free to comment without fear or favour.

A second advantage of anonymity is that behaviour that is frowned on or thought to be socially undesirable is more likely to be reported than if the question were asked by an interviewer. This is especially true when the information is sought by a health professional and the behaviour is regarded as unhealthy. For example, rates of cigarette-smoking during pregnancy reported in the postal survey were much higher than those reported to labour-ward midwives in a statewide survey carried out four years earlier.[14]

The disadvantages of anonymity included our inability to identify women who had not responded to the first copy of the questionnaire so that we could remind only those who had not already replied. The use of three mail-outs dealt with that problem, but at the price of almost trebling the printing and postage costs, not to mention annoying a few recipients of the second and then the third copy.

The assessment of the representativeness of those who responded, by comparing their characteristics with those of all women giving birth during the time period sampled, was necessarily restricted to the sort of information that is collected routinely, that is, social, demographic or reproductive factors. A more important question might be how representative the respondents were in terms of their dissatisfaction with care or their emotional well-being. Once again we could not assess this directly by, for example, telephoning a sample of non-responders — a widely used strategy[15] — but we could compare early, intermediate and late responders to the survey to see whether there were any trends in dissatisfaction or depression across the three groups. The responses, summarised in table 1.3, were extremely consistent and there were no significant trends. Although this was reassuring, it could not rule out the possibility that the responders and the non-responders differed in the extent of their depression or dissatisfaction.

Table 1.3 Comparing satisfaction with care and depression after birth in early, intermediate and late responders to the survey

	Early (%)	Intermediate (%)	Late (%)
Antenatal care			
Very good	59	58	59
Good	23	27	28
Mixed	14	12	16
Poor	0	2	0
Management of labour			
As liked	67	65	71
As liked in some ways	29	26	22
Not as liked	4	9	7
Active say in decision making			
All the time	43	44	45
Mostly	42	36	38
Sometimes	10	9	10
Not at all	3	9	1
Uncertain	3	2	6
Postnatal care			
Very good	68	69	65
Fairly good	31	30	34
Not very good	2	2	1
Depressed at 8-9 months	15	12	15

A more general limitation of postal questionnaires is that it is difficult for recipients to seek clarification from researchers. We did provide a telephone number and address to contact, for women who wanted clarification or to make a comment, and a few took advantage of it. It was only possible for the researcher to get back to the recipient with a query if the latter had provided her phone number or address for the purposes of taking part in further research. That was done where possible, but a few apparent inconsistencies remain unresolved. Even when careful piloting has been done to ensure that all items are readily understood, an item may not be interpreted in exactly the same way by everyone, especially across the diverse population of women giving birth. Thus postal questionnaires may end up with more items missed out or partially completed than questionnaires administered by an interviewer.[16]

The time and attention someone is willing to give a questionnaire depends on how important the events and experiences it deals with are to that person; how salient they are. We had no doubt that giving birth is one of the most memorable of human experiences. Women in all walks of life exchange birth stories and their detailed and consistent recall has been documented over periods of time beyond twenty years.[17]

While we had been reassured by the British methodological work that showed that a longer survey did not necessarily lead to worse completion, we did check that there was no significant increase in the proportion of unanswered questions from the beginning to the end of the questionnaire. The two questions with the highest proportion of missing replies were the one about total family income (6.8 per cent missing), always a sensitive issue in a questionnaire, and the one about how many times women had attended for antenatal care (7.2 per cent missing), a difficult question to answer, especially for women with more than the standard number of visits.

THE FOLLOW-UP STUDY

One major finding in the survey was the high rate of depression present in women eight to nine months after birth (see Chapter 6). Although there were many links between depression and the events and experiences captured in the survey, there were also many aspects of women's lives that the questionnaire had never been intended to explore. Women's additional comments had, quite explicitly, drawn our attention to some of them:

> I think the answers to your questions about how the mother is feeling now will be fairly useless since you do not know what sort of physical help the mother gets from extended family or friends, home help, child minding services etc (income won't tell you this); you do not know if the baby has been well, or frequently sick, or is disabled, or is a poor sleeper; you do not know the ages of the other children in the household; you do not know if the partner is usually present in the home.

We felt the need to explore the experience of motherhood as it affected both women who were depressed at the time of the original survey and those who were not. What did the two groups have in common? How did their lives differ? What changes had occurred between the time of the survey and our subsequent contact in both groups? Most of all we were interested in what women had to say about their experiences. How did women experience depression? What label did they give it? What help did they seek? Did they find it? What advice would they give to women in similar situations? These questions demanded a very different research approach.

The method for the follow-up study was an interview carried out in the woman's home. The women who were approached came from those (51 per cent) who had given their phone numbers or addresses at the end of the postal questionnaire. Of the 119 women who had scored as depressed in the original survey (a score above twelve on the EPDS), a slightly higher proportion (58 per cent) provided their phone numbers. It was decided to follow-up all these women and to compare them with a randomly selected group from the survey sample who had scored below 9 on the EPDS and had also provided their phone numbers. The latter group were women whose scores indicated they were definitely not depressed.

Were there any obvious differences between women who provided phone numbers and those who did not? Interestingly enough there were no differences in their scores on the EPDS or in overall satisfaction with care between the two groups. There were some, not unexpected, social differences: those who volunteered to take part in further research were more likely to have completed secondary education, more likely to have an above average family income, and less likely to be of NESB.

The follow-up study was undertaken 12 to 18 months after the original survey. Women were contacted by telephone and asked if they were interested in taking part in the study. The project was described as focusing on the experience of motherhood and on women's emotional well-being in the two years after birth. We talked about what would be involved, including the home interview and the completion of some questionnaires beforehand. Provisional appointments were made, and women were given telephone numbers for the researcher so that they could change the appointment time, or even change their minds about taking part, at any time.

Attempts were made to contact all 69 women whose scores on the EPDS indicated they were depressed at the time of the original survey (case group) and to contact an equal number of those with low scores (control group). Table 1.4 outlines the reasons for any non-inclusion in both groups. In the end, nine women in the potential control group did not need to be contacted as all women who had scored as depressed had a 'control' from the low-scoring group. The final sample was 45 women in each group. This was slightly smaller than we had hoped for, but larger than the minimum size we required (40 in each group) to give us the statistical power to identify relevant differences in scores between the groups on the standard questionnaires. The sample was too small for comparison of sub-groups, such as city and country women.

Table 1.4   Participation in the follow-up study

	Cases	Controls
Agreed to take part	45	45
Moved/unable to contact	18	9
Declined to take part	1*	5
Cancelled appointment	5**	1
Total approached	69	60

Cases: women who were depressed at 8-9 months after birth; EPDS >12
Controls: women who were not depressed, nor with a borderline score for depression, 8-9 months after birth; EPDS <9
* 'would be happy to do questionnaire but too busy for an interview'
** reasons for cancellation: surgery for breast cancer; glandular fever; new baby due in five weeks; 'working full-time and too busy at weekends'; 'too busy at present'; 'not up to it'

Women who agreed to take part in the study were sent five standardised questionnaires to be completed prior to being interviewed, including the EPDS,[18] a social support questionnaire,[19] a toddler temperament scale,[20] a measure of recent life events,[21] and a questionnaire on the experience of motherhood.[22] The rationale for including these was to enable some comparisons with populations studied elsewhere, and between the self-reports in the interview and standardised measures.

The home interview
A home-interview schedule was developed and all 90 interviews were undertaken by the authors. The median time for an interview was one hour and twenty minutes. The areas covered included partners' and women's participation in housework, child care and parenting; social and emotional support; 'timeout' from mothering; physical health factors (for women and children); women's own family and childhood; the role of paid work; expectations and experience of motherhood; and the experience of depression.

The interview followed a structured questionnaire in which some questions were pre-coded and others, more open-ended, were coded afterwards. A few questions included prompts: we asked women who had been depressed what factors they thought had contributed in their own case and followed this by prompting them with some putative factors they had not already mentioned.

The development of the home-interview schedule followed the same sequence as that for the postal questionnaire. The one difference was in the formal piloting phase, where an important component was to assess the feasibility and acceptability of interviewing women who had been depressed, and might still be. The Post and Ante Natal Depression Association (PaNDA) helped us by asking some of their members, who had recovered from a postnatal depressive illness and had a child in the toddler age-group, for permission for us to contact them.

All interviews in the study were taped with the women's permission, then transcribed by an independent party in preparation for coding and analysis. Listening to the tapes tells one more about the interview process than the transcripts alone. All the women had two-year-old children, many had older children, and some had new babies as well. Many of the children can be heard taking a vocal role in the conversation, sometimes switching off the recorder, but always playing a part. Occasionally the woman's partner or another adult family member was present, and although this hampered an intimate discussion it was not always possible to find an alternative.

Stephanie and Rhonda both returned from periods of maternity leave to work on the interview stage. Rhonda took Felix, the youngest of her three children, with her on most occasions, so sometimes it is his voice that can be heard babbling or crying on the tapes. Stephanie's youngest son, Keir, started attending a daycare centre just before she returned from leave. During the interviews women often asked about our own children, and in our approach to women asking them to participate we always mentioned to them that we had children ourselves. Stephanie was frequently asked who was minding Keir, and how she managed to leave a young baby in someone else's care. In Rhonda's case women often made comparisons between Felix and their own children, wondering how Rhonda managed to get two older children off to school and arrive in a country town two hours later seemingly composed.

It is not standard interviewing practice to demonstrate, as we did, an investment in the issues being studied. Scientific protocols demand that utmost efforts are made to ensure objectivity. Ann Oakley points out that this conventional interviewing code involves major contradictions for both interviewer and interviewee. Oakley calculated that during 178 interviews conducted by herself and a research assistant, 878 questions were asked of them by interviewees.[23] In our research, there was a relationship between the women we interviewed and ourselves. We did not want to turn women into objects of research by giving them no say in determining the process of the interviews, or no opportunities to check our understanding of what they were communicating. Nor would they have let us do so. We were invited into their homes, and the time they were prepared to give, and the detail in their stories, was dependent on their willingness to continue the dialogue between us. Our aim was to be a vehicle for documenting women's own accounts of their lives. We do not believe it is possible to do this using a formalised prescriptive interviewing practice.

The exchange of information about our children, and shared laughter at the happy and unhappy moments of motherhood, are a feature of the interviews. All interviews were done by one of the four authors, thus avoiding the common disjuncture between the collection of data — in this case women's own accounts of being a mother — and analysis. Interviewers cannot avoid some bias in conversations with interviewees; this project is no exception, but by doing the interviews ourselves and making clear our interest we hope the role that we played in the interviewing process will be apparent to the reader. Chapter 12 contains edited transcripts of three interviews, which give a sense of what the interviews were like, and show how the three authors who did the majority of the interviews approached this task.

Careful thought was given to how much we should know about the women before the interview. Since we wanted to ask women in the case group to verify whether they had felt depressed when we sent them the original questionnaire, it was necessary for the interviewer to know whether the woman was among the case or control group. We deliberately did not check other details on the survey forms before the interview. For example, we did not know how old the women were, whether they were married or single, or what type of birth they had. The standardised questionnaires, including the EPDS, were returned to us at the beginning of the interviews and we discussed their completion with women, but they were not coded until later. This meant we did not know women's scores on any of the questionnaires at the time of the interview.

A further aspect of our protocol was to inform women prior to the interview that the study was concentrating on women's experience of motherhood and emotional well-being in the two years after giving birth. After the interview, all the women were given an opportunity to talk about the issues we were investigating and the findings of the earlier study. Many women were not surprised when we told them that one in seven women had been depressed when we sent out the original survey eight to nine months after the birth, although women who had been depressed often commented on how alone they had felt with this experience.

In December 1992, once we had completed the analysis stage, we mailed to all the women who took part a pamphlet summarising our main findings. Since then, we have re-contacted them to tell them about this book, and to ask permission to use pseudonyms when quoting from their transcripts. Children's names and the names of women's partners have also been changed. There were eleven women in the case group, and five in the control group, whom we were unable to contact, and quotes from their transcripts appear without pseudonyms attached.

USING FACE-TO-FACE INTERVIEWS

This method lends itself well to the exploratory nature of the project and to our goal of listening to the 'missing voices'. The combination of highly structured and open-ended questions, and the detailed coding of the latter, allowed a combination of quantitative and qualitative approaches to be taken in the analysis.

In an interview there is every opportunity to seek clarification or extension of an answer, and there is no risk of questions being missed out or answered incompletely, as in the postal questionnaire.

The most important advantage lies in the detail; the richness and complexity of the material. The transcripts also illustrate the depth of thought women gave to the topics we raised with them. In discussing whether they were satisfied with their partners' contribution to housework or child care, for example, women consistently put this contribution into a context that took account of the long hours their partners typically spent at work: they were satisfied 'given the circumstances'.

One disadvantage of this method is its time-consuming and expensive nature. This was even more so than usual in the follow-up study since women were visited across the State. Another limitation is that the first approach to the interviewee, or the characteristics of the interviewer, might influence her responses in a way that is unlikely with a pre-coded postal questionnaire. Of course this can be a strength as well: women often appealed to 'our' shared experiences, not infrequently saying 'you know what it's like'.

USING STANDARDISED QUESTIONNAIRES

The key advantage of standardised questionnaires is that the extent to which they do measure what they were designed to has already been investigated. Eighty-eight completed sets of the standard questionnaires were coded, entered and checked by one of the authors, using the relevant scoring procedures for each questionnaire. Only two women (one case and one control) failed to return the questionnaires, a participation rate of 98 per cent.

The EPDS, which was incorporated into the postal questionnaire as well as being used in the follow-up study, has been compared with diagnoses made by psychiatric interview in three different communities in Britain.[24] At the time we first used the EPDS it had not been formally tested in Australia, but a recent formal validation has shown that it performs well here.[25]

The Toddler Temperament Scale had been specifically modified for use with Australian families and the expected findings for an Australian population have been defined.[26] The Experience of Motherhood Questionnaire was developed in Australia by one of the authors for use with mothers of two-year-olds.[27] The Life Experiences Questionnaire was chosen because it has been modified for use with women.[28]

Excerpts from all five scales are given in Appendix 3, with details about how they were scored. Their only obvious disadvantage was that they were sometimes perceived by women as 'boring', 'frustrating' or 'repetitive'.

USING THE COMMENTS AND THE TRANSCRIPTS

Almost one-third of the women who answered the postal questionnaire wrote comments on the final blank page. The women who added comments were not entirely representative of the women who replied to the questionnaire: they were more likely to have completed secondary education and less likely to be of NESB, and in these two ways were like the women who wanted to take part in further research and had supplied their telephone numbers. A more important difference was that women who made additional comments were more likely to be dissatisfied with the care they had received in labour and in the postnatal wards, and less likely to be critical of antenatal care than the total sample of respondents.

For these reasons the additional comments are mainly used to illustrate points arising from the quantitative analysis. Some comments gave a critique of the questions, usually in relation to the wider context of birth and parenting. Others elaborated on a question, for example, with respect to inconsistent advice over breastfeeding in hospital a woman added:

> Also you might want to look into the different opinions of relatives, friends, general doctors, specialists, nurses, midwives, clinic health sister who all have sound advice but also all disagree which makes the first few months with a baby very difficult for the parents.

The quotations from the transcripts are also used for illustration and, unlike those for the postal survey, they have names attached in most cases. Thus it is possible to follow the quotations of a particular woman through the book.

ASSESSING CHANGES OVER TIME
The 90 women who were part of the follow-up study completed the EPDS on two occasions, twelve to eighteen months apart. This enabled us to measure changes in emotional well-being over that time, and to identify new cases of depression that had arisen since the time of the postal survey.

We were also able to compare women's perceptions of the birth of the child when she or he was two years old, with those given eight to nine months after birth. Analysis of the child's temperament at two years also enables us to review the contribution of pregnancy and birth complications to infant temperament.

COMBINING RESEARCH APPROACHES
The different research methods utilised in these two projects allowed us to approach the experience of becoming and being a mother in a variety of ways and to assess the consistency of the findings across different approaches. They allowed us to listen to women's voices, contributed a wealth of detail to their stories, provided a reliable and valid means of measuring key constructs, gave a large descriptive data set for quantitative analysis, and added a longitudinal perspective, particularly to the description of depression. The commonality of the experience of motherhood, whether or not women were depressed, was as notable as the sometimes striking differences between these two groups.

READING THE BOOK
In the first half of the book we follow the 790 women who answered the postal questionnaire through their antenatal care, labour and birth, childbirth education, and the postnatal period, before pausing to look at depression in the year after birth. The second half of the book, based on the follow-up study, does not take a chronological path but deals with themes.

From this point on, most of the material in this chapter will be taken for granted. What we did and why we did it may be mentioned briefly, but the emphasis will be on the findings rather than the methods. Thus it may be helpful to refer back to this chapter when reading other sections. In addition, an account of some other research issues raised by our two studies is provided in Appendix 1. These are discussions about assessing satisfaction, the reasons for choosing a population sample, and the difference between population and clinical samples. Also included are details about coding the interview tapes and an account of 'causes' and 'risks'. A brief explanation of some of the statistical terms is given in Appendix 2, and more information about the standardised questionnaires appears in Appendix 3.

Judith Lumley, Stephanie Brown, Rhonda Small

The Survey of Recent Mothers

TWO

Care in Pregnancy

Pregnancy brings many changes to women's lives. For women having their first baby it is a time of transition between being a daughter and becoming a mother oneself. For all women pregnancy is a 'journey into the unknown'.[1] 'Will the baby be alright?' and 'Will I be able to cope?' are questions many pregnant women ask over and over again in the long waiting period before the baby is born. While pregnancy is not itself an illness, many women experience a range of symptoms during pregnancy — vomiting, backache, excessive tiredness, frequent urination — that would otherwise be viewed as signs of illness. Pregnancy also involves becoming a 'patient'. Although not 'sick', pregnant women are encouraged to attend for regular medical care, starting with an appointment within the first twelve weeks of pregnancy. These routine check-ups involve a range of diagnostic and screening procedures (such as blood tests, ultrasound examinations and so on) that are likely to be unfamiliar to many women, and for recently arrived migrants, a pregnancy may be the first point of contact with Australian hospitals and western health-care practices.

BECOMING A PATIENT

Maternity care in Australia combines elements of Canadian, United States and United Kingdom health systems. Pregnancy care is available to women on either a private or public basis. The three most common types of antenatal care are public hospital antenatal clinics, specialist obstetricians, or general practitioners in private consulting rooms. Medicare covers standard public hospital care including all antenatal visits and screening procedures (ultrasound, blood tests, fetal cardiotocography etc.) and is free at the point of service. Women attending public antenatal clinics are seen by resident and consultant medical staff, midwives, student doctors and student midwives. Some public hospitals also offer a midwives clinic where antenatal care is provided by a small team of midwives with medical back-up available if needed. A few public hospitals also offer team midwifery care in birth centres, where the same small group of midwives looks after a woman throughout her pregnancy and labour, again with medical back-up available.

Shared antenatal care is another option available to Victorian women. This involves a formalised co-operative arrangement between a maternity hospital and a general practitioner or community health centre. Occasionally care is shared between a specialist obstetrician, a general practitioner, and a hospital. Women who are enrolled in shared-care arrangements attend their local shared-care practitioner for most of their antenatal appointments, with visits to the hospital at specified times during their pregnancy or if complications arise. In most cases shared-care is fully covered under Medicare. A small number of midwives in Victoria work in private practice, providing personalised care throughout pregnancy, labour and birth and the period immediately after birth. There are no rebates under Medicare for private midwifery, and health insurance funds provide only limited reimbursement for women choosing this option.

More than half the women taking part in the survey attended a specialist obstetrician for antenatal care. Over a quarter were cared for by a general practitioner, and 17 per cent went to a public hospital clinic (see table 2.1). Sixteen women made other arrangements for antenatal care; six were cared for by birth-centre midwives; eight indicated that their care was shared between two sources (GP/obstetrician, GP/hospital clinic); and one woman attended a midwife in private practice. Only one woman reported that she received no antenatal care during her pregnancy.

Table 2.1 Provider of antenatal care

	No.	%
Specialist obstetrician	412	52.2
General practitioner	227	28.7
Public hospital clinic	131	16.6
Shared care	8	1.0
Birth-centre midwives	6	0.8
Private midwife	1	0.1
No one	1	0.1
No answer	4	0.5
Total	790	100.0

A comparison of the survey respondents with all women giving birth in Victoria in 1989, shows that the sample slightly over-represents women attending a specialist obstetrician and under-represents women who went to a public clinic. Data from the Health Insurance Commission (HIC) indicate that approximately 45 per cent of Victorian women attend a specialist obstetrician for antenatal care, compared to 52.2 per cent in our sample.[2] This difference is partly explained by the socio-demographic composition of the sample. As we will see below, younger women and single women, who were under-represented in our sample, are more likely to have attended a public clinic, while older women — over-represented in our sample — are more likely to have received antenatal care from a specialist.

It is difficult to estimate the proportion of women in Victoria currently receiving antenatal care from general practitioners. This is because data collected by the HIC does not differentiate between care provided during pregnancy and care provided during labour and birth. According to the HIC, 40 per cent of Victorian women having babies in 1989 were cared for as public patients during labour and birth. Some of these women would have attended a public hospital clinic during pregnancy, and others would have been cared for by a general practitioner. Among our sample, 50.7 per cent of the women who attended a general practitioner for antenatal care were looked after in labour as public patients.

The very small number of women taking part in the study who reported that birth-centre midwives provided most of their antenatal care is probably a true estimate. In 1989 around 1 to 2 per cent of births were in birth centres, but only some of the women who gave birth in birth centres would have been public patients cared for throughout their pregnancy and labour by midwives. A large proportion of the women choosing to give birth in a birth centre are privately insured and attend either a GP or specialist obstetrician for antenatal care. Shared antenatal care, on the other hand, was probably under-reported in our sample. In 1989 approximately 3 per cent of women in Victoria received shared antenatal care,[3] compared to only 1 per cent of our sample. It is likely that some of the women who listed a general practitioner as their provider of antenatal care were in fact participating in shared-care arrangements. Overall, then, the sample was reasonably representative in terms of the models of antenatal care available to Victorian women, with slight over-representation of women attending specialist obstetricians and under-representation of women attending public hospital clinics.

The vast majority of women in the study had their first antenatal check-up early in pregnancy (87.5 per cent attended in the first trimester), and regularly attended for routine visits throughout the pregnancy. Ten per cent of women attended for the first time between thirteen and 27 weeks of pregnancy, and less than 1 per cent after this time. Attendance for antenatal care is not routinely reported on the Victorian perinatal data collection forms, so it is not possible to check the representativeness of these figures. It is possible that the sample slightly under-represents women attending for antenatal care after the first trimester.

Just under half of the women in the survey (49 per cent) reported that they had between ten and fourteen antenatal visits; 13.4 per cent had between five and nine visits; and 29.7 per cent attended for antenatal care fifteen or more times during their pregnancy. Thus the vast majority of women attended antenatal check-ups at least ten times, and had their first check-up within the first twelve weeks.

The rationale for encouraging women to have frequent check-ups during pregnancy centres on the potential to prevent mortality and morbidity in babies, and to a lesser extent the prevention of maternal mortality. Since the 1940s standard antenatal management has focused on the following procedures: listening to the baby's heartbeat; measurement of fundal height; checking for high blood pressure, fluid retention and protein in the mother's urine; and monitoring the mother's weight gain. In the last two decades a range of more technical and highly specialised methods of monitoring the growth and health of the fetus *in utero* have been developed. These include ultrasound examination and monitoring of fetal growth; antenatal fetal cardiotocography (electronic monitoring of the baby's heartbeat); glucose tolerance tests; and prenatal screening and diagnosis (such as amniocentesis and chorion villus sampling). As a result, pregnant women today undergo far more routine tests and procedures than earlier generations of women.[4]

Almost all women in the study had at least one ultrasound examination during their pregnancy (92.4 per cent) and 33.9 per cent had two or more. More recent data show that in 1991–92, 97 per cent of pregnant women in Victoria had at least one ultrasound scan and 43 per cent had more than one scan (J. Yates personal communication). Ultrasound examination has thus become almost universal for childbearing women in Victoria.

Table 2.2 Explanations for ultrasound examination

	No.	%
Satisfied with explanation	685	95.1
Not satisfied	32	4.4
None given	3	0.4

Just under half our sample (49.2 per cent) reported having antenatal cardiotocography (fetal monitoring). This may be an over estimate. It was a great deal higher than we would have predicted, and it is possible that some women took this to refer to the small hand-held monitors, which use an ultrasound beam, that have almost replaced the 'ear trumpet' stethoscopes of old. No available statewide or national figures are available on the use of cardiotocography.

Almost all women who reported having an ultrasound examination or external fetal cardiotocography were happy with the explanations they received for why these procedures were done.

Table 2.3 Explanations for fetal cardiotocography

	No.	%
Satisfied with explanation	347	93.8
Not satisfied	18	4.9
None given	5	1.3

Table 2.4 What was good about antenatal care?

	No.	%
Women attending an obstetrician		
Regular check-ups	255	61.9
Getting information	217	57.7
Having an ultrasound	313	76.0
Total	412	
Women attending a general practitioner		
Regular check-ups	114	50.2
Getting information	89	39.2
Having an ultrasound	151	66.5
Total	227	
Women attending a public clinic		
Regular check-ups	88	67.2
Getting information	58	44.3
Having an ultrasound	94	71.8
Total	131	

Over 70 percent of women in the study listed ultrasound examination as one of the best aspects of their care during pregnancy. The ultrasound scan was rated more positively than several other aspects of pregnancy care, including information provided by care-givers, and the medical and nursing care given in check-ups, as table 2.4, which differentiates between women attending obstetricians, general practitioners and public hospital clinics, demonstrates.

Amongst the total sample, only 52 women (6.8 per cent) said that tests were not adequately explained, and 20 women (2.6 per cent) felt they had too many tests. One woman wrote on the survey form that some tests were 'unnecessary ... because the doctors didn't seem confident of their own opinions'. On the whole, though, most women seemed happy to comply with procedures used to monitor their pregnancy and the health of their baby, and were satisfied with the explanations given for the use of any procedures.

The aspect of antenatal check-ups that women rated most highly was being reassured that the baby was okay. Ninety per cent of women attending a specialist obstetrician, 80 per cent attending a general practitioner, and 72.5 per cent attending a clinic in a public hospital said that being reassured about the baby was one of the things they valued most in their antenatal care. Reassurance was also valued by women who experienced pregnancy complications, as the following annotation on the survey form by a woman whose baby was 'small-for-dates' indicates. She wrote that the good aspects of her care included:

> Reasonable care and good information when pregnancy showed as deviating from 'normal' pattern. Encouragement to get previous pregnancy records from —— hospital under Freedom of Information. Discussion of first birthing experience (by caesarean section) and encouragement that the outcome of this pregnancy could be quite different.

For women who attended a specialist obstetrician or general practitioner, being seen by the same care-giver at each visit also added to a positive experience of antenatal care; almost three-quarters of women who saw an obstetrician or general practitioner in pregnancy listed continuity of care as something they valued highly. Several women wrote comments on this section of the survey forms highlighting the benefits of getting to know one care-giver during pregnancy:

> The regular check-ups were friendly, personal and at no time did she do an internal. Also she visited me at my home — wonderful.

> [Having a] doctor one can feel at ease with who makes you feel special and is interested in you and is a good listener.

> [I had] consistency of care, thus building up a good rapport which helped me adjust to decisions in labour.

Public hospital clinics are rarely able to offer women the possibility of seeing the same care-giver at each visit. With the exception of the few public hospitals offering a midwives clinic, it is not uncommon for women to see a different set of faces each time they attend for check-ups. The potential for this to result in a lack of rapport between care-givers and patients, and for women to feel that they are never treated as an individual, has been well documented in other studies.[5] Summarising these studies, Jo Garcia noted that 'the recurrent images ... are of cattle markets and conveyor belts'.[6] Over one-third of the women in our study who attended a public clinic (35.9 per cent) complained about seeing a different care-giver at each visit. One woman commented:

> I sometimes felt that I had to remind clinic staff of tests required, for example that I had Rhesus negative blood, that I hadn't seen a doctor when they said I would. It just seemed a bit haphazard at times. The doctor (female) was too impersonal.

Another woman revisited the imagery in the British studies referred to earlier, simply writing 'I felt we were being treated like cattle'. In contrast, one woman compared her negative experiences in three previous pregnancies where she had attended public hospital antenatal clinics with her most recent pregnancy, during which she felt she had received more individual care from a specialist in private practice:

> I have four children, but only in my last pregnancy did I have private care. My second and fourth children were born in Victoria.
> Comparing the two pregnancies, my last was by far the better. I felt that it was more personal care from my doctor, rather than seeing a different doctor each visit and being pushed through because there were still more patients to see.

JUST ANOTHER PREGNANT LADY?

Most women looking back on their antenatal care eight months after the birth reported positive experiences. Table 2.5 summarises responses to the question 'On balance, how would you rate your antenatal care?' Eighty-six per cent of women described their care as either 'good' or 'very good', just over 13 per cent rated their care as mixed (good in some ways, poor in others), and less than one per cent said their care was poor.

While only a minority expressed some dissatisfaction with care in response to this question, less than half the women taking part in the study felt that care-givers had offered a personalised and caring approach. This highlights the importance in surveys of this kind of asking women specific as well as global questions about their experiences of medical care.[7]

Table 2.5 Overall rating of antenatal care

	No.	%
Very good	460	58.2
Good	214	27.1
Mixed (good in some ways, poor in others)	106	13.4
Poor	5	0.6
No answer	5	0.6
Total	790	

Although only a small number of women wrote comments about antenatal care on the survey forms, several women emphasised what it felt like to go to an antenatal appointment and find oneself rushed through without any opportunity to ask questions or raise matters of concern.

> My obstetrician took an average of 30 seconds for my check-ups — this was quite disconcerting.

> My doctor I feel views women as birthing machines, and that nothing is of any importance up until the moment of delivery. At this time he comes into his own, and is great. I think a machine could be devised to get the antenatal information that he sought — as effectively and warmly.

The time interval between pregnancy and receiving the survey form is probably one reason why women wrote fewer comments about antenatal care than about care in labour and birth. To avoid this possible bias, and to obtain a more detailed understanding of women's experiences of antenatal care, some studies have included a questionnaire filled out towards the end of pregnancy, and/or interviews with women before and after giving birth. Several studies based on 'in-depth' interviews have identified the quality of communication between care-givers and women attending for antenatal care as a cause for major concern.[8] Reid and McIlwaine's study of a random sample of 91 first-time mothers drawn from a small city hospital antenatal clinic in Glasgow, Scotland, showed that 39 per cent did not feel they were able to get all the information they wanted from doctors. Jo Garcia, summarising studies of satisfaction with antenatal care in the United Kingdom, points out that women face multiple problems in getting access to the sort of information they want during pregnancy; 'asking questions is often difficult and embarrassing', and when women do ask questions, the answers are sometimes empty reassurances that may be more upsetting than helpful.[9] While the system of providing antenatal care in the United Kingdom is different from that in Australia, these themes were echoed in some of the comments Victorian women wrote on the survey forms.

> Towards the end of my pregnancy I had a lot of fluid and he [doctor] seemed to treat it too casually. Sometimes he didn't even look at my feet which were so swollen I could hardly walk.

> The doctor was not concerned, [I was] just another pregnant lady.

> The GP let me go two weeks overdue without telling us anything.

> The doctor gave me little feedback. Sometimes he would tell me what my blood pressure or measurement was. I would have preferred he tell me each visit. I could have asked but I didn't want to appear an hysterical female.

The apparent mismatch between women's expectations of care-givers and what actually happened during their antenatal care is an indication of the different ways in which women and care-givers approach check-ups during pregnancy. While women are seeking to be told that everything is going well, doctors and nurses are looking for signs that something might be going wrong. From a consumer perspective, the organisation of medical care for pregnant women — whether via a range of personnel in a public clinic or from a private practitioner with a busy waiting room — may offer limited opportunities for a woman's *own* pregnancy and concerns about her *own* baby to be regarded as special and important.[10] From the perspective of care-givers working in overcrowded antenatal clinics or in busy private practices, the individual concerns of generally healthy pregnant women may seem trivial. The effect of this may be to discourage women from voicing their concerns at all.

Our survey, which was designed to cover the range of women's experiences through pregnancy, labour and birth, and the early postnatal weeks, did not allow detailed investigation of these issues. The questions we asked about antenatal care were limited to one global question asking for an overall rating of care, and two questions asking women to indicate whether particular items were things they regarded as 'good' or 'bad' aspects of their care. Discrepancies in the way women answered these questions suggest that the questions we asked did not adequately tap into the ways in which women thought about their experiences. For example, only 52.7 per cent of women attending specialist obstetricians, 44.3 per cent attending public hospital clinics, and 39.2 per cent attending general practitioners ticked the item to say that being able to get information was a good aspect of their antenatal care. On the other hand, fewer than 6 per cent of women attending any of the three main provider categories said that difficulty in obtaining information was a bad aspect of their care. It is difficult to estimate, on the basis of the survey, how many women had experiences that were similar to those of the women who chose to write comments. It is likely, however, that the proportion of women not happy with the information they received during pregnancy or the ways in which care-givers communicated information to them is higher than responses to the question asking women to indicate any bad aspects of their antenatal care seem to suggest.

ASSESSING THE ALTERNATIVES

As the foregoing analysis illustrates, women's experiences of antenatal care varied substantially according to whether they went to a specialist obstetrician, general practitioner, or hospital antenatal clinic. Women who attended an obstetrician in private consulting rooms were the most likely to be satisfied with their antenatal care, followed by women who went to a general practitioner. The least likely to be satisfied were women who attended a public hospital clinic (see table 2.6). Given the tendency of global questions relating to satisfaction with medical care to elicit high levels of satisfaction, the finding that almost one-third of women who attended an outpatients clinic for antenatal care were unhappy about some aspects of their care is a clear indication of problems in the way that care is provided.

Table 2.6 Satisfaction with antenatal care by primary care-giver

Care-giver	Very good/good No.	%	Mixed/poor No.	%
Specialist obstetrician	381	93.4	27	6.6
General practitioner	188	83.2	38	16.8
Public clinic	91	69.5	40	30.5

$\chi^2 = 19.76$, $p < 0.0001$

This finding is reinforced by comparisons between what women listed as the good and the bad aspects of their antenatal care. As we have seen, the extent to which women felt reassured, and the ease with which they were able to obtain information, varied significantly according to whether they attended an obstetrician, general practitioner or public clinic. Comparing the proportion of women who said that 'nothing was bad' about their antenatal care with their provider of care confirms that women attending a public hospital clinic were the least happy with their care; 62.1 per cent of women who saw a private obstetrician, and 58.6 per cent who saw a general practitioner, circled the response 'nothing was bad', whereas only 28.2 per cent of women who attended a public hospital clinic felt able to say this. Waiting times for appointments were a source of complaint amongst all three groups, but was much more common among women attending hospital antenatal clinics (58 per cent) than amongst women attending either a general practitioner or an obstetrician (around 20 per cent). While over one-third of the women who attended a public hospital clinic indicated that seeing a different care-giver at each visit was a bad aspect of their care, almost two-thirds of women who attended either an obstetrician or general practitioner regarded continuity of care as a good aspect of their care.

REAL OR IMAGINARY CHOICES?

To what extent are women free to choose between alternative antenatal care models? The existence of a number of different options for antenatal care tends to obscure the fact that not all women have access to the full range.[11] In practice, women's choices of care during pregnancy are restricted by the limited availability of some options (particularly in country areas), by guidelines that restrict access to birth-centre care and shared-care to women at low risk of obstetric complications, by their ability to pay for private health insurance, and by the information provided to women early in pregnancy about the range of options available. As Martin Richards notes, 'the notion of alternatives implies that there exists a comprehensive set of options to choose from and that the chooser is in a position freely to exercise choice in an informed way'.[12] Neither of these conditions is fulfilled in Australian maternity services at present.

Among the women in our study, those living in rural areas were much more likely to have attended a general practitioner (54.7 per cent) than those living in or near Melbourne (19.1 per cent). Metropolitan-based women, on the other hand, were most likely to have attended a specialist obstetrician; over 60 per cent of women living in the city were cared for by a private obstetrician, compared to just under one-third of country-based women (see table 2.7). City-based women were also more likely to have attended a public hospital clinic (19.1 per cent, compared to 10.8 per cent).

Although very small numbers of women reported attending a birth centre for antenatal care, the fact that all of these women were living in the metropolitan area probably accurately reflects the limited availability of birth centres in country areas. In 1989 only one country-based public hospital had a birth centre that offered midwifery care to public patients. Shared care, on the other hand, was used by small numbers of women in both city and country areas.

Table 2.7 Choice of antenatal care-giver in the city and the country

Care-giver	City No.	%	Country No.	%
Specialist obstetrician	325	60.2	68	32.1
General practitioner	103	19.1	116	54.7
Public clinic	103	19.1	23	10.8
Shared care	3	0.6	5	2.4
Birth-centre midwives	6	1.1	0	0.0

Sixty-two per cent of our sample had private health insurance. For the remaining 38 per cent, the high cost of hospital fees was a major barrier limiting their access to a specialist obstetrician or general practitioner. Although Medicare covers 75 per cent of the schedule fee for medical care provided by either a general practitioner or specialist obstetrician during pregnancy and confinement, women who are cared for by their own private practitioner in labour are automatically classified as private patients and incur full hospital charges in both public and private hospitals.

Shared care and birth-centre care are not available to women who have a high risk of developing complications during pregnancy or labour. For example, women who have had a previous birth by caesarean section are excluded from most birth centres. Other reasons for exclusion from birth centres include medical conditions such as diabetes and asthma, a prior premature labour or low birthweight infant, and more than two terminations of pregnancy. Some of these factors would also prevent women from gaining access to shared-care programs, particularly where close monitoring is required during pregnancy (for example, medical conditions such as diabetes). Where risk factors relate only to labour, for example, prior caesarean section, this may or may not be a reason for exclusion from shared care, depending on the policies of individual programs and practitioners.

Another option for providing antenatal care that is becoming more popular is a midwives clinic operating alongside a standard public hospital antenatal clinic. None of our study sample identified that they had attended a midwives clinic, although it is possible that some did so. This was not given as a precoded option on the survey form as midwives clinics were extremely unusual in

1989. By 1993 all three Melbourne teaching hospitals offered a midwives clinic, and some suburban and country public hospitals had also set up clinics along these lines.

Thus, while there is a range of options, including some in the public system that offer an alternative to standard clinic care, they are not universally available. Although the Ministerial Review of Birthing Services recommended the establishment of at least one birth centre in each health region (at the time there were eight health regions in Victoria) by 1993, there are still only four public hospitals that offer this option. The Ministerial Review also recommended that all Level III hospitals (specialist teaching hospitals) and Level II hospitals (larger suburban and country base hospitals) should offer a midwives clinic as an antenatal care option by the end of 1991. This has also been only partially implemented. For a majority of women without private health insurance, therefore, the main options in the city continue to be care in a public hospital clinic and to a lesser extent shared care, and in country areas care by a general practitioner as a public patient receiving standard labour ward care in labour.

IMPOSSIBLE TO PLEASE?

On one occasion when we presented these findings to a group of midwives attending a seminar for continuing education, a midwife who worked in a public hospital antenatal clinic commented that some women, young women in particular, were 'impossible to please'. When we spoke about the study at gatherings where obstetricians were present it was more likely to be assumed that 'middle-class' women or women having their first baby were those most often dissatisfied with their care. Table 2.8 summarises what we found when we looked at the associations between several sociodemographic characteristics (mother's age, marital status, family income, education, parity, country of birth) and satisfaction with antenatal care.

Several variables were associated with differences in satisfaction. Women who were socially disadvantaged in some way — because they were young, without a partner, living on a low income, or had immigrated from a country where English is not the main language — were the most likely to be dissatisfied. Parity (number of previous births) and women's level of education were not related to dissatisfaction, nor was there an association with whether women were pleased to be pregnant, would rather the pregnancy had happened a bit later, or would rather it had not happened at all. Women with private health insurance, on the other hand, were much more likely to rate their care as good or very good than women without it.

Table 2.8 Satisfaction with antenatal care by socio-demographic characteristics

	Very good/good %	Mixed/poor %	Statistical test
Maternal age			
15–19	72.7	27.3	χ^2 for linear trend
20–24	78.2	21.8	= 7.007
25–29	84.9	15.1	p = 0.008
30–34	87.7	12.3	
35–39	89.9	10.1	
≥40	92.9	7.1	
Marital status			
Single	65.4	34.6	χ^2 for linear trend*
Div./Sep.	75.0	25.0	= 9.148
De facto	82.6	17.4	p = 0.0025
Married	87.0	13.0	
Income			
<$20 000 pa	77.4	22.6	χ^2 for linear trend
$20 001–$30 000	84.5	15.5	= 16.19
$30 001–$40 000	87.4	12.6	p < 0.0001
>$40 000	92.9	7.1	
Secondary education			
Finished Year 12	88.1	11.9	χ^2 = 2.39
Less than Year 12	84.2	15.8	p = 0.12
Tertiary education			
Degree	86.2	13.8	χ^2 = 2.42
Diploma	90.2	9.8	p = 0.49
Apprenticeship	84.1	15.9	
None	85.1	14.8	
Parity			
0	86.5	13.5	χ^2 = 2.41
1	83.5	16.5	p = 0.49
2	88.8	11.2	
≤3	86.9	13.1	
Country of birth			
Australia	87.7	12.3	χ^2 = 16.96
Overseas (ESB)	87.8	12.2	p = 0.0002
Overseas (NESB)	71.7	28.3	
Insurance status			
Private cover	92.8	7.2	χ^2 = 46.99
Medicare only	75.3	24.7	p < 0.0001

* Marital status has been ordered to reflect increasing levels of partner support

These findings confirm the results of other studies that it is women who are the least well off financially, or who are socially disadvantaged in some way,[13] and in the Australian context lack private health cover,[14] who are most likely to be dissatisfied with their antenatal care. This raises the question of whether it is socio-demographic factors *per se* that lead to dissatisfaction or, given the strong association already noted between the provider of antenatal care and satisfaction, whether the associations between socio-demographic factors and satisfaction are accounted for by differences in the provider of care? In other words, are the associations between social factors and dissatisfaction independent of, or linked to, the issue of where women attended for antenatal care?

Table 2.9 Dissatisfaction with antenatal care by primary care-giver by socio-demographic characteristics

	Proportion of women rating their antenatal care as mixed or poor		
	Obstetrician %	GP %	Public antenatal clinic %
Maternal age			
<25 years	7.7	19.2	33.3
≥25 years	6.7	16.4	30.4
Marital status			
No partner	0.0	35.0*	46.2
Living with partner	6.9	15.0*	28.2
Income			
<$30 000pa	7.5	20.0	30.8
≥$30 000pa	6.4	12.0	23.8
Country of birth			
Australia	6.7	14.8+	26.2
Overseas (ESB)	6.1	14.3	23.1
Overseas (NESB)	7.7	43.8+	42.4
Insurance status			
Private health cover	5.0+	13.6	6.3*
Medicare only	16.1+	20.2	32.7*

* $p < 0.05$
+ $p < 0.01$

In order to assess the extent to which differences in socio-demographic characteristics were accounted for by differences in the care-giver attended during pregnancy, we stratified responses to the question requesting an overall rating of care, according to both the provider of care, and the significant socio-demographic factors of maternal age, marital status, country of birth, family income and health insurance. Table 2.9 summarises this three-way comparison. Our results confirm that the significant differences in satisfaction associated with these factors are explained by the restricted choices for antenatal care of women who are young, without a partner, on a low income, or of NESB.

Young women were much more likely to attend a public hospital clinic; 40 per cent of women under 25 years went to a hospital antenatal clinic, compared to 14 per cent of older women. Over half the older women attended a private obstetrician. Overall ratings of satisfaction with antenatal care did not differ between age groups. That is, young women attending a public hospital clinic were not more likely than older women to give a negative overall rating of their care. Young women who attended a public clinic, however, were more likely to complain about seeing a different care-giver at each visit (54.5 per cent) than older women (30.5 per cent), perhaps indicating that young women have a greater need of support during pregnancy than public clinics are on the whole able to provide.

Almost half of the women in the study who did not have a partner attended a general practitioner, almost one-third attended a public clinic, and around one-fifth a private obstetrician. In contrast, over half the women with partners attended a private obstetrician and fewer than one-fifth a public clinic. Women without partners were significantly more likely to be dissatisfied with antenatal care provided by a general practitioner (35 per cent) than women with partners (15.1 per cent). There were no significant differences in satisfaction with specific aspects of antenatal care associated with marital status within any of the provider categories.

When compared with Australian-born women, women of NESB were much more likely to have attended a public hospital clinic, much less likely to have attended a general practitioner, and rather less likely to have attended a private obstetrician. Women of NESB were significantly more dissatisfied with antenatal care provided by general practitioners (43.8 per cent) than Australian-born women (14.8 per cent). There were no country of birth differences in the other two provider groups. In all three provider groups, women of NESB were less likely to say they felt reassured, a difference which was significant for those who had attended a public hospital clinic (54.5 per cent versus 77.4 per cent) or a general practitioner (56.3 per cent versus 82.5 per cent).

Women returning the survey forms were almost evenly divided between those whose total family income was $30 000 or less a year, and those whose income was above this. Almost two-thirds in the higher income range attended a private obstetrician, compared with two-fifths of the others. Just over one-fifth of women with a high income, and almost two-fifths of women on lower incomes, went to a general practitioner for antenatal care. Only 11.1 per cent of women on higher incomes went to public hospital clinics, whereas 22.8 per cent of women on lower incomes did so. None of the differences in satisfaction by income between the provider groups was statistically significant.

As could be expected, the data confirmed that health insurance status is a major factor in where women go for antenatal care. Almost three-quarters of women with private health insurance went to a private obstetrician for most of their antenatal care; just under one-quarter went to a general practitioner, and a small group of sixteen women said they went to a public clinic. Two-fifths of the women who did not have health insurance attended a public clinic; a further two-fifths went to a general practitioner, some of whom were probably seen on a shared-care basis. The remaining one-fifth attended an obstetrician in private practice.

Women who had attended a private obstetrician were significantly more satisfied if they were privately insured, as were women who went to a public clinic. Insurance status was not significantly associated with satisfaction among women who attended a general practitioner.

Non-insured women who attended a private obstetrician were less likely than insured women who went to a specialist to regard their care-giver as caring and considerate (37.5 per cent versus 54.1 per cent) or to have felt reassured (78.6 per cent versus 93 per cent), and more likely to have complained that care was not individualised (11.3 per cent versus 2.7 per cent), that tests were not explained (11.3 per cent versus 3.3 per cent) and that it was difficult to get information (9.4 per cent versus 3.3 per cent).

On inspection the small group of women with private health insurance who attended a public antenatal clinic (n=16) were not a homogenous group. It is possible that at least some of this group had not correctly understood the question regarding who provided their antenatal care. Women without insurance who attended a specialist obstetrician for antenatal care (n=56) were atypical in a number of ways: they were more likely to be single (3/56), to be young (10/56 were under 25 years), to have an income below the median (29/56), and not to have planned the pregnancy (16/56). They did not differ in education or parity, were not more likely to be of NESB, and were not more likely to have been admitted to hospital during pregnancy. Possibly their greater dissatisfaction with antenatal care stemmed from the fact that they would have had more out of pocket expenses to pay for both their medical and hospital care than other women attending a specialist. The converse might also be true — women who have paid a large amount for private health insurance may be reluctant to be critical in the light of this financial investment. The survey does not enable us to sort out the possible pathways to dissatisfaction amongst this group beyond these speculations.

Table 2.10 Odds ratios for associations of antenatal care provider and social characteristics of respondents with dissatisfaction with antenatal care

Characteristic	Unadjusted OR	[95%CI]	Adjusted OR*	[95%CI]
Provider (obstetrician/public clinic)	5.05	[2.86-8.92]	4.07	[2.20-7.53]
Maternal age (25+/under 25)	2.53	[1.24-5.16]	1.37	[0.61-3.06]
Marital status (partner/other)	2.67	[0.93-7.63]	1.27	[0.35-4.64]
Income (more than $20 000 p.a./ $20 000 or less p.a.)	2.61	[1.37-4.94]	1.34	[0.61-2.95]
Country of birth (Aust/NESB)	2.27	[1.17-4.41]	1.67	[0.81-3.46]

* Adjusted for other variables in the table

When we submitted these findings to a journal for publication, one of the reviewers suggested that we confirm our analysis using logistic regression. This is a method of statistical modelling that makes it possible to sort out the relative contributions of a range of factors to a specified outcome, in this case dissatisfaction with antenatal care. Using a computer software package called Egret we entered all the socio-demographic factors associated with dissatisfaction (being young, without a partner, on a low income, of NESB), together with the provider of care, into a logistic model comparing women attending a specialist obstetrician with those attending public hospital clinics (see table 2.10). None of the socio-demographic factors made any additional contribution to dissatisfaction beyond the contribution made by the provider of care. This confirmed our conclusion that in the Australian context the caregiver women attend for antenatal care is the most salient factor determining their likelihood of satisfaction.

THE INVERSE CARE LAW

The findings reported in this chapter consistently point to major problems for women without private health insurance and for women receiving antenatal care in public hospitals. Although a majority of women are happy with antenatal care, almost one-third of women attending a public clinic were unhappy about some aspects of their care. There is thus an 'inverse care law' applying to the way in which Victorian maternity services provide care to pregnant women. The women most likely to be in need of sensitivity from care-givers — women who are in some way socially disadvantaged — are the least likely to have access to more individualised maternity care. Public antenatal care — the only choice available to many — fails to meet women's expectations regarding continuity of care, individual concerns and information requirements, or waiting times for appointments. With a population-based sample of women in the Lothian district of Scotland, Claudia Martin has demonstrated a clear inverse relationship between lack of continuity of care and satisfaction; the greater the continuity the more likely women were to rate their care highly.[15] Randomised trials of antenatal care options that offer care by a small team of midwives, including one conducted in a Sydney teaching hospital, have also demonstrated higher levels of satisfaction with antenatal care among their experimental groups than among women randomised to standard antenatal care.[16] The findings of this study might encourage Australian public hospitals to implement antenatal care options that provide women with greater continuity in the care-givers they see during pregnancy and labour.

Stephanie Brown, Judith Lumley

THREE

Thoughts About the Birth Eight Months Later

Elsewhere in the world pregnancy is still a major health hazard for women; almost two-thirds of a million women die each year from complications arising from pregnancy, labour and birth, and in the subsequent six weeks from illnesses made worse by pregnancy.[1] Maternal deaths are now very rare in Victoria, occurring in around one in ten thousand births.[2] While this threat to women's health has largely been eliminated in western countries, morbidity in the period after birth is still very common. Backache, urinary stress incontinence and frequency, haemorrhoids, depression and anxiety, extreme tiredness, and frequent headaches and migraines are problems for many women in the weeks and months after birth. One of the few studies that has investigated women's health after childbirth found that 83.1 per cent of women in a large population-based sample in the United Kingdom had experienced one or more of these problems for at least six weeks.[3] For around one-third of women giving birth in Victoria, the first few weeks, and sometimes longer, are made even more difficult by having to recover from either a caesarean section or a birth with forceps. Despite the obvious need for such studies, we in fact know very little about how women cope with the symptoms they experience after childbirth, or how much the birth and procedures in the context of the birth contribute to the incidence and severity of health problems in the ensuing weeks and months.

We had several interests in documenting women's views about their childbirth experiences. The first and primary aim was to investigate how satisfied Victorian women were with the care they received in labour and at the time of birth. A second and related aim was to document what actually happened to them: whether the birth occurred at term, how long they were in labour, whether their labour was induced or spontaneous, whether they used pain relief, whether forceps were used, whether they had an episiotomy or tear, and so on. A third aim was to assess women's emotional well-being eight months after birth. And a fourth was to investigate whether there was a relationship between birth events and experiences and satisfaction with care or emotional well-being at the time of the survey. The design of the questionnaire did not enable us to obtain a picture of women's physical health after childbirth, although this was investigated in the follow-up study.

This chapter documents what women said about what happened to them in labour and birth. A very brief overview of maternity care options in Victoria and current patterns of intervention (for example, how many women had a caesarean section, how many used pain relief) precedes this analysis. Readers who would like to know more about current patterns of care in Victoria can find this information in *Having a Baby in Victoria: Final Report of the Ministerial Review of Birthing Services*.[4] The question of an association between birth events and experiences and depression is discussed in Chapter 6. A discussion of the preferences women expressed regarding where they would like to give birth were they to have another pregnancy, and the primary care-giver(s) they would most prefer to be present at the birth concludes the chapter.

WHERE TO GIVE BIRTH?

Almost all women in Victoria give birth in hospital in a conventional labour ward or operating theatre. In 1989 between 1 and 2 per cent of women gave birth in a birth centre, and less than 1 per cent at home. This is consistent with the pattern of care in other States, for example, between 1985 and 1987, 0.5 per cent of births in New South Wales occurred at home,[5] and in 1992, 2.4 per cent of births in New South Wales were in a birth centre.[6] Amongst our sample, 42 women (0.5 per cent) planned to give birth in a birth centre, and of these sixteen were transferred to a standard labour ward following complications that arose in pregnancy or labour, and 26 gave birth in a birth centre as planned. Three women planned to give birth at home and only one did so.

Data on all births in Victoria, including rates of use of a range of procedures, are collected routinely by midwives at the time of birth, and reported to the Victorian Perinatal Data Collection Unit. Our study asked women to provide some of the same information, and also asked about a few procedures that are either not routinely recorded on Perinatal Data Collection Forms (for example, whether they were given an enema or shave), or that validation of the data collection has shown are under-reported by midwives (for example, whether they had an episiotomy or a perineal tear requiring stitches). The questions we asked about the birth enabled us to compare the women who returned the survey forms with all women giving birth in Victoria in the survey weeks. This confirmed that women returning the questionnaire were representative in terms of their method of birth (vaginal, caesarean section, forceps), which was an important finding for our subsequent analysis of the survey. (See Chapter 1 for further discussion of the comparison between our sample and women who gave birth in the survey weeks.)

Figure 3.1 Operative Delivery Rates: Inter-country comparisons

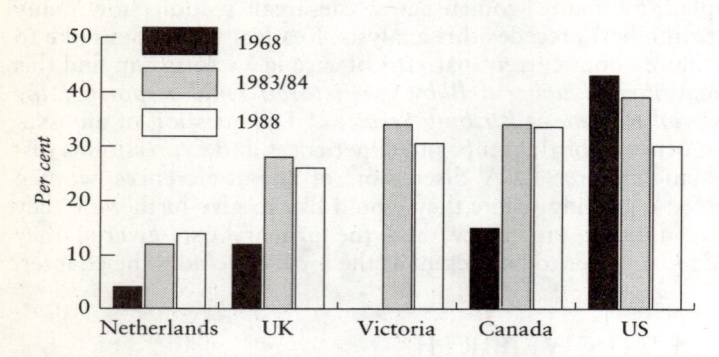

[Bar chart showing operative delivery rates (per cent) for 1968, 1983/84, and 1988 across Netherlands, UK, Victoria, Canada, and US. Approximate values: Netherlands: 4, 12, 14; UK: 12, 28, 26; Victoria: —, 34, 30; Canada: 15, 34, 33; US: 43, 39, 30.]

(Source: I. Chalmers et al., *Effective Care in Pregnancy and Childbirth*, Oxford University Press, Oxford, 1989; World Health Organization unpublished data on regional variations in obstetric practice)

Almost one in three women in our sample (and the same proportion of all women giving birth in Victoria in 1989) had operative deliveries (caesarean section, forceps and vacuum extraction), over half of these by caesarean section. Inter-country comparisons show that Australia has one of the highest rates for operative delivery in the world, comparable with the United States and Canada (see figure 3.1). Throughout the western world, rates of many obstetric procedures have risen steadily over the last two decades.[7] There has been widespread discussion of the reasons for this, and much misinformation in the way in which the issues are debated. For example, while rates of caesarean section have increased in almost every year since data began to be collected by the Perinatal Data Collection Unit in 1982, rates of induction and use of forceps have declined during this time.[8] Nevertheless, the rates of induction and forceps delivery in Victoria are still well above the rates recommended by the World Health Organization's Joint Interregional Conference on Appropriate Technology for Birth held in Fortaleza in Brazil in 1985.[9] This level of specific detail is rarely aired in public debate on the question of appropriate technology for birth. Media coverage of the issues often concentrates on the perils or the benefits of modern technology, rarely considering both sides. Women are alternately encouraged to make use of all that modern technology has to offer in the way of pain relief and intervention to speed the process of labour, or dissuaded from using this technology at all by articles condemning the over-medicalisation of birth and encouraging a return to 'natural' childbirth methods.

The Ministerial Review of Birthing Services in Victoria argued that the emphasis in discussion of intervention should be placed on the 'appropriateness' of particular procedures, rather than on 'non-intervention' or the 'reduction of intervention'.[10] From this point of view, the questions that need to be asked about current obstetric practice relate more to the effectiveness of procedures than to whether or not rates of intervention are rising or falling. Are outcomes for mothers and babies improved by the use of a given procedure? Are there any negative outcomes associated with its use? Is there sufficient evidence to answer these questions? In 1989, as a result of collection of information from all reported randomised trials of obstetric procedures, a compendium was published summarising the available evidence on the effectiveness of a vast range of obstetric procedures.[11] The authors provide a list of the procedures for which there is firm evidence of improved outcomes; those requiring further evaluation; and some still in use in many places, that 'should be abandoned in the light of available evidence', including 'shaving the perineum routinely' and 'failing to provide continuity of care during pregnancy and birth'.

Figure 3.2 Pathway to the point of first intervention in labour and birth: 100 Victorian women 1989

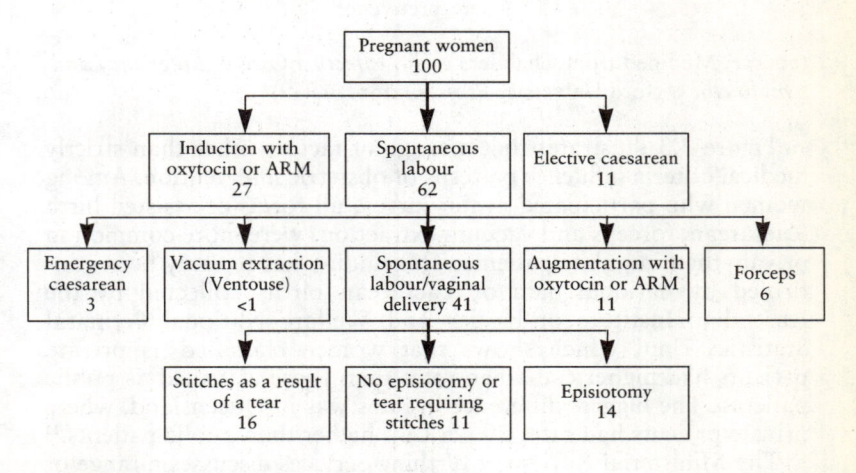

```
                        Pregnant women
                             100
         ┌───────────────────┼───────────────────┐
         ▼                   ▼                   ▼
   Induction with       Spontaneous        Elective caesarean
  oxytocin or ARM          labour                 11
        27                   62
   ┌─────┼─────────┬─────────┬─────────┐
   ▼     ▼         ▼         ▼         ▼
Emergency  Vacuum   Spontaneous  Augmentation   Forceps
caesarean extraction labour/vaginal with oxytocin   6
    3    (Ventouse) delivery 41   or ARM
           <1                       11
         ┌────────────┼────────────┐
         ▼            ▼            ▼
   Stitches as a  No episiotomy or
   result of        tear requiring    Episiotomy
     a tear          stitches             14
      16               11
```

(Source: Survey of Recent Mothers, 1989)

We do not know how much patterns of obstetric intervention are influenced by the availability of evidence regarding their effectiveness and indications for their use. We do know that most, if not all, women giving birth in Australia today do so with some form of intervention by health professionals. Only 11 per cent of the women who took part in the 1989 survey gave birth vaginally without experiencing major obstetric procedures; that is without their labour having been induced or augmented, the birth having been assisted by forceps or vacuum extraction, or stitches being required as a result of an episiotomy or tear.[12] Figure 3.2 depicts the pathway to the point of first intervention in the labour and birth experiences of 100 women.

Figure 3.3   Factors influencing the decision to intervene
___

Clinical preference

Commercial interests		'Need'
Fee-for-service payment		Culture
Status protection		Clinical experience
Fear of litigation	Decision	Client experience
Need to use equipment	to	Scientific evidence
Need to use drugs	intervene	Risk assessment
Need to fill beds		Tradition
Use techniques		Fashion
Fill buildings		Place of care
Use personnel		Care provider

Client preference

(Source: Modified from Chalmers et al., *Effective Care in Pregnancy and Childbirth*, Oxford University Press, Oxford, 1989)

Figure 3.3 illustrates that a range of factors other than strictly medical criteria influence patterns of obstetric intervention. Among women who participated in the survey, all forms of assisted birth (caesarean, forceps and vacuum extraction) were more common in private than in public patients. This finding has recently been confirmed by national data on caesarean births collected by the Australian Institute of Health and Welfare National Perinatal Statistics Unit, which shows that women classified as private patients had higher caesarean rates than those classified as public patients. The biggest difference in rates was in Queensland, where private patients had rates 50 per cent higher than public patients.[13]

The Ministerial Review of Birthing Services discusses a range of other factors, including regional differences and country of birth, which may influence patterns of intervention, and notes the wide variation in the use of procedures between different hospitals. The Review Committee was unable to explain this, and concluded that the factors influencing the decision to intervene were subtle and difficult to quantify.

The Ministerial Review also notes that there is no apparent relationship between variations in practice and differences in the outcome of pregnancy as far as death rates for infants are concerned. When rates of intervention in different hospitals with the same case-mix and level of services are plotted against standardised perinatal mortality rates at the same hospitals, there is no significant association between lower standardised rates, and higher or lower intervention rates.[14]

The main procedures experienced by women who took part in the study were as follows:
- 174 (22.4 per cent) women had their perineum shaved after arriving at the hospital;
- 214 (27.6 per cent) women had an enema;
- 217 (28 per cent) women had their labours induced using oxytocin or by artificial rupturing of the membranes;
- 253 (32.6 per cent) women had their labours augmented (speeded up) with oxytocin or artificial rupturing of the membranes;
- 90 (11.6 per cent) women had an elective (planned in advance) caesarean section;
- 52 (6.7 per cent) women had an emergency caesarean section;
- 100 (12.9 per cent) women had forceps to assist the birth;
- 16 (2.1 per cent) women had vacuum/suction to assist the birth;
- 269 (34.7 per cent) women had an episiotomy;
- 197 (25.4 per cent) women had a tear requiring stitches.

These figures are based on the total sample, including in the denominators women who had an elective caesarean section.

There is little information available to pregnant women on the relative frequency of obstetric intervention. One woman who had a caesarean birth commented:

> Caesarean births are not dealt with satisfactorily in childbirth preparation classes and are glossed over in most literature — even your own research only asked three questions regarding caesareans and yet questions 28,29,30,32,37 and 39 were applicable. Women who have caesareans have special needs — how about asking us about our anaesthetics and our pain and our after care?

It is also doubtful that many women are in a position, especially once labour has started, to have much influence over what procedures are used. Some women returning the survey forms complained that they were denied access to pain relief when they wanted it; others felt that procedures such as episiotomy were performed without adequate indications for their use.

> I wanted epidural pain relief, but it was denied, and I'm very bitter about this.
>
> There is one thing that sticks in my mind and that is when the baby was born I wasn't able to touch her properly until they had sewn up my episiotomy cut, which both my husband and I agreed was not needed. A comment was made by the doctor who said 'Seeing I had one episiotomy with my first child, he had better do another one'. More explanation of why I was cut would have settled my mind.

MEASURING SATISFACTION

Being in labour, whether for the first time or for the fifth, involves many unknowns. It is not possible to predict how long it will continue, whether it will be an 'easy' or a difficult birth, whether the baby will enter the world strong and healthy or will need resuscitation and special care. This sense of uncertainty was reflected in women's comments about their experiences of labour.

> My labour didn't go as I had imagined it to be. The baby showed signs of stress after contractions, therefore matters were somewhat taken out of my hands. The last hour was full of rushed procedures. This feeling of not being in control was no fault of the doctor or nursing staff.
>
> The birth of my last baby was induced and I didn't feel I got enough information about this. It took from 10 a.m. to 3.30 p.m. before I actually felt anything happening. By then I felt I was in for a long labour like my last one (16 hours). Once things started happening I was not very well informed as to what stage I was up to. My labour (bad pains and pushing) lasted only half an hour. This was a real shock and it took me a long time to realise that it was over — and I had given birth. If better informed I think I would have coped with this better. Both my babies were posterior, so it seemed strange for the two labours to be so different. I had not read or heard about this except to expect my second labour to be a little shorter.

These two comments reflect different sorts of experiences. The first woman, although she felt things were out of her control, was happy with the care she received. The second woman similarly felt things happened in an unexpected sequence, but she felt more could have been done to help her deal with the turn of events.

Much has been written about the difficulties and advantages of assessing satisfaction with care using postal questionnaires. As noted in Chapter 1, the main advantages are that it enables whole populations to be sampled, and is relatively inexpensive. Comparisons of women's reporting of events with medical records show that women do accurately recall what happened during pregnancy, labour and birth. Questions that remain unanswered concern the difficulty of defining and measuring satisfaction in a meaningful way.[15] As the two quotations above demonstrate, women who experience adverse events in labour may feel positive or negative about their care. It is difficult to know how women come to give meaning to their childbirth experience, and how they relate their own interpretations of events to the sorts of questions that can be asked in a postal questionnaire. It is generally acknowledged that pre-coded scales asking for an overall rating of care probably provide an under-estimate of the extent of dissatisfaction with particular aspects of care.[16] For this reason, the survey included both a global question asking women to rate their care in labour and birth as either 'as they liked', 'as they liked in some ways, and not in others' (mixed) or 'not as they liked', and more specific questions about access to information, helpfulness of care-givers, whether anyone was present at the birth they would have preferred not to have been, and the role women played in making decisions concerning their care. We have also made use of the comments women wrote on the survey forms to illustrate quantitative analysis of coded responses.

Madeleine Shearer argues that asking women to rate their satisfaction with care when they may perceive that the alternative to the procedures they experienced would have entailed unacceptable risks to their unborn infant is highly contradictory.[17] The complexity of women's thinking about the events of their labour and birth is well illustrated by the comments appended to the survey forms. Seventy-one women (9 per cent) offered further information about their labour and birth on the blank page at the end of the survey. This compares to sixteen women (2 per cent) who wrote about antenatal care, and seventy (9 per cent) who commented on care they received in hospital postnatal wards. On the basis of this, it seems clear that the birth was still of great importance to women eight months later. Like the women quoted above, the comments women made about their labour reflect a desire to clarify and explain, to give us a better basis on which to interpret their responses to our questions. This is possibly also one of the reasons why women who were dissatisfied with their care were more likely to write comments.

As noted when we described the methods employed in the two studies, surveys have the disadvantage of providing no opportunity for researchers to seek clarification from the participants, and little opportunity for participants to clarify questions or describe in detail the context of their experiences. However, women completing this questionnaire often made concerted efforts to enable us to understand their interpretations of events. This seemed particularly so in relation to the events and experiences of labour.

THE GLOBAL PICTURE
The global question about women's intrapartum care (care given in labour and birth) was worded as follows:

Overall do you feel your labour and delivery were:
managed as you liked
managed as you liked in some ways, but not in others
not managed as you like?

This question was taken from the questionnaire designed by the Institute for Social Studies in Medical Care in England.

Two-thirds of women (67 per cent) reported that their labours and births were 'managed as they liked'; 27 per cent said their care was mixed, and 6 per cent said their labour was not managed as they would have liked. Circling either of the latter two responses was taken as an indication of dissatisfaction.

Comparing this with the rating of antenatal care, it is clear that many more women felt unhappy with the care they received in labour and birth. Figure 3.4 represents this comparison: 86 per cent of women were satisfied with their antenatal care, whereas only 67 per cent were satisfied with the care they received in labour and birth.

Figure 3.4 Satisfaction with care: antenatal versus intrapartum

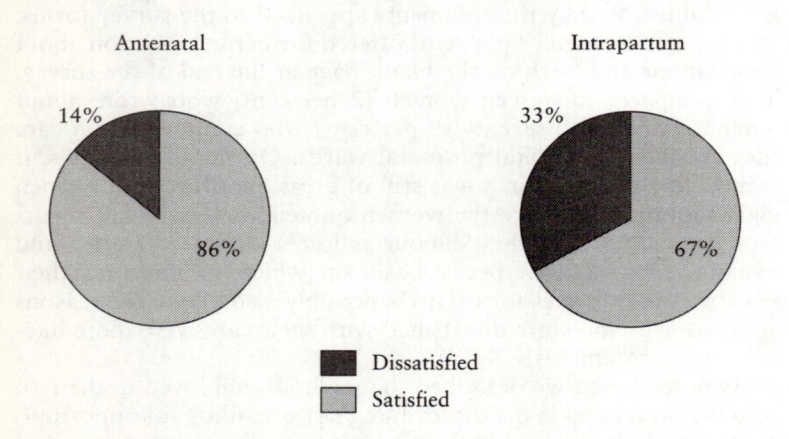

Since this is probably an underestimate of the proportion of women who were dissatisfied with specific aspects of their care (see earlier discussion this chapter and Appendix 1), the finding that one in three women was unhappy with her intrapartum care, particularly when contrasted with the much smaller proportion of women unhappy with their antenatal care, raises serious questions about the ability of maternity services in Victoria to provide the care that women want in labour.

It should be noted here that questions about satisfaction with birth were not asked of women who had an elective caesarean section, so this comparison and the analysis that follows is based in a sub-group of the sample (n=690) who had either a vaginal birth or an emergency caesarean section.

In contrast to the marked association between socio-demographic factors (being young, without a partner, of NESB, having a low family income) and dissatisfaction with antenatal care, none of these social factors was associated with dissatisfaction with care in labour and birth. Three other socio-demographic factors were associated with dissatisfaction. Primiparous women — women having a first birth — were more likely to be dissatisfied (39.8 per cent) than women having a second or subsequent birth (29.0 per cent); women who had not completed secondary school were more likely to be dissatisfied (36.6 per cent) than women with a higher level of education (28.8 per cent); and rural women were more often dissatisfied (39.6 per cent) than city women (30.5 per cent). Whereas private health insurance made a significant difference to satisfaction with antenatal care, women with private insurance were not more likely to be satisfied with their care in labour and birth than women without it.

These findings challenge common assumptions about the factors that promote dissatisfaction with care in labour. The idea, widely promoted by professional associations during the Ministerial Review of Birthing Services, that it is mainly middle-class, more highly educated women (driven by 'unrealistic expectations' of childbirth) who are critical of maternity care is not only unsubstantiated, but the reverse would appear to be the case. Women who had completed more years of formal education were more likely to be satisfied, not less.

It comes as no surprise that women having their first baby were more likely to be dissatisfied. First labours tend both to be longer and involve more frequent complications. Whether it is parity (number of births) alone, or a combination of factors that contribute to the greater dissatisfaction of first-time mothers is a question we shall return to later.

The finding that country women were more often dissatisfied with their intrapartum care than city women we had not anticipated, although it confirms comments made in public meetings in country areas during the Ministerial Review about the more limited choices available to country women, and about conservative attitudes encountered by some rural women. Comments written on the survey forms reinforced these themes.

> I would like to mention that in —— [country town] it's only in progress now to have private care in a private hospital. Till now we have had no choice, so us paying for 100% [private health insurance] coverage has been wasted to a certain degree. ... Also in the base hospital, there is only one way of giving birth. That's lying on a table. There is no birthing chair and they do not allow any other means of delivery.

Of course, not all women living in country areas had bad experiences, and some women felt they benefited from more personalised care made possible by the smaller size of country hospitals.

> I feel that the care I received during labour and delivery was excellent, partly because I gave birth in a smallish country hospital. The care was personal and the facility was small and easy to relate to.

The finding that health insurance status was not associated with satisfaction also confirmed an impression gained from Ministerial Review consultations and submissions that being a private patient confers no significant protection against being dissatisfied with care in labour, although women who are private patients clearly benefit from the continuity of care they receive in pregnancy (see Chapter 2). A majority of women planning a pregnancy do take out private health insurance (62 per cent of our sample), presumably believing it will enable them to afford the best available care. A number of women commented on why they had chosen to be private rather than public patients. One woman with three children wrote

> I feel it is necessary to have private care to allow me to get the type of care I need. I believe midwife based care is best, but here I opt for a private consultant obstetrician to ensure consistency of care.

The fact that women who had private health insurance were not more satisfied with their care in labour than women who were public patients, although they were more satisfied with their antenatal care, is an important finding of the survey. It calls into question the capacity of maternity services to provide the sort of care women are seeking during labour, even when services are provided by the woman's chosen practitioner.

Why is it that the calculation women have made — at considerable financial cost — that they will be better cared for if they have their own private obstetrician or general practitioner does not appear to result in these women being happier with care in labour and birth? There are several things we need to know in order to answer this question. How many of these women were actually cared for in labour by their chosen practitioner? Were some women happy with the care provided by their doctor, but not happy with the midwives who looked after them while they were in labour? What other factors apart from the care-givers attending women in labour contribute to satisfaction with care?

DOCTOR OR MIDWIFE, OWN DOCTOR OR OWN MIDWIFE — DOES IT MAKE A DIFFERENCE?

There were 479 women in our sample who had private health insurance. Sixty-five of these had an elective caesarean section, so they are excluded from this analysis. Almost 80 per cent of the women who had private health insurance and did not have an elective caesarean said their own obstetrician or general practitioner was present during their labour. There were 80 women who were privately insured who said their own doctor was not present during labour; eight of these noted that their doctor's locum was present instead.

Although a few women commented on the survey forms that they were disappointed their own doctor was not present for the birth, women whose own doctor was present were not more likely to be satisfied with their care than women whose own doctor was not present. Nor were they more likely to be satisfied than women who anticipated that their doctor would be present, but then found he or she was unable to.

In the question about who was present during labour, we did not differentiate between whether women were cared for by a specialist obstetrician or a general practitioner. To examine whether there is a similar gradient in satisfaction between women looked after by specialists and women cared for by general practitioners to that noted in relation to antenatal care, we looked at women's rating of their intrapartum care according to whether they attended an obstetrician, general practitioner or public hospital clinic during pregnancy. The proportion of women unhappy with their intrapartum care was very similar across the three groups; roughly one-third of women were dissatisfied with their intrapartum care in all three provider categories. Figure 3.5 shows how this contrasts with the strong association noted earlier between women's satisfaction with their care in pregnancy and who provided this care.

The survey also showed that there was no association between satisfaction and whether it was a doctor, a midwife, or a doctor and midwife working together who provided 'hands on' assistance when the baby was born. Further analysis shows that there are no differences between women attending an obstetrician, general practitioner or public clinic in how kind and understanding care-givers were perceived to be during labour; how satisfied women were with explanations given by care-givers — both midwives and doctors — about events during labour and birth; or in women's perception of the helpfulness of midwives during this time. Women who had attended a private obstetrician (87.1 per cent) or general practitioner (88.9 per cent), however, were more likely to say that the doctor who attended them in labour was helpful, than women who attended a public hospital clinic (72.7 per cent). The group of women who attended a specialist obstetrician were also more likely to say that they had an active role in decisions made about their care in labour (88.3 per cent) than women who attended a public clinic (76.4 per cent).

Figure 3.5 Satisfaction with care: by provider of care

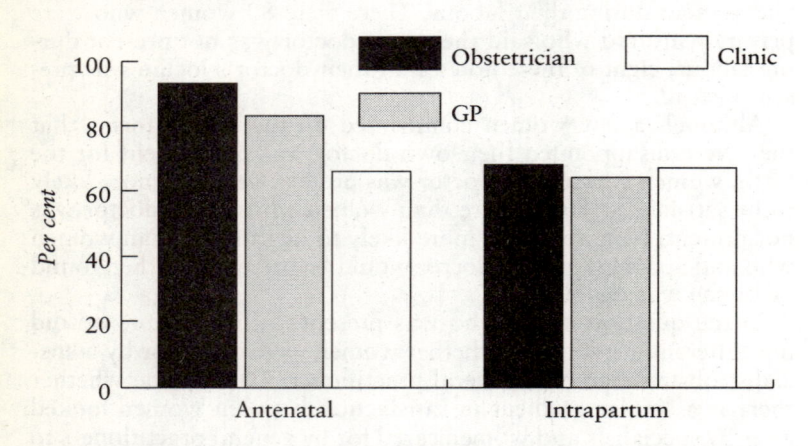

Thus it seems that being attended by a private practitioner makes only a small difference to satisfaction with care in labour; a difference so small that it is not apparent in women's overall ratings of their care. Nor does it seem to make a major difference to women's satisfaction whether or not a doctor, a midwife, or a combination of care-givers assists them with the birth.

PREGNANCY AND REPRODUCTIVE HISTORY
Very few factors related to the current pregnancy or past reproductive history were associated with satisfaction with intrapartum care. By far the strongest association was with dissatisfaction with antenatal care. Just over half of the women (54.6 per cent) who rated their antenatal care as mixed or poor were also dissatisfied with their intrapartum care, although this only amounted to 25.6 per cent of all the women who were unhappy with their care in labour. No other factors related to the current pregnancy, such as whether or not women were pleased to be pregnant, being hos-

pitalised for a period of the pregnancy, or having attended or not attended childbirth education classes (see Chapter 4) were associated with satisfaction. Three reproductive history factors were associated with dissatisfaction. Fifty per cent of women who had had a prior caesarean section, and 32.2 per cent of women who had not, were dissatisfied with their intrapartum care for the current pregnancy. Having a previous premature birth (47.7 per cent) or a previous breech birth (54.5 per cent) were associated with similarly raised levels of dissatisfaction. There was no association between satisfaction and a history of pregnancy loss (stillbirth, spontaneous or induced abortion), having had a previous low birthweight infant, or prior forceps delivery.

INTRAPARTUM EVENTS

What was labour like for the women in the study? How did they feel when they went into hospital? Did they see any familiar faces among the labour-ward staff? Who was present during their labour? Did they anticipate that their labour would be more or less painful than it was? Were they given an epidural or other forms of analgesia? Did they use other methods of pain relief — standing under the shower, music, relaxation exercises? What position were they in when the baby was born — lying on the bed, on hands and knees, sitting propped up, squatting? Was the decision about what position to be in left up to them or determined by their care-givers? Was the room they were in comfortable and homelike, brightly or dimly lit? Did people knock before they entered the room? Was anyone present they would have preferred not to be?

Unless they are unconscious or heavily drugged, women generally have very vivid memories of the events occurring in their labours, even recalling them clearly twenty years later.[18] From the replies to the survey, we know the answers to many of the above questions, though not all of them. We do not know how many women were greeted by a familiar face when they went into hospital — although it is likely that very few were — or how many different people were involved in each woman's care. A handful of women wrote comments on the end of the survey form addressing these issues.

> Even though I have a good gyno. once again I felt rather let down during labour. A midwife attended right through until she felt there were complications and she called my doctor. The midwife was exceptional all the way through — very caring and very informative, but I felt she was doing the job I was paying my doctor for. I have known my doctor for quite a while and was looking forward to a familiar face during labour — it wasn't there until the last half hour of delivery and so I was very thankful I had a good midwife.

Being a public patient I saw a variety of doctors during my pregnancy, none of whom was present at the birth. This made it impossible to discuss a birth plan in advance. I thought the labour ward was badly understaffed at night — our midwife was just a flash racing in and out only when absolutely necessary. In the morning I was told I should have 'made more noise' to get attention sooner!

I couldn't have done it without the constant support of my husband throughout the labour — midwives changed, the doctor came and went, but he was always there.

The recurring theme in these accounts is the desire to be cared for by people who are known and trusted by the labouring woman — not surprising, given the many other 'unknowns' women have to deal with at this time. For most women, entering hospital to have a baby means getting to know and become accustomed to an unfamiliar environment. All mammalian species are known to look for a safe and quiet place to give birth.[19] The environment of modern hospitals — bright lights, a hospital bed in the middle of the room, strange personnel coming in and out, other women in labour crying out and making strange noises — while it may be the safest place to be in one sense, may not for some women feel like a very secure one at all. Knowing the people who are around you is one way in which this strangeness and unfamiliarity can be lessened.

In 1977 it was rare for Victorian hospitals to allow partners unrestricted access to labour wards. Most required formal consent by a doctor, and some only allowed partners to be present when the doctor was in the room.[20] By 1982 this had become a non-issue — all restrictive policies had been removed. Among our sample, fathers were present during labour in 92.8 per cent of cases. Of the 50 women not accompanied by a partner, 22 had a relative or friend with them for all or most of the time they were in labour. A further 65 women (9.3 per cent) had both their partner and a relative or friend with them while they were in labour. In all, 96 per cent of the women who experienced labour were accompanied by their partner, a relative or a friend.

By 1989 it had clearly become accepted practice for fathers and other relatives and friends of women giving birth to be present in labour wards. This shift in policy and practice has occurred without any rigorous evaluation of its impact on women, or on the actions of carers. Although it is assumed to be beneficial, it remains unclear from the available evidence that this is always the case.[21] Keirse et al. have drawn attention to observational studies of father-attendance that 'suggest that in some settings neither active support nor supportive companionship is manifested'.

From the comments written on the survey forms it seemed clear that the issue of emotional support may not be the only factor requiring further investigation. Some women had clearly relied on their partners to provide basic physical care when labour wards were busy or short staffed, one woman commenting that she would have fallen out of bed had her partner not been present.

> The birth of my child could have turned into a disaster (cord around the neck) — the hospital was short staffed and as I had a quick birth and was handling contractions they never worried to check me. My cervix wasn't checked on arrival or even later and they had no idea my baby was nearly there. My water broke, the head appeared and the baby was born in minutes. My husband had to leave the room to find a midwife — there was no one around at the nurse's station. When they finally came, it was a bit of a panic. The hospital (private) was badly understaffed.

> I was not impressed with —— hospital. I had my first child at —— [another] hospital and it was great. I expected the same concern and treatment second time around. This did not happen. I was left unattended during labour and if it was not for my husband being with me I don't know what may have happened. Yes they were *very busy* on the day, but I believe you pay good money to deserve better, and besides the money I thought it was hospital policy to have a midwife with you for most of the labour. On two occasions my husband caught me falling out of bed. [emphasis in original]

With the current pressure on hospital budgets, and associated reduced staffing levels, the potential for the presence of a woman's partner to be used as a surrogate staff member at times when labour wards are busy needs careful monitoring.

While some women complained about lack of staff available to assist them, others had too many. One woman complained that there were so many people in the room at the time her baby was born that her partner was pushed into the background.

> I had a breech birth and I never found out about her position till my water was broken. I didn't carry much fluid, nor did I put on the 12 kg required. This birth was a shock as my other was normal. I had my husband and mother there. Yet at the last minute my mother was asked to leave while four students came in to watch the birth which I thought stunk. I was unprepared for a breech birth and would rather have had my mother with me. I understand students have to learn but I knew nothing about a breech birth and the more strange faces scared me. I had two midwives, my GP, an obstetrician for an emergency caesar if necessary, a paediatrician, four students and my husband. Ten counting me and that was far too many for the size of

> the room. My husband was pushed to the back for students to watch. With my first birth, my husband helped deliver. This time he was last in line to get to hold her there were so many people in front of him.

This woman's experience raises the issue of unwanted people being present at the birth. This was less common than is sometimes imagined. Thirty-nine women (5.7 per cent) said that there were persons in the room with them during labour who they would have preferred not to be there. In eleven cases the unwanted persons were student doctors or student midwives. More often it was hospital staff or the woman's own doctor, and in a few cases women mentioned relatives that they would have preferred were not there, including in one case a woman who said she wished her husband had not been present. Several women noted that it was just one particular doctor or midwife they did not like, and that other staff were helpful and considerate.

Two out of five women (42.3 per cent) in the sample found their labour more painful than they expected, with women having first births being much more likely to say this. Sixty-one per cent of primiparous women said that the pain they experienced with contractions was worse or much worse than they had expected, compared to 36 per cent of women having their second or subsequent baby. Over 71 per cent of women used some form of pharmacological pain relief. Use of pain relief was more common among first-time mothers (85.7 per cent) than among women experiencing second or subsequent births (63 per cent). The main types of pharmacological pain relief used by women are summarised:

- 365 women (53 per cent) used nitrous oxide (gas and oxygen);
- 334 women (48.5 per cent) used pethidine;
- 159 women (23.1 per cent) were given an epidural;
- 20 women (2.9 per cent) were given a general anaesthetic.

Unfortunately, the questionnaire did not ask about other methods women used in order to cope with pain. Of the 195 women who did not use pharmacological pain relief, 73.8 per cent said they had not wanted any; one woman noting that she 'did not want the after effects'. Of the remaining women, half said there was not enough time for them to be given any pain relief, and half said pain relief was not offered to them. Eight women wrote comments about pain relief at the end of the questionnaire. Four of these argued that pain relief should be more readily available to women who want it.

> I think epidurals should be offered as an option far more readily than they presently are. Childbirth may be a natural experience, but it is also an extremely painful one. Current opinion has it that women who give birth naturally (i.e. at home, with no pain relief or

surgical/medical intervention) are in some way superior to those who seek medical help. Women are made to feel guilty for being unable or unwilling to manage birth without artificial help. Yet no one says men should have prostate operations without the aid of anaesthetics because it's more natural that way.

Other comments regarding pain relief pointed out that pain relief does not always work, and may have disabling side effects as well. For instance, one woman wrote

> The only pain relief I had was pethidine, although I would hardly call it 'pain relief'. I was still in *agony*, but I felt really spaced out. I couldn't even estimate how long I was pushing. I wish now I had asked for an epidural, but at the time I didn't even think to ask. I didn't feel in control at all. [emphasis in original]

Two out of three women having their first baby said that pain relief was unsuccessful (not even partially successful); among women having later births, 17 per cent noted that pain relief was not successful.

The question people most often ask after 'Was it a boy or a girl?' and 'How much did she/he weigh?', is 'How long were you in labour?' This is a difficult question to answer. Does it mean from the time you first noticed contractions that seemed a bit unusual; when they became regular (sometimes they are never regular); when they became 'painful'; when you decided to go to hospital? It is just as difficult to obtain precise estimates of the time women spend in labour when taking this information from hospital records as it is when asking women for this information in a postal questionnaire. We did ask women to give us an estimate of how long they were in first stage, although we were well aware of these difficulties. The question asked women to tell us how long it was from the time when pains became strong and regular, and/or they rang up the hospital, until they started pushing down or had a caesarean section. Using this definition, the majority of first-time mothers were in first-stage labour for between two and twelve hours (67 per cent), another third were in first-stage labour for more than twelve hours, and 2 per cent for less than two hours. Women having second or subsequent births experienced slightly shorter labours. A third were in first stage for less than two hours (34 per cent); 80 per cent spent between two and twelve hours; and only 6 per cent spent any longer than this amount of time.

Most women held their babies soon after birth, although 19 per cent of first-time mothers and 12 per cent of multiparous women were unable to do so.

The survey leaves several important questions unanswered. In particular, we know little about how women felt about the environment in which they gave birth, whether they were attached to equipment that prevented them from moving around or getting into positions in which they were more comfortable, what position they were in when they gave birth, and how many people (and changes of shifts) looked after them during labour.

WHAT DIFFERENCE DO BIRTH EVENTS MAKE TO SATISFACTION?

As well as looking at whether or not women experienced individual procedures, we calculated a score for obstetric intervention based on the scoring system developed by Elliot and co-workers.[22] This provided a score for every woman weighted to take into account both the number and types of procedures she had experienced. For example, two points were given for an episiotomy, six for a general anaesthetic and ten for a caesarean (details of the scoring system are given in Appendix 3). The median score on this scale was four, with a range from nought to 25. The relationships between intrapartum events, including the total score for obstetric intervention, and women's global rating of their care are presented in table 3.1. The table shows the proportion of women experiencing each event who were dissatisfied with their care, distinguishing between first-time mothers and women having a second or subsequent birth.

Table 3.1 Relationship between intrapartum events and dissatisfaction with care in labour and birth by parity

	First births				Subsequent births			
	%	(% dissat.)	OR	[CI]	%	(% dissat.)	OR	[CI]
Labour induced								
No	66	(34)	1.00		70	(30)	1.00	
Yes	35	(50)	1.95	[1.1-3.4]	30	(27)	0.83	[0.5-1.4]
Labour augmented								
No	53	(32)	1.00		69	(29)	1.00	
Yes	47	(47)	1.93	[1.1-3.3]	31	(30)	1.08	[0.7-1.7]
Length of labour								
< 2 hours	2	(33)	1.00		34	(22)	1.00	
2–12 hours	67	(39)	1.3	[0.2-14.8]	80	(29)	1.42	[0.7-3.0]
> 12 hours	31	(42)	1.45	[0.2-16.8]	6	(52)	3.75	[1.2-11.4]

	\%	First births (% dissat.)	OR	[CI]	%	Subsequent births (% dissat.)	OR	[CI]
Birth								
Spontaneous vaginal	62	(31)	1.00		89	(27)	1.00	
Emergency caesarean	11	(52)	2.43	[1.0-5.8]	5	(53)	2.97	[1.1-8.2]
Forceps	27	(54)	2.61	[1.4-4.8]	7	(39)	1.73	[0.7-4.1]
Episiotomy								
No	49	(30)	1.00		67	(28)	1.00	
Yes	51	(49)	2.26	[1.3-3.9]	33	(33)	1.27	[0.8-2.0]
Obstetric procedure score								
0-4	48	(28)	1.00		71	(13)	1.00	
5-9	23	(43)	1.97	[1.0-3.9]	20	(35)	3.72	[1.9-7.2]
10+	29	(57)	3.35	[1.8-6.4]	9	(44)	5.41	[2.3-12.5]
Held baby soon after birth								
Yes	81	(37)	1.00		89	(27)	1.00	
No	19	(52)	1.85	[1.0-3.6]	12	(52)	3.02	[1.6-5.8]
Primary care-giver at the birth								
Doctor	77	(44)	1.00		61	(29)	1.00	
Midwife	12	(28)	0.51	[0.2-1.2]	28	(29)	0.98	[0.6-1.6]
Midwife/doctor	8	(20)	0.32	[0.1-1.1]	6	(29)	0.99	[0.4-2.7]
Other	3	(44)	1.03	[0.2-5.0]	6	(28)	0.94	[0.3-2.5]
Pain relief								
None	15	(18)	1.00		37	(21)	1.00	
Gas and O_2	64	(42)	3.22	[1.3-9.1]	23	(37)	2.26	[1.4-3.8]
Pethidine	70	(44)	3.46	[1.4-9.8]	36	(35)	2.08	[1.2-3.6]
Epidural	24	(48)	4.01	[1.4-11.8]	5	(33)	1.27	[0.3-4.0]
General anaesthetic	4	(55)	5.3	[1.0-29.2]	1	(83)	19.06	[2.0-908.6]
Success of pain relief								
Very/partly successful	37	(31)	1.00		83	(33)	1.00	
Not at all successful	63	(51)	2.35	[1.3-4.4]	17	(38)	1.23	[0.6-2.5]
Experience of pain								
As expected or better	39	(25)	1.00		64	(20)	1.00	
Worse or much worse than expected	61	(47)	2.75	[1.5-5.2]	36	(46)	3.47	[2.2-5.6]

Both experienced and first-time mothers were more likely to be dissatisfied if they had a caesarean section; used pethidine, nitrous oxide, or general anaesthesia; found the pain worse than anticipated; had a high obstetric procedure score (above the median of four); or could not hold the baby soon after birth. The following factors were associated with dissatisfaction in first-time mothers but not in women having their second and subsequent birth: induction, augmentation, epidural anaesthesia, forceps, and episiotomy. Being in first stage for longer than twelve hours was associated with dissatisfaction among multiparous women, but not among women having their first baby.

Many of the women dissatisfied with their care experienced intervention during their labour and birth, but was their dissatisfaction a direct result of undergoing specific procedures and the ways in which their care was altered by their use, or was it simply that they had more protracted and difficult labours that tended to leave women feeling dissatisfied with their care?

> I really felt that the birth I had was traumatic and painful. I had prepared to have a normal birth, but being overdue I had to have my waters broken and a drip inserted in my arm and then because my baby had pooed inside me (I've forgotten the posh word) I had a monitor attached inside me to the baby. So although my contractions started without the use of the stuff in the drip I felt like I was tied down to all these tubes. I think my negative feeling to all this was one of the reasons for the traumatic birth. I felt I couldn't do what I wanted during contractions (i.e. walk, shower, etc.).

Having dealt with something they had not (could not have?) expected, in an unfamiliar environment, surrounded by unfamiliar faces, attached to a monitor and unable to move around, it is not surprising that women who experienced greater intervention were less satisfied with their care. Other studies have also documented an association between exposure to intervention and dissatisfaction with care.[23] Another group of studies reports that women are more negative about the birth itself (rather than the care they received) when they have experienced intervention.[24] Josephine Green and her colleagues argue that the care women received, whether they were able to get enough information, and the extent to which they were able to influence decisions about their care and maintain a sense of 'being in control' are more important to women's satisfaction with their birthing experience than intervention *per se*.[25] Before discussing what our survey data suggests in relation to this question, we need to look at the individual relationships between access to information, women's views of care-givers, the role women played in decisions regarding their care, and overall satisfaction with intrapartum care.

INFORMATION AND VIEWS ABOUT CARE-GIVERS

The questions we asked about access to information and satisfaction with the care provided by care-givers were:

> *In general during labour and delivery did the nurses and midwives [a separate question referred to doctors] explain what was happening, or would you have liked more information from them?*
>
> *Did you find that the doctor/midwife [asked separately] was helpful?*
>
> *Would you describe the way you were looked after in labour and delivery as very kind and understanding, fairly kind and understanding, or not very kind and understanding?*

The responses of first-time mothers and experienced mothers to these questions are shown in table 3.2. Both groups were much more likely to be dissatisfied if they thought that they had not obtained sufficient information from care-givers, and if they thought that midwives and doctors had provided only some, little, or no help. Women who described their care-givers as only fairly or not at all kind and understanding were also more likely to be dissatisfied with their care overall, irrespective of parity. The magnitude of these associations is particularly striking. Lack of information was associated with a four-fold to six-fold increase in dissatisfaction. Women who did not regard their care-givers as being very kind and understanding were four to five times more likely to rate their care negatively, and the odds of dissatisfaction increased two-fold to eight-fold when women assessed care-givers as only sometimes or not at all helpful.

These findings were reflected in the comments women wrote on the survey forms. Women who felt their care-givers put effort into explaining things described how much they valued this; information being withheld prompted negative comments.

> The doctor who delivered my baby was fantastic. He explained everything about each stage during labour to myself and my husband. After delivery he stayed and helped me to try to breastfeed.

> [In labour] My blood pressure soared. I wasn't able to walk around or actively participate in the labour. What annoyed me was that the doctor was seemingly aware of this problem but neglected to inform me *at all* at any of my visits, in fact said I was good. The nurses said he was aware of the problem. [emphasis in original]

> I found the doctor only explained when asked, he didn't give any details other than what was asked for. I would have liked him to talk and explain more.

Table 3.2 Relationships between access to information and views about care-givers and dissatisfaction with care in labour and birth by parity

	First births				Subsequent births			
	%	(% dissat.)	OR	[CI]	%	(% dissat.)	OR	[CI]
Informed of pain relief options before labour								
Yes	87	(39)	1.00		67	(24)	1.00	
No	13	(44)	1.22	[0.6-2.7]	33	(40)	2.09	[1.3-3.3]
Information from doctors								
Enough	80	(33)	1.00		86	(23)	1.00	
Wanted more	20	(74)	5.76	[2.7-12.7]	14	(64)	6.14	[3.0-12.7]
Information from midwives								
Enough	79	(32)	1.00		86	(24)	1.00	
Wanted more	21	(67)	4.33	[2.2-8.6]	14	(63)	5.50	[2.9-10.3]
Helpfulness of doctors								
Very/fairly helpful	85	(38)	1.00		85	(24)	1.00	
Some, little or no help	15	(64)	2.95	[1.3-6.6]	15	(56)	4.03	[2.05-8.0]
Helpfulness of midwives								
Very/fairly helpful	93	(37)	1.00		93	(26)	1.00	
Some, little or no help	7	(83)	8.52	[2.3-46.8]	7	(75)	8.55	[3.4-24.4]
Kindness and understanding of care-givers								
Very kind and understanding	79	(32)	1.00		78	(22)	1.00	
Fairly kind/not very kind and understanding	21	(73)	5.78	[2.9-11.9]	22	(55)	4.35	[2.6-7.3]

Care provided by care-givers was also the subject of both grateful and critical comments. The following annotations were typical of women who had positive experiences.

> I had my baby in —— hospital under the care of Dr ——. I have nothing but praise for everyone concerned in the birth of my baby.

> Midwives are the ones with a feel for the situation, be it mother, father, pain, anguish — anything. They are excellent in my view.

A few women noted that they appreciated the care of a particular person, but were less positive about others.

> Had changeover of staff — in both cases one excellent nurse each time, others I didn't care for.

> I had a student midwife with me during my labour and a fully qualified one coming in and out. I would have much preferred the fully qualified midwife with me all the time and she seemed to know more about what was going on and made me feel at ease every time she came near me.

While some staff had the capacity to make women feel 'at ease', others were criticised for 'being too cold and clinical', 'making jokes about a woman who is in pain', 'not answering' questions, or simply not being there when they were needed, as in the following example.

> In my opinion, the midwife should not have waited 15 minutes to attend me. I had said that I had to push and 15 minutes is too long to wait especially for a third baby. As a result the doctor missed the birth, and the midwife did not even 'catch' the child when he was born. He just shot out and landed on the bed. Because the doctor did not make the birth I did not have an episiotomy and subsequently tore quite badly. It seemed that the midwife was more interested in catching up with her paperwork than attending to patients.

WOMEN'S ROLE IN DECISION MAKING

A further dimension of the experience of childbirth concerns the extent to which women are able to influence decisions about their care and the actions of those around them. The survey included two questions relevant to this issue: a general question regarding the role women saw themselves as having in decision making, and a question about the presence of anyone at the birth whom they did not want to be there. Since many women who attended consultations and sent in written submissions during the Ministerial Review of Birthing Services talked in terms of wanting to have an 'active say' in decisions regarding their care, we worded the first of these questions as follows:

> *Do you feel you were given an active say in making decisions about what happened in your labour?*
>   *yes, in all cases*
>   *yes, in most cases*
>   *only sometimes*
>   *no, not at all*
>   *uncertain*

The relationships between women's responses and their overall satisfaction are shown in table 3.3. Not having an active say in decisions was associated with a six-fold increase in dissatisfaction among women having their first baby and a fifteen-fold increase among women having a second or subsequent baby. Unwanted people being present at the birth was associated with a three-fold increase in dissatisfaction among multiparous women, and a two-fold increase among first-time mothers, although the latter finding just failed to reach significance.

Table 3.3 Relationship between women's role in decision making and dissatisfaction with care in labour and birth by parity

	First births %	(% dissat.)	OR	[CI]	Subsequent births %	(% dissat.)	OR	[CI]
Given an active say in decisions about what happened in labour								
In all cases	39	(24)	1.00		46	(11)	1.00	
In most cases	38	(38)	2.02	[1.1-3.9]	39	(33)	3.95	[2.2-7.2]
Only sometimes	14	(74)	9.39	[3.6-25.2]	7	(77)	26.91	[9.5-79.4]
Not at all	6	(73)	8.94	[2.3-41.1]	4	(88)	57.33	[11.6-533.9]
Uncertain	3	(50)	3.25	[0.6-18.6]	3	(71)	20.48	[5.2-94.9]
Unwanted people present at the birth								
No	93	(39)	1.00		95	(27)	1.00	
Yes	7	(61)	2.49	[0.9-7.4]	5	(55)	3.23	[1.2-8.7]

Women might have meant many things when they chose among the five options concerning their participation in decisions regarding their care. Having an 'active say' might mean being given an opportunity to choose between options, being able to decide when certain action will be taken, being given information as to why decisions were made, having the right of veto, or all of these depending on the circumstances at the time. Several women wrote about situations in which they felt their wishes had not been respected, including this mother of twins:

> I had too many people in the room at the time of the births. I was forced to stay on my back for hours with monitors all around and inside my body ... I was given repeated vaginal examinations while on my back which is agony when carrying two babies. I never got to hold my babies after the birth so I just felt I was a machine.

This woman's experience echoes the description given earlier by the woman whose mother was asked to leave while four students watched her give birth to a baby in breech position. Other comments pertaining to how decisions were made included the following critical comments about women's own preferences about the management of labour and pain relief being overridden:

> The midwives on duty at the time we were in labour ward were not very helpful — if anything, they were critical and argumentative over my decision to have an epidural for pain relief.

> I feel that trends in medical opinions or doctor's personal preferences regarding the management of labour, pain relief, etc. in the hospital labour ward play too great a part in determining how your child is born. The doctor is not giving birth and if the mother is capable of making an informed decision relating to the birth, she is the one who should make this.

Other women who felt their views had been respected described how much they valued this:

> My first child was an emergency caesarean following 14 hours labour, failed forceps and failed epidural delivery. The support I was given by my doctor to deliver naturally, despite the fact that he advised against it, made the birth of my second child fantastic ... The respect I was shown by the medical profession in letting me determine my fate is something I was really grateful for.

> [In] this hospital I was much freer to do what I wanted than the hospital where I had my first child (3 years ago). [I was] able to give birth in unusual position — everything was for my comfort rather than the doctors' or midwives' convenience.

SORTING OUT ASSOCIATED FACTORS

Are these factors — having an active say in decisions, getting the information you want from care-givers, having only people you want present at the birth, feeling that care-givers are helpful, kind and understanding — more important to women's overall satisfaction with care than the types of procedures they experience, or the length of time they are in labour? To what extent does being a first-time mother alone account for dissatisfaction? One way to explore these questions is to fit all the factors associated with dissatisfaction together in the one logistic model. In this way is it possible to see how various aspects of women's experiences are related, and to determine the extent to which each contributes to dissatisfaction.

Using the computer software package, Egret, we entered all the social factors (being a first-time mother, not having completed secondary education) and birth events and experiences associated with dissatisfaction (having a high obstetric procedure score, a long first stage of labour, unwanted people being present at the birth, not having an active say in decisions, not having enough information, pain being worse than expected, care-givers being unhelpful, being unable to hold the baby soon after birth) into a logistic regression model with dissatisfaction as the outcome being investigated (see table 3.4). Data on the helpfulness of midwives and doctors were pooled to give one measure of the helpfulness of care-givers. The same was done to create a single measure of access to information. Rather than include individual procedures, we used the weighted intervention score dividing the sample into two groups according to whether the score was greater than or equal to five, or less than five (the point closest to the median). Although living in the country was associated with dissatisfaction, place of residence was left out of the analysis because there were many women who had not filled in their postcode, which did not allow us to code this information. One hundred and forty-seven women were excluded from the analysis because of missing values for at least one item, leaving 543 women included. Those excluded were not more or less likely to be dissatisfied than women remaining in the analysis (χ^2 =1.5, 1df, p=0.22).

Of the ten factors we put into the model, only five remained significantly associated with dissatisfaction after adjusting for all the others. These were: having an active say in decisions sometimes or not at all; wanting more information; pain being worse than expected; care-givers being some, little or no help; and not having completed secondary school.

To give a more precise estimate of the contribution these factors made to dissatisfaction, two further models were fitted. In the second model we entered parity and the intervention score, and then the five factors from the first model that had contributed to dissatisfaction. Parity and the intervention score were entered first because both of these factors have direct biological implications for women's experience of childbirth. In this model, being a first-time mother and having a higher intervention score do not exert any additional influence on satisfaction after adjusting for the five other variables. The model showed that being a first-time mother and having a higher score for intervention did not contribute to greater dissatisfaction.

Table 3.4 Odds ratios for associations of parity, education, birth events and experiences with dissatisfaction with care in labour and birth

	Unadjusted odds ratio	[CI]	p	Adjusted odds ratio	[CI]	p
Given an active say (sometimes or not at all/always or in most cases)	11.46	[6.4-20.4]	<0.001	7.35	[3.9-14.0]	<0.001
Access to information from caregivers (wanted more/enough)	5.7	[3.6-8.9]	<0.001	2.55	[1.5-4.5]	<0.001
Experience of pain (worse or much worse than expected/ as expected or better)	3.98	[2.7-5.8]	<0.001	3.13	[2.0-4.9]	<0.001
Helpfulness of care-givers (some, little or no help/ very or fairly helpful)	4.73	[2.8-7.8]	<0.001	1.94	[1.0-3.9]	0.05
Obstetric procedure score (greater than or equal to 5/ less than 5)	2.24	[1.5-3.3]	<0.001	1.38	[0.9-2.2]	0.20
Held baby soon after birth (no/yes)	2.32	[1.4-3.9]	<0.001	1.54	[0.8-2.9]	0.20
Unwanted people present at birth (no/yes)	2.97	[1.4-6.3]	0.004	2.22	[0.8-6.1]	0.12
Length of first stage of labour (12 hours or more/ less than 12 hours)	2.01	[1.3-3.2]	0.004	1.33	[0.7-2.5]	0.36
Parity (0,1+)	1.69	[1.2-2.3]	0.006	0.86	[0.5-1.4]	0.55
Education (less than year 12/completed year 12)	1.57	[1.1-2.3]	0.016	1.56	[1.0-2.4]	0.05

In the third model, we deliberately excluded women's rating of pain because of its strong association with intervention (χ^2 for linear trend = 33.27, p<0.0001). In this model, reported in table 3.5, a higher score for intervention was associated with close to a twofold increase in dissatisfaction. Being a first-time mother continued to exert no significant additional influence on dissatisfaction after adjusting for the other factors. To explore the relationship between reporting of pain and intervention further, women's rating of their intrapartum care and the weighted intervention score were stratified according to whether pain was worse than expected, as expected, or better than expected. Among the group who reported experiencing worse pain than expected, an intervention score of five or higher was associated with a four-fold increase in dissatisfaction (OR=3.90 [1.8-8.3]), indicating that for this group of women intervention has a highly significant effect.

Table 3.5 Adjusted odds ratios for associations of parity, obstetric procedure score, role in decision making, access to information and helpfulness of care-givers with dissatisfaction with care in labour and birth

	Adjusted odds ratio	*[CI]*	*p*
Parity			
(0,1+)	1.17	[0.8-1.8]	0.48
Obstetric procedure score (greater than or equal to 5/less than 5)	1.73	[1.1-2.7]	0.015
Given an active say (sometimes or not at all/yes, in all or most cases)	7.31	[4.0-13.5]	<0.001
Access to information from care-givers (wanted more/enough)	3.11	[1.8-5.3]	<0.001
Helpfulness of care-givers (some, little or no help/very or fairly helpful)	1.94	[1.0-3.7]	0.04

WHAT DO WOMEN WANT?

These findings suggest that access to information during labour, relationships to care-givers, the extent of women's involvement in decisions about their care, and exposure to intervention are critical to women's satisfaction with care. The high odds of dissatisfaction associated with wanting more information, care-givers being only some help or not at all helpful, and not having an active say in decisions indicates that these factors may be best thought about as individual components of satisfaction. The fact that each remained in our first model after adjusting for other factors suggests that women may rate their care negatively for any one of these reasons. Our data lend only partial support to the conclusion of Green et al. that being a first-time mother is an additional factor leading to lower satisfaction.[26] Parity alone did not exert a significant influence on any of the logistic models we developed. However, for certain key variables, such as involvement in decision making and exposure to intervention, first-time mothers were much more likely to be dissatisfied even when they had apparently similar experiences.

The greatest increase in odds of dissatisfaction in each of the models we developed was associated with not having an active say in making decisions about what happened in labour. Some obstetricians who saw the survey in the course of our obtaining approval from hospital ethics committees suggested omitting this question from the questionnaire. Although we included 'uncertain' as a category of response, it was contended that women would be unable to answer the question. Another view, with which we disagree, held that if women completed the question, their responses would be biased because of its wording. These responses from practitioners highlight the degree of tension surrounding the issue of women's participation in decisions regarding their care — tensions that from our data clearly exist for women as well as obstetricians. There is a need to research these issues further, in particular to explore what women from different backgrounds understand by the phrases 'having an active say' and 'feeling in control', and what factors contribute to good and bad experiences in individual settings.

INTERVENTION — AT WHAT SOCIAL COST TO WOMEN?

An important set of questions relates to whether the dissatisfaction accompanying more intense intervention is a correlate (unavoidable?) of a more complicated and therefore more painful labour, or whether it has more to do with aspects of the procedures themselves or the ways in which care may be altered by their use. The survey offers several clues in answer to these questions. First, the fact that having a longer labour was not associated with dissatisfaction among first-time mothers suggests that the reasons why intervention is associated with dissatisfaction in this group are not solely related to having more complications in labour. Second, the multivariate analysis confirms that many factors, and not just the amount of pain experienced, determine women's overall satisfaction with care.

The five factors entered into our original model that remained significantly associated with dissatisfaction (not having an active say in decisions, wanting more information, care-givers not being helpful, pain being worse than expected, and not having completed secondary school) demonstrate the importance of relationships with care-givers. Although intervention did not add to this model, it remained significant when pain was left out of our third model. This result together with the finding that women who rate their pain as worse than expected were much more likely to be dissatisfied if they experienced greater intervention, suggests that in the Australian context, intervention *per se* is important to women's overall satisfaction in addition to and separately from their relationships with care-givers, access to information, and role in decision making. The fact that intervention carries with it an increased risk of dissatisfaction irrespective of these factors adds further weight to an already convincing body of evidence for questioning current patterns of obstetric intervention.[27]

DID THE SURVEY INFLUENCE POLICY DEVELOPMENT?

The aim of all research on women's satisfaction with maternity care must ultimately be to influence what happens in practice settings. This study was unusual among reported studies because it was directly linked to a process of policy review. Having access to a reliable source of data from a largely representative sample of Victorian women enabled us to counter several stereotypes about what makes women dissatisfied, and about how representative views expressed in public meetings and submissions were. The circulation of stereotypes about women who are dissatisfied with their care often operates to discredit the critical feedback when it is given.[28] The survey did not substantiate the idea that it is mainly middle-class and more educated women who are critical of maternity care. Women of higher socio-economic status may have been more likely to attend public meetings and contribute written submissions, but in response to the survey they were not more likely to be dissatisfied than women with less formal education or lower total family income.

Although some individual practitioners took issue with the survey methodology and its findings, no members of the Ministerial Review Committee or any of the professional practitioner bodies were openly critical of the evidence on which the report was based. This is in direct contrast to recent events in the United Kingdom, around the House of Commons Health Committee Report on Maternity Services,[29] where professional bodies were critical of the report, arguing that it lacked a representative basis for making claims about consumer views.

The survey findings also influenced the deliberations of the Ministerial Review by illustrating that it tends to be during labour and birth that women encounter difficulties in relation to their care, rather than during pregnancy. The much greater dissatisfaction of women with their intrapartum care than with their antenatal care encouraged the review team to tailor recommendations for improvements in this area. This feedback from women is reflected in the guiding principles accompanying the recommendations regarding models of care, and underpinned the priority given to models providing continuity of care, such as team midwifery, multidisciplinary team care, birth-centre care, and community-based midwifery.

Our findings reinforce the arguments contained in the Review of Birthing Services that Australia's current mix of private and public services leaves a substantial minority of women unhappy with aspects of their care. The question of whether alternative models, such as those suggested in the Review of Birthing Services, would lead to better social outcomes for mixed populations of women requires further research. Although the numbers of women participating in non-standard models of care in 1989 were very small, our findings show that women who chose to give birth in a birth centre (including women who were subsequently transferred out of the centres) experienced lower levels of intervention. This is shown by the distribution of scores in the two pie-charts in figure 3.6.

While 73 per cent of women who planned to give birth in a birth centre had a score for obstetric procedures of less than five, only 56 per cent of women who were booked into labour wards had a score this low. When women at higher risk of complications are excluded from the analysis, it does not alter the finding that women planning to give birth in a birth centre have lower intervention rates.

Women who gave birth in a birth centre were also more likely to be satisfied with their care; 92 per cent of birth-centre patients said their care was 'as they liked', compared with 66 per cent of women who gave birth in a labour ward (OR = 6.17 [2.23-23.65]). Women who were transferred from a birth centre were not more or less satisfied with their care than other women giving birth in a labour ward although, with only sixteen women in the transfer group, we had little power to detect a difference.

These findings are important since they demonstrate the success of birth centres as a strategy for lowering intervention rates, and for achieving high levels of satisfaction with care. Birth centres have also been successful in encouraging women to see benefits in early discharge, an issue considered in Chapter 5. An important question for hospital administrators and service providers is how many women would choose to give birth in a birth centre if one were available to them. In the final section of this chapter, we look at what women said about where they would like to give birth, and the care-givers (doctor or midwife) they would like to assist them.

Figure 3.6 Labour ward versus birth centre: obstetric procedure score

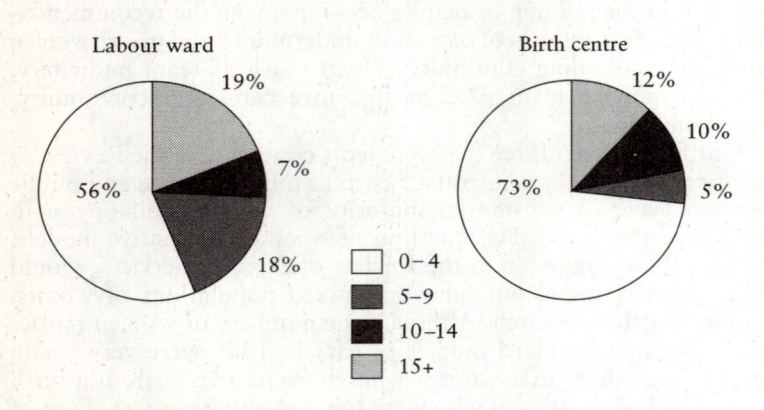

Labour ward
- 56% 0–4
- 18% 5–9
- 7%   10–14
- 19% 15+

Birth centre
- 73% 0–4
- 5%   5–9
- 10% 10–14
- 12% 15+

(Comparison based on where women planned to give birth)

LOOKING FORWARDS AND BACK

Women's preferences for where they would like to give birth were significantly different from what they experienced in 1989. Although 97 per cent had given birth in a hospital labour ward, this was the preferred place for only 76.3 per cent. One in every five women (20.3 per cent) would have liked a birth-centre birth and 3.3 per cent would have liked to give birth at home.

It would not have been surprising if the preference for birth-centre care had been more common in women living in Melbourne, since at the time of the survey there was only one birth centre outside the metropolitan area. Other commentators have also noted the tendency for health service users to assume that 'what is must be best'.[30] We had been told by health professionals attending Ministerial Review consultations that it was only middle-class women who were interested in birth-centre care. Counter to this, the survey showed that maternal age, marital status, income, education, health insurance status, residing in the country or the city, being born in Australia or elsewhere, or having a first or subsequent birth did not predict who would have a preference for birth-centre care.

Women's preferences regarding the primary care-giver at the time of birth were as follows: 77 per cent wanted a doctor, 16 per cent wanted a midwife, and 7 per cent preferred a combination of a doctor and midwife. Midwife care was more commonly the preference of women on lower incomes, women without a partner and women without private health insurance (these factors clearly being related).

At present very few women in Victoria are able to gain access to maternity services that offer either birth-centre or midwifery care (where midwives are the primary care-givers). Possibly the major difference between birth-centre care, and team midwifery based models of care, in particular, and more conventional labour-ward care is that women are offered the opportunity of getting to know the midwives who will care for them in labour before labour begins. Over half the women who took part in the study had seen the same care-giver throughout their pregnancy, but in labour almost all women, whether public or private patients, had encountered midwives and sometimes doctors, students and other personnel whom they had never met before. With changing shifts they might also have met another new set of faces, and if they experienced complications or a long labour, as we have seen, they sometimes found themselves surrounded by multiple extra personnel while their partner was pushed to the back of the room. The challenge for maternity-service providers is to find ways of overcoming the current level of discontinuity and fragmentation in the way that care is provided. Birth centres and team midwifery care, in so far as they offer greater familiarity with a small number of midwives, and an environment in which the use of obstetric procedures tends to be less frequent, are two options worthy of wider implementation by hospitals.

Stephanie Brown, Judith Lumley

FOUR

Childbirth Classes: Making a Difference?

Why *do* women and their partners attend childbirth preparation classes? At the time antenatal classes became established, 40 to 50 years ago, preparation was seen as the key to acquiring the 'correct' ideas about childbirth, so that freed from fear and anxiety, a natural, and therefore good, birth would follow.[1] The goals were accordingly straightforward: to reduce the need for drugs in labour; to improve labour itself by reducing fear, tension, anxiety and thus pain; and to reduce the need for intervention and operative delivery.

It is much more difficult to know what the goals of childbirth preparation classes are today. There is general agreement that classes aim to prepare women and their partners for childbirth and early parenting, but beyond that there is as much diversity of content as there is diversity of style and structure.

The Ministerial Review of Birthing Services painted this picture:

> The content may stress the physiological side of pregnancy and birth or take a broad view encompassing social and emotional aspects as well. There may or may not be discussions of options for care during pregnancy and birth. A focus may be placed on natural childbirth methods; or there may be more emphasis on preparing women for all possible eventualities; or indeed, there may be a focus just on psychological and psychodynamic issues. Different courses will place different emphasis on breathing techniques for labour or exercise during pregnancy. The benefits and risks associated with various forms of intervention in pregnancy may or may not be discussed.[2]

We looked elsewhere for consensus on the current goals of childbirth preparation classes and found it in one of the other State reviews *Maternity Services in New South Wales*.[3]

This listed the goals of childbirth preparation classes as follows:
- Promote confidence and fitness in the mother
- Increased flexibility in managing the labour — physically and mentally

- Reduction in the need for analgesia and/or need for intervention resulting from its use
- Increased satisfaction with self in birth process
- Improve physical health outcomes for mother and baby
- Reduce levels of stress in new parents
- Promote bonding between mother and infant
- Increase numbers of mothers breastfeeding successfully — to at least six months of age
- Reduce risk of child abuse
- Increase satisfaction with parenting and the development of the functional family

This list has much in common with the summary provided by Simkin and Enkin in their review of the effectiveness of antenatal classes: the use of psychological, or physical, non-drug methods of preventing pain in labour; good health habits; stress management; anxiety reduction; enhancement of family relationships; feelings of 'mastery', enhanced self-esteem and satisfaction; successful infant feeding, smooth postnatal adjustment and family planning. All aim to enhance the woman's sense of confidence as she approaches childbirth.[4]

One woman's comments encapsulated many of those ideas:

I think this good birth experience helped me settle into caring for this baby much more easily than with my first one. I really owe most of the encouragement I received in pregnancy and labour to the prenatal classes run by ——. They got me *mentally* prepared (and boy, did I need it!) and I was ready to stick up for myself if I should need to. My husband was also better prepared because I was and was a terrific help and encouragement.

Despite the diversity of style and content childbirth educators in different continents *do* seem to have shared goals and expectations. Whether those are the goals of new parents when they book into classes we do not know.

SURVEY OF RECENT MOTHERS
The specific questions asked about childbirth education were:

Did you go to any childbirth preparation or parenthood classes during your recent pregnancy?

Who were the classes run by?

If you are married or have a partner that you live with on a permanent basis did that person attend classes with you?

Approximately how many people altogether usually attended the classes you went to?

Those who had not attended were given a list of possible reasons (eight plus 'other — please specify') and invited to circle all those which applied.

There were three other questions elsewhere in the questionnaire asking women to rate each of a variety of sources (books, films, family members, friends, childbirth classes, doctor, midwives, talking with other people pregnant at the same time) as extremely helpful, very helpful, some help, little help or no help. We asked this in relation to 'understanding and dealing with pregnancy', 'understanding and dealing with labour and birth', and in relation to 'preparing you to cope with life with a new baby'.

CHILDBIRTH EDUCATION

Childbirth education is available in a variety of settings. Public hospitals and some community health centres provide classes that are almost always free. Public and private hospitals commission fee-paying classes for women in private care. The classes are likely to be staffed by physiotherapists, midwives, or a combination of the two, with obstetricians or anaesthetists occasionally contributing to one or two of the classes. There is also a range of childbirth education organisations with independent childbirth educators from a range of backgrounds. Private classes are also offered by individual childbirth educators, mostly physiotherapists.

Classes differ not only in the setting, the cost, and the background of the childbirth educator, but in the size of classes, the competence and skills of the teacher, the class format — from small-group discussions emphasising a participative approach to lecture-style presentations — and, as mentioned above, the class content.

Who Attends Classes?

Almost half of the women who replied to the questionnaire had attended classes in the current pregnancy. If they had not done so the most common reason was that they had attended them in a previous pregnancy. For this reason most of the following analysis is restricted to the 300 women who were having their first child. Eight of them did not complete the question about childbirth preparation, so the effective sample was 292, of whom 245 (83.9 per cent) attended classes. It was usual for partners to attend classes as well: 71.1 per cent always did and 20.2 per cent sometimes did.

The most common reasons for not attending classes given by women having their first child were that they did not feel classes would help (19); others concerned the time of day when classes were held (15); the distance to travel (7); the lack of local classes (3); their expense (3) or the fact that they were booked out (3).

Only two women said they did not know about classes. As women were invited to circle all the factors that applied the total reasons exceeded the number of women (47).

Table 4.1 Social differences between women who did and did not attend childbirth preparation classes

	Attended No.	(%)	Did not attend No.	(%)	
Maternal age					
< 20	7	(2.9)	4	(8.9)	χ^2 for
20–24	39	(16.2)	14	(31.1)	linear trend
25–29	102	(42.3)	17	(37.8)	8.25
30–34	77	(32.0)	8	(17.8)	p = 0.004
35–39	15	(6.2)	2	(4.4)	
40 +	1	(0.4)	–		
Marital status					
Married	210	(86.8)	32	(71.1)	χ^2 = 7.09
Living with partner	20	(8.3)	7	(15.6)	p = 0.024
Other	12	(5.0)	6	(13.3)	
Residence					
Metropolitan	184	(78.3)	29	(67.4)	χ^2 = 2.38
Other	51	(21.7)	14	(32.6)	p = 0.12
Left school					
< Yr 12	127	(53.1)	33	(73.3)	χ^2 = 6.26
Yr 12	112	(46.9)	12	(26.7)	p = 0.012
Family income					
< $20 000	29	(12.4)	13	(34.2)	χ^2 for
$20 001–30 000	63	(27.0)	10	(26.3)	linear trend
$30 001–40 000	48	(20.6)	8	(21.1)	11.09
> $40 000	93	(39.9)	7	(18.4)	p = 0.0009
Health insurance					
Yes	165	(68.2)	15	(33.3)	χ^2 = 19.64
No	77	(31.8)	30	(66.7)	p = 0.0001
Antenatal care					
Public clinic	42	(17.6)	24	(53.3)	χ^2 = 29.2
General practitioner	49	(20.5)	9	(20.0)	p = 0.0001
Obstetrician	148	(61.9)	12	(26.7)	

The high attendance rate is very similar to that reported in Western Australia (81 per cent) from a similar population survey carried out in conjunction with its review of obstetric and related services.[5] It is almost identical with a postnatal survey carried out in the Hunter region of New South Wales.[6] Childbirth preparation is clearly a cultural norm for first-time mothers in Australia.

There were marked social differences between women who attended classes and those who did not. The latter were younger, poorer, more likely to have left school before completing secondary education, and less likely to be married (table 4.1). Although attendance was less common among women living outside the metropolitan area this difference was not significant. There were too few women of NESB (31) to compare them with Australian-born women. Only one-third of the women who did not attend classes had private health insurance and over half of them were public hospital clinic patients. The characteristics of women who did not attend classes have a great deal in common with the women who were under-represented in the survey (young women, single women, women of NESB) so the attendance rate at classes for first-time mothers in our survey will be a slight over-estimation of rates in the whole population.

What Classes Did Women Attend?
More women attended public hospital classes (54.5 per cent of attenders) than private fee-paying hospital classes (26.4 per cent). The remaining 19 per cent who went to classes held independently of the hospital comprised 4.1 per cent attending private physiotherapist classes, 7.4 per cent at community health centres, 4.5 per cent at Childbirth Education Associations, with very small numbers in any other category. Simkin and Enkin point out that curricula for classes may be similar and there may be little difference in the information taught or the skills imparted. They go on to comment: 'Nevertheless, there may be great differences in the attitudes that are encouraged. As a general rule community-sponsored childbirth education classes are structured to incorporate the interests of parents into the curriculum; hospital-based classes may be required and expected to explain existing policies to parents, not to question, nor to offer alternatives, nor to help parents decide their own birth plans'.[7] This assertion would be disputed by many childbirth educators and observers who see as many differences within the broad categories of hospital-based and community-based classes as between them, but it is an important assertion. We were unable to test it since the numbers in totally independent classes were too small: the power of the survey to compare the experiences of women who had attended them with women attending hospital classes was inadequate.

Most classes were run as small groups: 43.8 per cent of women attended classes of fewer than fifteen people; 33.8 per cent attended classes of fifteen to 25 people. Only 17.4 per cent of women went to classes of more than 25 people. Large classes were seen to have major drawbacks:

> Both my husband and I felt these classes were far too big.
> If they were smaller they would be a lot more personal. All films shown during these classes portrayed groups of no more than eight who knew each other and made an effort to keep in contact during their stay in hospital and after their return home. I was very disappointed to learn that was not to happen at our classes. Any questions that were posed were answered but I would have preferred a much smaller group so that detailed discussion could follow.

Satisfaction With Classes
Women who attended childbirth preparation classes rated them highly in terms of helping them understand and deal with pregnancy. Classes were rated as extremely helpful or very helpful by 62.9 per cent of those who attended hospitals' public classes, 65.6 per cent of those attending private hospital classes, and 75 per cent of those attending independent classes. The proportions rating classes as very helpful or extremely helpful in understanding and dealing with labour and birth were lower: 57.8 per cent, 53.4 per cent and 62.2 per cent. Satisfaction with classes in relation to preparing women for life with a new baby was much lower: 30.3 per cent of those attending public hospital classes, 15.6 per cent of those attending private hospital classes, and 15.2 per cent of those attending independent classes were rated as extremely or very helpful. Public hospital classes were significantly more likely to receive a high rating when compared with the other two ($\chi^2=7.35$, $p=0.01$) in relation to preparing for life with a new baby.

Relative dissatisfaction with childbirth education as preparation for parenthood was a feature of the comments added to the questionnaire.

> We felt that all effort was directed towards the actual birth. Certainly all the reading and energy was centred on the actual birth which was active and drug free. Not nearly enough is said about breast feeding, (particularly difficulties that may be experienced) and what to expect *at home* with a new baby and no support. [emphasis in original]

> Antenatal classes: I think more attention should be given to parenthood skills rather than child birth; and [people] informed of available resources for new parents.

Antenatal classes should concern themselves more in teaching parents how to care for and cope with new babies as most women today are geared to work — not have babies — and so do not have the practical knowledge of the early stages of child rearing.

Childbirth educators point out the difficulty they perceive in preparing first-time mothers for life with a new baby. It is as if the magnitude of the birth itself — long awaited, desired, feared, unknown and unknowable — blocks out the future.

PAIN AND PAIN RELIEF

The prevention of pain in labour has always been one of the cornerstones of childbirth preparation and one of the few outcomes of antenatal classes to have been confirmed in randomised controlled trials.[8] Thus we were particularly interested in the comparison of women who attended classes and those who did not with respect to pain and pain relief. The findings are shown in table 4.2. There were some significant differences. Women who had not attended childbirth preparation classes were much more likely to say that pain relief had not been discussed with them before labour, suggesting that this topic is not raised with women during their antenatal care but is left to childbirth educators.

The same proportion of both groups used some form of pharmacological pain relief (83.7 per cent and 86.6 per cent), but those who had not attended classes were more likely to have received an epidural anaesthetic (37.2 per cent versus 20.4 per cent) and less likely to have used gas and oxygen (48.8 per cent versus 65.3 per cent). As effective use of the mask that delivers gas and oxygen is much easier with some practice beforehand, this is a difference we might expect. The use of pethidine was very similar in the two groups (65.1 per cent versus 69.9 per cent). Sally Redman and colleagues in their Hunter region study also found no differences in the use of pethidine and epidural anaesthesia between women who had attended classes and those who had not.[9] Thus these two recent population-based studies show no association of class attendance with a key 'desired outcome'. Having a drug-free labour was mentioned by one-third of women in one of the few papers to have asked women why they wanted to attend classes.[10]

There were no differences between attenders and non-attenders in the success of pain relief: just over one-third reported pain relief as very successful (37.1 per cent and 37.0 per cent). There were no differences either in their ratings of the pain and discomfort of labour. About half of the women in both groups described the pain as worse than expected, with one-third regarding it as much worse than expected.

Table 4.2 Pain in labour and pain relief

	Childbirth classes				
	Attended		Did not attend		
	No.	%	No.	%	
Pain relief not discussed before labour	17	(7.9)	15	(34.9)	$\chi^2 = 24.07$, $p < 0.0001$
Pain relief					
Pain relief given in labour	188	(86.6)	36	(83.7)	
Gas and O_2	141	(65.3)	21	(48.8)	$\chi^2 = 4.12$, $p = 0.04$
Pethidine	151	(69.9)	28	(65.1)	
Epidural	44	(20.4)	16	(37.2)	$\chi^2 = 5.67$, $p = 0.017$
General anaesthetic	9	(4.2)	2	(4.7)	
Success of pain relief					
Very	68	(37.0)	13	(37.1)	
Partly	90	(48.9)	17	(48.6)	
Not at all	26	(14.1)	5	(14.3)	
Pain and discomfort in labour					
Much worse than expected	73	(33.8)	14	(32.6)	
A little worse	47	(21.8)	6	(14.0)	
About what expected	37	(17.1)	6	(14.0)	$\chi^2 = 2.58$, $p = 0.28$
A little better than expected	15	(6.9)	6	(14.0)	
Much better	16	(7.4)	4	(9.3)	
Uncertain	28	(13.0)	7	(16.3)	

THE EVENTS OF PREGNANCY AND LABOUR

Table 4.3 summarises the two groups of women in relation to the procedures they experienced during pregnancy and labour. Just over half of the women (51.2 per cent) who did not attend classes had labour induced, compared with only 30.1 per cent of those who did attend.

The use of other interventions and procedures was strikingly similar in the two groups of women. There was no evidence that childbirth preparation was associated with lower rates of monitoring or intervention. This finding should not surprise. As Madeleine Shearer pointed out in an editorial in *Birth*, 'the attitudes and policies of labour and delivery personnel utterly swamp the effects of prenatal education'.[11]

Table 4.3 Procedures used in pregnancy and labour

| | \multicolumn{4}{c}{Childbirth classes} |
| | Attended | | Did not attend | |
	No.	%	No.	%
Single scan	141	(57.8)	28	(60.9)
> 1 scan	92	(37.7)	15	(32.6)
Non-stress testing	139	(57.0)	25	(54.3)
Cervical suture	20	(8.2)	7	(15.2)
Amniocentesis	9	(3.7)	2	(4.3)
Shave	63	(25.8)	12	(25.5)
Enema	80	(32.9)	9	(20.0)
Fetal monitoring	150	(61.7)	26	(63.4)
Induction	65	(30.1)	22	(51.2)*
Augmentation	98	(45.4)	21	(48.8)
Forceps/vacuum	65	(26.5)	11	(23.4)
Episiotomy	107	(43.7)	25	(53.2)
Stitches	162	(66.1)	36	(76.6)
Elective caesarean	27	(11.0)	4	(8.5)
Emergency caesarean	24	(9.8)	5	(10.6)

* $\chi^2 = 7.11$ $p = 0.008$
(Denominators change slightly between procedures because of missing values)

In the early years of childbirth preparation, when standard care involved large amounts of medication, the effect of reducing drug use by antenatal classes sometimes flowed on to reducing other interventions as well, notably the use of forceps, especially in the United States. Such an effect would not be expected here, since there was no evidence that class participation was associated with important differences in anaesthesia or analgesia. In contrast, women whose care was provided in a birth centre were shown to have significantly lower rates of pharmacological pain relief and lower rates of intervention. This emphasises the importance of care-givers and context, rather than classes, in patterns of intervention.

Preparing women for labour is intrinsically difficult: 'the variability of the event is one of its striking features. Labours can be long, short, painful, exhausting, exciting; everything from "orgasmic" to "torture in solitary confinement". Both the quality of the experience and the observed details of the birth cover a wide range of outcomes within one culture'.[12] Antenatal classes were criticised in the survey both for saying too much about possible complications and for providing too little information about what might go wrong.

> The classes were very negative, talking about everything that could go wrong, showing pictures (photos) of episiotomies etc. (which I had), which in my opinion are not really necessary and [are] depressing.

> I also felt that I was not prepared for a difficult birth as the films made it look as though it would be 3 or 4 pushes and presto — baby arrives, not 3 hours or so of hard pushing. Maybe it's just me but the classes, although not there to frighten, did however, fail in warning about what might have happened.

SATISFACTION WITH INFORMATION

The questionnaire contained nine questions about satisfaction with access to information through pregnancy, birth and the postnatal period. There were no differences between women who had attended childbirth preparation classes and those who had not on any of the following ratings:

- Being able to get information was a good aspect of antenatal care.
- Difficulty in getting information was a bad aspect of antenatal care.
- Satisfaction with the explanation given for carrying out ultrasound scans, non-stress testing, cervical suture or amniocentesis.
- The nurses and midwives explained enough about what was happening during labour and delivery.
- The doctor explained enough about what was happening during labour and delivery.
- Satisfaction with the explanation given for delivering the baby by (elective) caesarean.
- Different nurses gave me different advice about feeding.
- Helpful advice and support given over feeding the baby.
- Easy to find out what I wanted to know about my own and the baby's condition, treatment and progress.

Research on childbirth preparation in the Hunter region of New South Wales has shown that classes are successful in increasing the knowledge of both women and their partners.[13] Educators hope that this learning process facilitates access to information during pregnancy and birth, but there was no evidence in the survey to support this, and written comments provided equivocal support for increased knowledge leading to better decisions:

> I think the more educated people are about pregnancy and birth the better they will be able to make their own decisions. I was lucky to have such a great pregnancy and birth. I think you need to make sure you understand your doctor and his/her methods and be able to trust them. My Dr was very natural all the way through. Even though I enjoyed giving birth there was no way I could have totally prepared for the experience. Classes etc. helped but you must experience it to understand it fully.

> Water leaked and had a show Monday. Continued to visit Dr until Thursday after which I went into labour but was sent home till Friday night (daughter born Saturday). This neglect of my condition was contrary to what I had been taught in antenatal classes I attended.

The first woman quoted above did link information to better decision making within a context emphasising a relationship of trust with her doctor. The second had information that made her unhappy with her doctor's care, but this did not help her to get satisfactory information from her doctor. At the time of the survey she reported her experience in 'what was bad about antenatal care'.

Table 4.4 compares women who attended classes and those who did not in relation to their overall satisfaction with care in pregnancy, labour and after birth; their confidence about looking after the baby when they left hospital, and their emotional well-being at the time of the survey.

Only one measure was significantly different between the groups: women who had not attended childbirth classes were more than twice as likely to rate their antenatal care as mixed or poor. This was confirmed in a series of more specific questions on antenatal care: they were less likely to say that nothing was bad (37.0 per cent versus 59.9 per cent); more likely to say that they had seen different staff at each visit (23.9 per cent versus 6.7 per cent) and more likely to complain about long waits at antenatal visits (41.3 per cent versus 25.3 per cent). These were characteristic responses of all women receiving care in public hospital clinics, as discussed in Chapter 2, so the group difference in this regard can be explained by the fact that most women who did not attend classes received their antenatal care in public clinics.

None of the responses to the other questions, including one about having an active say in decision making, differed between the groups, although more women who had not attended classes gave 'uncertain' as their response to this question. Redman and her colleagues included four questions about satisfaction dealing with issues of control, being involved in decisions, length of labour, pain and 'staff having time to deal with my problems'. None of these was significantly different between women who had attended classes and those who had not.[14]

Table 4.4 Satisfaction with care, confidence and emotional well-being

	Childbirth classes				
	Attended		Did not attend		
	No.	%	No.	%	
Antenatal care					
very good/good	214	(89.2)	35	(74.5)	χ^2=7.37
mixed or poor	26	(10.8)	12	(25.5)	p=0.007
Labour and delivery					
managed as liked overall	127	(58.8)	28	(65.1)	
in some ways, not others	71	(32.9)	11	(25.6)	
not managed as liked	18	(8.3)	4	(9.3)	
Active say in decision making					
in all cases	85	(40.3)	16	(43.2)	
in most cases	86	(40.8)	11	(29.7)	
sometimes	30	(14.2)	5	(13.5)	
not at all	10	(4.7)	5	(13.5)	
uncertain	4		4		
Care in labour					
very kind and understanding	154	(77.4)	33	(89.2)	
fairly/not very kind	45	(22.6)	4	(10.8)	
Care after birth					
very kind and understanding	160	(66.4)	24	(55.8)	
fairly/not very kind	81	(33.6)	19	(44.2)	
Feelings about looking after the baby on your own at home					
very confident	49	(20.2)	11	(24.4)	
fairly confident	134	(55.4)	23	(51.1)	
definitely anxious	59	(24.4)	11	(24.4)	
Emotional well-being* (8–9 months)					
EPDS >12	33	(13.8)	8	(18.2)	
EPDS ≤12	207	(86.3)	36	(81.8)	

*EPDS   Edinburgh Postnatal Depression Scale

One criticism of antenatal classes is that they promote unreal expectations about birth in a way that leads, inevitably, to disappointment and dissatisfaction. One of the women quoted earlier made just that observation. It is important to emphasise that there was no evidence in the survey to support that criticism. Women who attended classes were not, on any criterion, more dissatisfied with and critical of their care.

No differences were detected between those who attended classes and those who did not, in relation to the woman's feelings of confidence about looking after the baby on her own at home, or to depression at the time the survey was carried out, eight months after birth. These were the only survey questions relating to possible longer-term benefits of childbirth preparation to emotional well-being and confidence.

Table 4.5 Health behaviours in pregnancy and after birth

	\multicolumn{4}{c}{Childbirth classes}	
	Attended		Did not attend		
	No.	%	No.	%	
Attended all planned antenatal appointments					
Yes	225	(93.4)	36	(80.0)	Fisher (2-tailed)
No	16	(6.6)	9	(20.0)	p=0.0077
Cigarette smoking in pregnancy					
None	199	(81.6)	21	(44.7)	χ^2 for trend
1 to 9	25	(10.2)	12	(25.5)	25.55
10 to 20	19	(7.8)	13	(27.7)	p<0.00001
21 to 40	1	(0.4)	1	(2.1)	
> 40	0	–	0	–	
Alcohol consumption in pregnancy					
None	114	(46.5)	30	(63.8)	χ^2 (none vs any)
occasional (<1/week)	108	(44.1)	14	(29.8)	= 4.71, p=0.03
3 to 7/week	21	(8.6)	3	(6.4)	
2 to 3/day	2	(0.8)	0	–	
Breastfeeding from birth					
Yes	198	(91.7)	25	(67.6)	χ^2=17.48
No	18	(8.3)	12	(32.4)	p=0.00003
Breastfeeding at 3 months					
Yes	152	(62.0)	18	(38.3)	χ^2=9.11
No	93	(38.0)	29	(61.7)	p=0.0025

HEALTH PROMOTION AND HEALTHY BEHAVIOURS

Does attendance at childbirth preparation classes increase the likelihood of what Simkin and Enkin call 'good health habits'?[15] There were four relevant behaviours included in the questionnaire and in table 4.5 their prevalence is compared across the two groups. Women who attended childbirth classes were less likely to have missed any planned appointments for antenatal care, less likely to have smoked cigarettes in pregnancy, more likely to have begun breastfeeding and more likely to have been breastfeeding three months after birth. By contrast, they were also more likely to have consumed alcohol in pregnancy.

Although it is possible that childbirth preparation classes might have contributed to the breastfeeding outcomes, these five differences consistently reflect the social differences between attenders and non-attenders, most strikingly the higher smoking rate but lower alcohol use of poorer, less well-educated and unmarried women. Redman et al. reported no significant difference in breastfeeding at the time of hospital discharge, but a higher proportion of smokers among non-attenders. They carried out statistical modelling and concluded that the differences in smoking behaviour were fully accounted for in a logistic regression model by the sociodemographic differences between attenders and non-attenders at classes.[16]

PROFESSIONALS OR PEERS?

Women who did not attend classes more often rated their friends or sisters as extremely helpful or very helpful in preparing them for understanding and dealing with pregnancy (52.3 per cent versus 36.5 per cent), and less often rated written material as very helpful (59.6 per cent versus 73.5 per cent). They were more likely to rate mothers as extremely helpful or very helpful in preparing them for labour and birth (27.9 per cent versus 17.7 per cent), and to rate friends and sisters likewise (44.2 per cent versus 27.9 per cent). No such differences were apparent in the section dealing with sources found to be helpful in preparing for life with a new baby where family and friends were highly regarded by all women.

The higher ratings of family sources as helpful in relation to pregnancy, labour and birth that were made by women who did not attend classes may reflect a more limited access by them to either professional or independent sources of information and support. It is however reminiscent of the preferences for family and community sources over professional sources described by St Clair and Anderson among inner-city women attending public prenatal clinics (or having no prenatal care) in Baltimore.[17]

Our study, like most of its predecessors, compares women who chose to attend childbirth preparation with those who did not. Its strength is that it was population-based, rather than being based on a single hospital or an individual series of classes. The survey was independent of those who had provided care and those who had provided education and preparation. Had major differences been found between the two groups of women it would be difficult to be confident about the possible causes. As differences (in pain, pain relief, interventions, satisfaction, and emotional well-being) were virtually non-existent, it can be inferred that attendance at antenatal classes is not, in Victoria at this time, associated with differences in those outcomes mentioned above.

The same criteria apply in evaluating the effectiveness of childbirth education as in assessing whether social support in pregnancy reduces the incidence of low birth weight infants, or whether epidural anaesthesia results in more long-term backache than other forms of pain relief. The two groups being compared must differ *only* in whether or not they received the intervention: in all other respects they must be equivalent. The best way, probably the only way, to ensure that they are comparable is by asking the participants to agree to be allocated to one or other group by random assignment. This 'gold standard' for assessing whether an intervention has the desired effects, the randomised controlled trial, is often perceived to be at the other extreme from research that respects the individual participant's role and contribution to a research project. This is a misunderstanding of what trials have to offer.[18]

It is depressing to discover that in the long march of childbirth preparation so few trials of its effectiveness even in relation to pain relief, let alone its more subtle benefits and possible side-effects, have been carried out. Now that two large Australian studies have failed to find any differences in outcomes between women attending and not attending childbirth preparation classes there is a challenge for educators to identify the benefits and join in trials to see whether they can be demonstrated.

We agree with Simkin and Enkin that there may be indirect effects of childbirth education that change the culture and the environment of hospitals. We find it much harder to agree with them that 'Once a critical mass of mothers becomes aware of the options that are available to them, major changes in obstetrical practice may ensue'.[19] The critical mass is already exposed to childbirth education, at least in Australia, with no evidence that this has resulted in a change for the better in obstetric practice.

When randomised trials are designed it will be important for them to address the interesting question: why do people attend and express satisfaction with classes? Is it just another example of 'what is, must be best'?[20] Are there long-term benefits to participating couples or families, not yet studied? Do people go in order to meet others caught up in the excitement and uncertainty of becoming a parent? How far do clients and educators share the same goals and desire the same outcomes? If they do, are there specific styles and forms of preparation which best meet certain individual needs?

Judith Lumley, Stephanie Brown

FIVE

Thrown into a New Job

When women commented on childbirth education (see Chapter 4) there was a clear sense that preparing to care for a new baby had not come easily and that official or formal preparation had been found wanting. Researchers have noted the small amount of attention paid to the in-patient stay after birth, compared with research on antenatal care or the management of labour.[1] This is a surprising omission given the sudden and complex changes to relationships and responsibilities which occur at this point, not to mention the dramatic physical changes in the weeks after birth. In the light of this we were particularly interested in women's experiences during the postnatal hospital stay. Did they feel 'cared for' in hospital? Was feeding the baby satisfying for both mother and baby — and their care-givers — or was it a source of anxiety and frustration? Were babies separated from their mothers? Did women manage to rest in hospital? Was it easy to find out what was happening, especially for women with a sick baby?

CHANGING THE RULES IN THE POSTNATAL WARD

Twenty-five years ago, one major Melbourne hospital allowed only the husband and grandparents to visit the mother for the first five days after birth. The baby was brought to the mother for feeds only, was not allowed out of the ward nursery during visiting hours, but could be 'viewed' by approved visitors. The visitors held up a card inscribed 'Please show me Baby (surname)' to authorise the nursery staff, on the other side of a glass window, to hold the (wrapped) baby up for inspection.

Fifteen years ago, it was most unusual for babies and mothers to be together in postnatal wards, or even in single rooms. Standard practice was for the baby to spend most of the time in the nursery, being brought to the mother's bedside for feeds. A 1977 survey of Melbourne hospitals[2] reported that 'rooming-in' was the usual form of care in only 18 per cent of them. The definition of rooming-in at that time was that the mother and baby were together, with the mother looking after the baby during the main part of the day, except during visiting hours. By 1984, the proportion of hospitals where rooming-in was usual had risen to 41 per cent.[3]

By the time of the 1989 survey a complete transformation had taken place: 86.9 per cent of babies were beside their mothers all or most of the time, and 6.9 per cent were beside them some of the time. So, by the criteria of the 1970s and early 1980s, almost 94 per cent were rooming-in. Only 6.2 per cent of babies were separated from their mothers. Most of these (38/48) were in a nursery because they were sick. Almost 40 per cent of them were of low birth weight. A substantial proportion of their mothers (29 per cent) had been admitted to hospital during pregnancy. Hence, by 1989, only major health problems kept babies and mothers separated in hospital.

In 1977 only half of the hospitals had allowed fathers to hold their babies without any restrictions.[4] Almost 10 per cent regarded this as a dangerous practice and forbade it altogether. A typical hospital rule at that time was that 'fathers are permitted access to babies' — the language is very telling — 'during a specific half-hour each day, when there are no other visitors and no children are present'. By 1982 no hospitals had a policy restricting access by fathers to the ward nursery.[5] Along with this shift to rooming-in and a more family-centred style of maternity care has come a profound relaxation of rules about visitors.

POSTNATAL CARE

> My second child was born at a private hospital which I found to be fantastic. My baby and I couldn't have had better care, and I could get my strength back before going home after the casearean. The nurses would do as little or as much as I wanted them to do with the baby.

> I enjoyed my stay in hospital, was thankful for the support of my doctor and nursing staff.

> ... but I must say I was very disappointed with the stay in hospital. I was only pleased that it was my second child. If it were my first I think I would have been thrown off by motherhood. Having the child beside you 24 hours a day since birth gives you no rest at all.

Unfortunately, the experience of the third of these women was characteristic of those who commented on postnatal care. One in three women (32.7 per cent) was dissatisfied with the care she received, rating it as not very kind and understanding or only fairly kind and understanding. Women in the study were even more dissatisfied with two specific aspects of their care: only 50.1 per cent of them reported that they had received helpful advice on and support over feeding, and a similar proportion (53.6 per cent) had enough rest and sleep during their hospital stay, issues which will be discussed in more detail later. British research into postnatal care has come up with almost identical criticism, similarly affecting large proportions of women.[6]

Dissatisfaction with postnatal care was unlike dissatisfaction with antenatal care in that family income, age, education, city or country residence, being of NESB, being a first-time mother or having other children, receiving care from a specialist obstetrician, a general practitioner, or a public hospital clinic made no difference to the likelihood of being unhappy with one's care. Women who were not married were more likely to be dissatisfied (43 per cent) than married women (31.3 per cent), and there was a small difference in dissatisfaction levels between women with private health insurance (29.0 per cent dissatisfied) and those without (38.3 per cent).

There were, however, strong associations between dissatisfaction with postnatal care and dissatisfaction with care in other phases of pregnancy and birth. Half the women who had rated their antenatal care as poor or mixed were not satisfied with postnatal care, though this group made up only 23.8 per cent of those who were dissatisfied. Similarly, women whose labour had not been managed as they would have liked were much more likely to be dissatisfied with postnatal care (47.6 per cent), though, once again, this group of women accounted for fewer than half of those who were dissatisfied.

Women who were dissatisfied with postnatal care were less happy with their length of stay after birth than other mothers: 14.3 per cent compared with 8.7 per cent felt their stay was too long; 11.1 per cent compared with 5.2 per cent felt it had been too short. Being dissatisfied with postnatal care was also powerfully associated with lack of confidence about looking after the baby on leaving hospital.

Most women (90 per cent) found it easy to get information about themselves or their baby's health during their hospital stay, 8.6 per cent found it rather difficult, and only 1.6 per cent very difficult. There were some important exceptions to this. Almost one-quarter (23.7 per cent) of women whose babies were in the nursery reported difficulty in finding out what they wanted to know.

> All the nursing staff ... in the postnatal ward and special care nursery were wonderful.

> My daughter stopped breathing 3 hours after she was born. Whilst 'it's a common problem' is a little reassuring, I would have appreciated a better explanation seeing as how she spent 3 days in an oxygen crib.

Women under 25, those having a first baby, and those of NESB were also significantly less satisfied with access to information.

Other social differences (education, family income, private health insurance, care-giver, and area of residence) were not important.

Rest and Sleep

The main factors which we had presumed might interfere with rest and sleep in the postnatal ward were listed as possible explanations on the questionnaire. The responses were:
- other babies crying 333 (42.2 per cent)
- own baby crying 273 (34.6 per cent)
- own visitors 187 (23.7 per cent)
- being woken up early in the morning 178 (22.5 per cent)
- other people's visitors 138 (17.5 per cent)

It is notable that the women who did not get enough rest each reported two or three reasons; that one's own baby crying was almost as important as the crying of other babies and that women's own visitors were more often a factor than other people's visitors.

To this formidable array of complaints were added another 172 annotations about being 'unable' to rest or sleep. Only a few of these (12 per cent) dealt with the mother's own health or that of the baby: kept dreaming about [the] painful birth; worrying the baby would stop breathing; sore breasts, leaking milk; some 5 per cent mentioned being in a state of excitement: being high as a kite and rooming in with three others in the same condition; being excited and on a 'high'. There were also a few specific negative comments about the hospital beds and the temperature of the wards.

The dominant criticism was of noise: vacuum cleaners, television sets, snoring, other mothers and their visitors, staff noise at night, buzzers and telephones, not to mention less common noises, such as adjacent building construction work and the arrival of ambulances. Along with complaints about constant noise came complaints of constant movement, activity and lights during the night.

> Visitors allowed in, out of visiting hours, talking at the tops of their voices and about 10 around the patient's bed.

> A snoring woman [and] an inexperienced breast feeding mother turning on the light all the way through the night trying to feed.

> Incessant activity in my room — cleaners, tea lady, nursing staff 'have you bathed your baby yet?' etc.

> Nurses who came in at 2 to 3 am and whispered too loud.

The other key phrases in the complaints were 'hospital routines' and 'interruptions', the former often being a polite way of describing the latter.

> I felt being woken up to change bed linen in the mornings in hospital was unnecessary and annoying when I had been up with my baby a lot during the night.
>
> Being woken up for temperature checks ...
>
> Rigid routines by cleaning staff constantly interrupting sleep and feeding hours.

The context for these comments was the now established norm of rooming-in, which also received specific comments — one in favour and twenty opposed:

> Rooming-in at night was compulsory — would have liked baby in nursery.
>
> [Rooming-in] was the only part of the care in hospital that mothers were upset about. There should be a choice whether you want your baby in with you at all times or whether you'd like a break and leave the baby in a nursery for an hour. This is not so anymore! I left hospital a day early so I could get some rest and put the baby in a room of his own.
>
> Nurses made me do everything myself.

Rooming-in, once permitted only rarely and reluctantly, appears to have become an oppressive and compulsory hospital routine. Have the changes in postnatal wards been a pyrrhic victory? Before drawing that conclusion it must be recognised that *no* woman in the survey wanted her baby to be in the nursery all the time or even most of the time. Very few women had experienced the sort of separation from their babies that was once routine, and one of the few who did described the separation as totally preventing her from sleeping. It was the non-existence of any other option, for any part of the day or night, that lay at the heart of the complaints about rooming-in.

One group of women for whom rooming-in presents particular problems is women from South East Asia.[7] For South East Asian communities, the confinement period is intended to provide mothers with rest, warmth and an opportunity to recuperate in order to promote the mother's long-term health and well-being. Their strong cultural beliefs about the importance of rest after birth, the need to avoid physical activities such as walking around, carrying heavy loads, and doing household tasks conflict with current hospital expectations for mothers to be up and about, doing postnatal exercises, being active very soon after birth, and caring for their babies themselves. These cross-cultural differences in belief and practice are compounded by language and communication barriers between immigrant women and their care-givers, so that women often end up feeling neglected while staff end up perceiving mothers as lazy or uncaring.[8] Similar conflicts have been described for Asian mothers and hospital staff in Britain[9] and the US.[10]

Infant Feeding Then and Now
Changes in feeding practices over the past fifty years have been profound. From 1945 rates of breastfeeding in Victoria fell steadily, reaching their lowest point in 1971. Records kept by the Maternal and Child Health Service show that in that year only 26 per cent of babies were breastfed at three months of age and only 9 per cent at six months.[11] In the twenty years that followed the decline was reversed with a steep increase to today's relatively high levels.

Yet a reader of baby manuals or nursing or paediatric texts from the 1960s and 1970s could be forgiven for thinking that the majority of women were breastfeeding at that time. Health experts expected that women would choose breastfeeding. At the same time, there were both hospital practices (such as exposure to more drugs in labour and separation from babies after birth) and social norms that militated against successful breastfeeding.

Feeding babies on demand was permitted in only 14 per cent of Melbourne hospitals in 1977.[12] It was 'actively supported' by hospital staff in 87 per cent of the same hospitals by 1984.[13] Feeding was regulated not only with respect to its frequency, but also in the minutiae of cleaning ('sterilising') the nipples before and after each feed, the duration of suckling in minutes per side, graduated over the first five days, and the techniques of expressing milk after each feed. Giving babies bottles in the nursery at night was customary in 1977: it was breastfeeding at night that was contentious.[14] Even in 1984, 20 per cent of hospitals reported that staff routinely gave night formula feeds in the nursery.[15] 'Top-ups' (complementary formula feeds) by day were not at all unusual.

In 1977, once home, babies were believed to need additional fluids. Solids were introduced early, sometimes within the first few weeks. Breastfeeding in public was much less acceptable than it is today. As recently as 1972 one of the authors of this study was asked by a young Maternal and Child Health nurse to go into a separate room to feed her nine-week-old baby instead of feeding him in the presence of other mothers and toddlers at a playgroup.

In the 1989 survey 60.5 per cent of babies were fed on demand during their hospital stay, 19.1 per cent were fed on demand but not more often than every two hours, 9.8 per cent were fed every three hours and 10.6 per cent were fed every four hours. Where feeds were three- or four-hourly the decision was made by the mother in half the cases and by the hospital in the rest. Hospitals were more likely to have made the decision if the mother was having a first child, was under 25 years of age, or unmarried.

Almost nine of every ten women (87.8 per cent) in the survey had begun breastfeeding at birth; 64.3 per cent were breastfeeding three months later, and 49.6 per cent were breastfeeding at six months. These figures may be a slight over-estimate of the true population rates because the groups of women less likely to reply to the questionnaire were also the groups with lower than average rates of breastfeeding (young women, single women, women of NESB).

The factors associated with still breastfeeding at three and six months were mostly social ones: maternal age between 25 and 39, being married or formerly married, born in Australia or in another English-speaking country, having private health insurance, a family income above the median, formal education to the end of secondary school or beyond. Country–city differences and differences by number of births were minimal.

There were biological factors of importance as well. Twins, low birthweight babies (less than 2500 grams) and babies who had been admitted to a nursery after birth were less likely to be breastfed, as might have been expected. It was a little more surprising that high birthweight infants (more than 4499 grams) were less likely to be breastfed at three months and that not quite so large but still big babies (more than 3999 grams) were also less likely to be breastfed at six months. Women with very high scores for obstetric intervention (fifteen or more: the median was four) had breastfeeding rates of 57.5 per cent at three months and 41.1 per cent at six months, compared with rates of 64.5 per cent and 51.1 per cent for women with scores under fifteen. Mothers in their late thirties and early forties were less likely to be breastfeeding, despite a social profile that would have predicted that they would be.

One of the strongest associations with bottle-feeding was cigarette-smoking. While non-smokers had breastfeeding rates of 91.6 per cent at birth, 69.1 per cent at three months and 55.8 per cent at six months, the corresponding rates for women who smoked more than twenty cigarettes a day were 75.0 per cent, 45.9 per cent and 18.9 per cent. Although the social factors associated with smoking have many similarities with those associated with bottle-feeding, there are some inconsistencies. Women of NESB had lower rates of breastfeeding but very low rates of smoking: women living in the country had longer durations of breastfeeding but high rates of smoking. The most striking association of cigarette smoking by far was being unmarried. Under one-quarter of married women were smokers, but the proportion rose to more than half among women who were single, separated or living with a partner but not married.

Feeding: Advice and Support
Although a majority of women are now breastfeeding their infants at three months of age, infant feeding is not always easy and straightforward.

> I have five children, the first born in 1970. I found the care and advice given to the mother-to-be today to be extremely good and caring...This is the first baby I have breastfed. Years ago we were encouraged to bottle-feed. Thanks to today's midwives and nursing staff I find it a great experience and bonding. Only wish they'd been around 20 years ago.

> I gave up the right to breastfeed my baby when she was three weeks old because nobody *showed* me how to feed her properly. Not one person told me to have the nipple as well as the brown circle in the baby's mouth ... so *please* give first time mothers a go, get midwives who have had babies to tell first time mums how to feed their babies properly. [emphasis in original]

> One of the most distressing things in the hospital after the baby was born was to do with feeding. I had 101 different bits of advice and did not sort out the problems until I got home.

> I didn't really have the hang of breastfeeding and ended up with mastitis. I found that ringing the —— Birth Centre and Nursing Mothers was really no help and I ended up at the —— hospital ... I think mastitis is a serious ailment and I was very distressed by the extreme pain and temperature. I discovered that my GP knew practically *nothing* about breasts in general and there seems to be a great void in the area of breastfeeding. [emphasis in original]

The spectrum of opinion about the advice, help and support provided in hospital over breastfeeding is fairly represented in the above comments. A few people reported good experiences, but critical and negative accounts were much more common. This was quite consistent with the replies to the question on advice and support over feeding, in which half of the women did not find staff very helpful. There were no social differences in relation to this question: everyone, regardless of age, income, education, marital status, health insurance status, area of residence, care-giver, birthplace and language background was equally dissatisfied.

Complaints about hospital policies implementing compulsory demand feeding and some hospitals' refusal to allow any complementary feeds were reminiscent of the complaints about compulsory rooming-in, with which they were often linked:

> Rooming-in at night, demand feeding and wouldn't give baby bottle at night [prevented rest and sleep].

> Comp. feeding was not allowed — baby was frantic for the first few days.

The major complaint was that 'different nurses gave me different advice about feeding', with almost two in every three women (62.5 per cent) describing this as a problem. It was a worse problem for women having their first child, 71.2 per cent of whom reported it, but more than half of those with other children (56.8 per cent) also complained about it. There was a significant increase with increasing family income: four out of five women in the highest income category (more than $40 000/yr) having a first child had complaints about inconsistent advice.

Over 40 per cent agreed with the statement that 'they were just left to get on with feeding'. This reaction was not restricted to women with previous children, though they were more likely to agree with the statement than women having a first child (47.2 per cent versus 32.5 per cent). It was slightly more common among women without private health insurance, and also among the small group of women who were bottle-feeding. A number of women commented that while they had coped with both inconsistent advice and being left to get on with feeding by themselves because they already had children, they had concerns about what it was like for first-time mothers.

Almost one in three women felt that bottle-feeding was frowned upon. This was more likely to be stated by women who were bottle-feeding.

> I was quite concerned at the attitude of staff towards bottle-feeding. My baby was bottle-fed soon after birth because of low blood sugar and then put into an isolette because of a wet lung. I tried expressing and making up the rest with formula. My milk was not much as not stimulated by baby. After becoming very distressed myself and not knowing when baby would come out of the isolette I decided to bottle-feed. And then I felt quite guilty because of midwives' attitudes to this making me feel as though I was harming my baby by *artificially feeding* as they called it. The stress I felt was great and uncalled for. [emphasis in original]

Mothers' Ill-Health After Birth

Many women mentioned in passing their tiredness, exhaustion, and common physical problems such as sore breasts, pain from stitches, and leaking milk. A few women had more serious physical problems, and all felt that their problems had been trivialised or ignored at the time:

> The student doctor did my stitches. For three days after the birth I complained about 2 certain stitches ... nurse told me to expect a little discomfort and live with it. After not being able to urinate other than in bath I demanded they be looked at. They were not done correctly and were taken out.

> Baby was left with me one night, 36 hours after the caesarean when I had just had a pethidine drip removed, for me to feed with no nursing staff ... impossible for me to hold right, change breasts ... I felt totally stranded.

> After the birth I bled a lot — had a blood transfusion. But when I asked why I bled so much [I] was told it's just one of those things, which doesn't seem satisfactory to me because there must be a reason why I bled so much. Also a couple of days after I'd had the baby I passed a huge blood clot (I thought it was my kidney or something because I was so paranoid about everything HA HA). She said my placenta was whole — so what would that have been? Who knows? I must say no one can prepare anyone for birth, it's a real nightmare and having stitches and piles and sore breasts and a squawking baby and blood transfusions is not my idea of a good time! However when I look at my baby and see how wonderful he is I know it was worth it.

Rules, Guidelines and Flexibility in the Postnatal Ward
The one aspect of care that remains the same is the plethora of inconsistent advice, and that too comes from inflexibility and intransigence. Advice, it seems, is rarely offered in the form of suggestions — 'try this' — but as a confusing series of solutions, given with inappropriate certainty by the parade of passing experts. As one woman wrote on her questionnaire:

> Also you might want to look into the different opinions of relatives, friends, general doctors, specialists, nurses, midwives, clinic health sister who all have sound advice but who all disagree which makes [the] first few months with a new baby very difficult for the parents.

When reflecting on the complaints that women made 20 to 30 years ago about postnatal care, and those that are heard today, we came to see that what they had in common was the lack of flexibility and the insensitivity to individual preferences and needs. What linked past and present was the absence of choice. Twenty-five years ago women were not permitted access to their babies outside feeding times: now 'rooming-in' with them is compulsory. A statewide survey of recent mothers in Arizona demonstrated that the most potent factor in dissatisfaction with postnatal care was not having one's choices honoured.[16]

We would not like to under-estimate the benefits of changed practices in the postnatal wards. There is a more relaxed attitude towards feeding, which is one of the factors contributing to much higher rates of breastfeeding. The experience of fathers and their contact with new babies is enormously improved. However, we did end up with concerns about the need for mothers' recuperation after birth and with a sense that this is not given a high enough priority.

LENGTH OF STAY: ARE FEARS ABOUT SHORTER HOSPITAL STAYS JUSTIFIED?

One topic that became a magnet for concerns about postnatal care was the question of how long women should (or could) stay in hospital after birth. When the Ministerial Review of Birthing Services was established in June 1988, one of its terms of reference being to consider the question of shorter lengths of stay in hospital after birth, there was quite vehement reaction both from women and service-providers. This was due in part to beliefs that shorter lengths of stay were to be considered simply for their cost-cutting potential, in part to concerns about the possible detrimental effects of shorter hospital stays for women and their babies, and in part to anger that women themselves might have no say in deciding how long they should stay. There was also concern about whether shorter stays, if introduced, would be accompanied by the provision of appropriate domiciliary midwifery services.[17] What constitutes an appropriate length of hospital stay after birth, and thus what is meant by 'early discharge', are culturally determined. In Australia at the time this was five to seven days.

In Australia in recent years there has been a fall in the provision of community-based support services (such as household help) to women after birth, with a resetting of first priority to the elderly. In this context, the notion that more women might be discharged earlier than day five was bound to raise concerns among women and their care-givers. In particular, fears were expressed that shorter stays could result in lower breastfeeding rates, a higher incidence of postnatal depression, and women feeling less confident about caring for their babies when they left hospital.

Opinions about who would be disadvantaged by shorter lengths of stay varied. Women having a first child, it was believed, would suffer because they would not develop the confidence to be gained by continual access to expert advice in hospital. Women who had other children might not get enough rest if they went home early to the demands of caring for other children. And it was often stated that staying for five to seven days benefited all women because it released them from household duties. A five to seven day stay in hospital was a firmly established cultural norm — one based on strongly held beliefs that women should stay in hospital to gain confidence, get rest and establish feeding.

There were also concerns that large numbers of women were already being 'sent home' early (mostly on day three or four) without domiciliary midwifery support and before they were happy to leave. A media campaign on this issue can be traced through the major newspapers in late 1989 and early 1990. Indeed, from about the middle of 1988 a number of maternity hospitals in Victoria *were* being encouraged to reduce their average lengths of obstetric stay for uncomplicated vaginal births through a specific State–Commonwealth funding initiative.[18]

On the other hand, a shorter hospital stay and early discharge has been regarded as a part of a recognition of pregnancy and birth as states of health rather than illness, and as a response to consumer pressures for more family-centred maternity care and less family separation. Earlier establishment of lactation, promotion of parent–infant attachment, and reduction of postnatal depression are further reasons given for the consideration of early discharge programs.

The dissatisfaction of recent mothers with many aspects of postnatal care in hospital also suggests that there may be a place for shorter lengths of stay — if only as a solution to the twin problems of inconsistent advice over feeding and intrusive noise.

The three relevant questions in the survey were:

How long did you stay in hospital after the birth of your baby?

In your opinion was your stay:
  too long
  about right
  too short?

When you had to look after the baby on your own at home, did you feel:
  very confident about this
  fairly confident
  definitely anxious about this?

Research on length of stay after birth has interpreted early discharge as leaving hospital anything from twelve to 72 hours after birth.[19] Given the cultural context of length of stay in Victoria, between five and seven days, women's length of stay has for the most part been grouped for purposes of analysis into stays of less than five days and stays of five days or more.

Table 5.1 shows the distribution of lengths of stay after birth in the survey, which was largely representative of Victorian women's lengths of postnatal stay in that year. About one-quarter of all women left hospital before the fifth day, most of these on the third or fourth day. Stays of nine or more days were not uncommon, with 13 per cent of women staying that long.

Table 5.1 Postnatal length of stay: the survey versus all Victorian women giving birth in 1989 (stillbirths and neonatal deaths excluded)

	Survey sample		Victorian women 1989	
	No.	%	No.	%
<24 hours	13	1.7	1711	2.7
24-48 hours	15	1.9	1894	3.0
3-4 days	152	19.7	13546	21.2
<5 days	180	23.3	17069	26.9
5-6 days	277	35.8	24315	38.3
7-8 days	215	27.8	15819	25.0
9+ days	101	13.1	6235	9.8
5+ days	593	76.7	46369	73.0
Total	773	100.0	63438	100.0

Some characteristics of women who were significantly more likely to go home before the fifth day were predictable: women who had a spontaneous vaginal birth were more likely to go home early than those who had an assisted delivery. Women who had other children at home were also more likely to go home early. Women attending birth centres were another group who would be expected to leave hospital early and more than half of them did: 57.7 per cent of those who gave birth in a birth centre and 41.5 per cent of those transferred from birth centre care left before the fifth day; 46.2 per cent of the former actually left within 48 hours, as did 28.6 per cent of those who had been transferred.

There were some groups whose earlier discharge was more surprising. More than one-third of women cared for in public hospital clinics (37.2 per cent), more than one-third of those without private health insurance (36.8 per cent), and 27.6 per cent of those whose family income was below $30 000 a year left hospital before the fifth day. Obviously these three groups overlap to a large extent. All of them include many women with heightened needs for practical and emotional support after birth, coupled with little or no capacity to buy the extra assistance they might need.

Satisfaction with Length of Stay
The majority of women — 82.3 per cent — were happy with the length of their hospital stay after birth. Of women dissatisfied with their length of stay, a somewhat greater percentage thought that it had been too long (10.6 per cent) than too short (7.1 per cent).

A number of socio-demographic variables (marital status, education, income, rural or metropolitan residence, or whether the mother was Australian-born or from a NESB) provided no clue to satisfaction with length of stay. Women under 25 years of age were the only group more likely than average to have felt that their stay was too long (17 per cent versus 9.8 per cent of other women).

By contrast, there were several groups of women over-represented among those who believed their stay had been too short: women without private health insurance (10 per cent) compared with those who had insurance (5 per cent); women who were public hospital clinic patients (14.7 per cent) compared with those in the care of an obstetrician or general practitioner (5.4 per cent), and those whose delivery was assisted by forceps (11.1 per cent) compared with those who had a caesarean (4.4 per cent). Women who were depressed at the time of the survey, eight to nine months after the birth, and women who said they had felt definitely anxious about looking after the baby at the time they left hospital were also more likely to believe their stay had been too short.

Among those who felt their stay had been too short only women without private health insurance and public hospital clinic patients had in fact had a short stay. These were the groups least likely to have a choice about their length of stay.

Breastfeeding
Breastfeeding rates for women leaving hospital before five days (early leavers) and those leaving later (traditional stayers) showed no significant differences either in the proportion who breastfed from birth (86.5 per cent and 88.2 per cent) or in rates of breastfeeding at one week (84.3 per cent and 84.8 per cent) or at three months (62.9 per cent and 65.6 per cent) or at six months (50.6 per cent and 51.0 per cent).

Confidence
Just over one in every ten women indicated that when they left hospital they had felt definitely anxious about looking after their baby at home. Women having their first baby were much more likely than other women to feel anxious (24.5 per cent versus 2.1 per cent). This was also true for women under 25 years of age, 19.3 per cent of whom were definitely anxious compared with 9.6 per cent of older women. Another group who were definitely anxious were women who had a forceps delivery (20.2 per cent). These three fac-

tors — first child, young age and use of forceps — were all strongly related to one another. The strongest association was with length of stay: the longer a women spent in hospital after the birth, the more likely she was to be definitely anxious when she left (see table 5.2). Does spending more time in hospital serve to decrease a woman's self confidence to look after her baby? Or do women lacking confidence tend to stay longer?

Table 5.2   Confidence to care for baby on going home

Postnatal length of stay	Very/fairly confident No.	%	Definitely anxious No.	%
<48 hours	28	100.0	0	0.0
3–4 days	144	95.4	7	4.6
5–6 days	247	89.5	29	10.5
7+ days	270	85.4	46	14.6

χ^2 for linear trend = 14.005, p = 0.000

The mother's marital status, income, education, place of residence, or country of birth (whether English-speaking or not) was not associated with her degree of confidence about looking after the baby.

Emotional Well-Being at the Time of the Survey

There were no significant differences between the 'early leavers', 11.9 per cent of whom were depressed at eight to nine months, and the 'traditional stayers', 16.4 per cent of whom were depressed. However, women who went home very early (less than 48 hours after the birth) were much less likely to be depressed (7.1 per cent) and women who had stayed nine days or more were much more likely to be depressed (20.2 per cent). Another paradox was that women who were depressed were more dissatisfied with the care they received in the postnatal wards.

Health Insurance Status

Women without private health insurance were both more likely to go home early and to feel that their hospital stay had been too short. Interestingly, however, the women without private insurance who went home before day five were not significantly more likely than their counterparts staying longer to say that their stays were too short (11.2 per cent versus 9.2 per cent). Even when they did think their stay was too short, they were certainly not more likely to be anxious about caring for their babies — of the 107 public patients who went home before day five, only six were anxious and four of the six thought that their length of stay was about right or too long! Nor would going home early appear to have affected their emotional well-being at eight to nine months after birth: 13.2 per cent of public patients who went home before day five were depressed, compared with 17.8 per cent of public patients who went home on day five or later.

First Births
Although women having their first babies comprised 87.8 per cent of the women who felt anxious at the prospect of caring for their babies at home, they were not significantly more likely than women with other children to say that their hospital stay had been too short (8.6 per cent versus 6.3 per cent). Furthermore, the 30 first-time mothers who did go home before day five were less likely to be anxious than those who stayed longer (10 per cent versus 26.3 per cent).

Unresolved Issues
While this study is reassuring about Victorian women's satisfaction with their length of stay in hospital after birth, there are some important gaps in our knowledge and understanding about the issues. We do not know what contributed to women's satisfaction (or dissatisfaction) with their length of stay. Which of the women who left hospital before day five had domiciliary midwifery care? Were these women more or less satisfied with their length of stay than those who did not? We also know almost nothing about the extent and availability of practical support from family and friends. Nor do we know to what extent women actively chose their length of stay or had it chosen for them, nor what role choice plays in satisfaction with length of stay.

> The nursing staff had no consistent approach to advice to new mothers ... I left hospital exhausted from rooming-in, very anxious about caring for my baby and actually sick from an infected episiotomy wound. I would ideally have stayed longer to recover my health but couldn't stand the place any longer.

This woman circled the response 'about right' for her length of stay, but her comment makes it clear that 'about right' was a compromise between 'too long' in some ways, and 'too short' in others.

Questions such as these are only likely to be satisfactorily explored by controlled trials where different patterns of postnatal care in conjunction with early discharge can be evaluated. One pattern of postnatal care that could well be included in such an evaluation would be own choice of length of stay.

Unwarranted Concerns?
The fact that the majority of women were satisfied with their length of stay lends support to the conclusion that at the time of the survey women and their care-givers were for the most part choosing appropriately who should go home early. The findings are rather different from those in a study carried out in Britain a few years before in which 40 per cent of women said they would have liked to leave hospital sooner than they had.[20] Changes to hospital funding in Victoria from July 1993 seem likely to encourage earlier discharge for women after uncomplicated births and it would be unwise to conclude that the situation will be the same in the second half of the 1990s as it was at the time of the survey.

Concerns raised in the Ministerial Review of Birthing Services about the effects of shorter lengths of stay were not borne out in the survey, which supported findings from other research on early discharge that women who left hospital early were, if anything, more likely to breast feed,[21] less likely to be depressed,[22] more likely to feel confident[23] and to have fewer maternal concerns[24] than women having traditional hospital stays. Most early discharge studies include only those women who *choose* to leave hospital early, though two of the studies just cited were randomised controlled trials.[25]

The fact that women without private health insurance were both more likely to go home before day five *and* to feel that their stays were too short, supports concerns raised in the Ministerial Review about some public patients being sent home before they would otherwise have chosen to go. It would certainly appear that at the time of the survey some public hospitals were targeting public patients to help reduce their average length of obstetric stay.

> My baby was five days old when I left hospital and it wasn't my choice. I'm thankful I had extra aftercare because I feel that with three young children it was necessary ... Many mothers now choose to stay only one or two days — that is their choice. I also believe on the other hand that if mothers wish to stay longer it should also be their choice. Unfortunately, being in a public hospital that is not so.

> With subsequent children rest and relaxing is very important before you go home with your new child. The time you spend in hospital is very often the only time you get alone and unhassled to get to know your child. Once home with the rest of your family there are too many commitments and pressures to relax and enjoy your baby as

much as you would like to. Problems that apply to your first birth can also apply to other births — engorgement, cracked nipples etc. Therefore I think that *all* new mothers should be able to stay in hospital for 4–6 days after the birth of their child *if they wish to do so*, no matter if they have private health insurance or not. [emphasis in original]

Policy Questions
This study adds to other evidence that suggests that shorter postnatal stays, particularly for women who choose them, but possibly even for some who do not, are not disadvantageous and may be associated with significant benefits.

Promoting earlier discharge — whether because of changes to hospital funding or because of beliefs about potential benefits to mothers and babies — is likely to be most successful if carefully targeted. This would not appear to be happening currently. Given that 10.6 per cent of women thought that their stays were too long, there is untapped potential for reducing length of stay by encouraging women to go home when they feel ready rather than necessarily adhering to the traditional five to seven day stay.

Unless women have the opportunity to think about an alternative and to plan for this in advance, they are unlikely to choose to go home early. If there is to be pressure for shorter stays then attention needs to be given to the issue well before birth. Systematic discussion with women during pregnancy concerning the potential benefits of going home early would be one way of beginning to question the conventional wisdom of a longer stay for everyone. A program of antenatal preparation that emphasises women's ability to manage their new babies at home, with support, may also serve subtly to promote a woman's confidence in her own abilities as a mother as well as to challenge the idea that confidence is gained through access to 'expert' advice at the hospital bedside — a notion called into question by the findings of this study.

Promoting and expanding birth-centre care with early discharge is also likely to be a fruitful strategy, as our findings indicate that birth-centre clients, even when transferred, tend to go home much earlier than other women. Some of them would have liked their stay to be even shorter:

> 24 hrs is the stated time that must be spent in the birth centre post delivery — this should be more flexible and allow parents and babe to leave when ready prior to the 24 hours — even if only a couple of hours post delivery.

Another felt her short stay had been a bad choice:

> I had my baby at the —— Birth Centre and even though the care was
> excellent I really needed another day in hospital to recover. Coming
> home after 24 hours was a mistake for me.

Findings of the survey also show an unmet demand for birth-centre care, which suggests that this strategy is likely to be acceptable as well as effective (see Chapter 3).

While we understand why women say that the only determining factor in the length of hospital stay after birth should be the woman's own choice, this 'right to choose' has to be recognised as having a strong component of cultural expectation — 'What is, must be best'.[26] Hospitals may be unable, in the current funding climate, to accommodate preferences that do not reflect a major health factor. After all, shorter hospital stays did not result in the feared detrimental effects for the women who experienced them.

Further research is required to determine the exact nature of benefits to women and to explore further the elements of women's satisfaction and dissatisfaction with the length of their hospital stays, including the role that choice plays in satisfaction.

AFTERWARDS: GOING HOME

The most highly rated professional source of help for coping with a new baby was the local Maternal and Child Health nurse, rated so by 61.7 per cent of women generally and 72.2 per cent of those from a NESB.

> I would add a point here about the benefit of Maternal and Child
> Health Centres. I have been lucky enough to have had some nice,
> reassuring sisters at mine ... it is important to know that they're there
> when you need them.

Traditional family and peer sources were at least as important as professionals, maybe more so. The woman's own mother and her friends and sisters were rated highly by two-thirds of the women in the survey (66.5 per cent). The absence of such help made women feel very vulnerable:

> Once home with a few littlies I became unwell ('flu); there is NO
> support available (unless one has family or friends who are willing
> *and* able to help). This is very frightening. [emphasis in original]

A few women also drew attention to the support provided by their partners:

> I am so fortunate that I have a loving and caring husband towards
> myself and our children. I am so lucky!

> A wise, understanding and supportive husband.

A similar number mentioned support groups, especially the Nursing Mothers' Association and clubs for mothers of twins, though the comments about these groups were not universally positive.

Whatever assistance is available new mothers are, as one mother wrote, 'thrown into a new job that you're not really prepared for — and it's a 24 hour job, too!'

> No one can really prepare you for having a baby at home after birth. Especially the full-time responsibility. Only experience can teach you.

Judith Lumley, Rhonda Small, Stephanie Brown

SIX

One in Seven: Depression after Birth

LABELLING DEPRESSION
When we began discussing postnatal depression it became apparent that there was substantial confusion about the term itself and about its implications. Most people agreed that this term did not include the condition known as 'the baby blues' — a very common, mild and transient period of mood swings and unhappiness occurring about the third, fourth or fifth day after birth.[1] Most agreed that the very rare and much more serious postpartum psychosis,[2] which affects about two women in 1000 after birth, should be regarded as a separate entity. The disputed questions were whether there was some other disorder in the year after birth that warranted the label 'postnatal depression': if there was, how common and how severe was it, and to what extent could it be specifically linked to the events and experiences of pregnancy and birth? Within that last question lay another disputed issue: were the relevant aspects of birth the complications and ill-health of the mother and the baby or, as one commentator asked, 'Is obstetric technology depressing?'.[3]

The understandable wish to reduce the over-medicalising of life events and experiences has led many people to be concerned about the use of the term 'depression' in relation to new mothers. Terms such as 'postnatal stress', 'postnatal distress' or 'lack of emotional well-being' have been used instead, with the added intent of emphasising the continuity and overlap between these experiences and those of everyday motherhood. Unfortunately, this re-labelling runs the risk of down-playing the seriousness of what is going on and of misrepresenting its severity, intensity and sometimes prolonged duration. It also minimises the continuity between this disorder and women's mental health and well-being at other stages of their lives, including their experiences as mothers of older children.

IDENTIFYING DEPRESSION
Reviews of publications about depression after birth have drawn attention to the very different ways in which depression has been

assessed.[4] Sometimes women were asked a single question about their feelings, in other studies the overall clinical impression of an experienced general practitioner was the criterion, in another group of studies the assessment was by means of a standardised questionnaire or a self-completion scale, and in others by formal and well standardised diagnostic interviews. Despite these different approaches there is substantial agreement that depression in the first year after birth affects 10 to 20 per cent of women.[5]

Given the design of the Survey of Recent Mothers there was no alternative to using a self-completion scale for assessing depression. The one we chose, the Edinburgh Postnatal Depression Scale (EPDS) is relatively brief and simple. It consists of ten statements, each with four possible answers, and the woman is asked to underline the one that comes closest to how she has felt over the past seven days. (A sample of the questions, with more detail about the scoring and the average scores is given in Appendix 3.)

The EPDS was developed specifically for the assessment of depression after birth.[6] It does this by omitting those questions about changes in sleep patterns, appetite, rest, waking, and the presence of other bodily symptoms that are difficult to interpret in the context of motherhood. Waking early in the morning, having a much greater appetite, feeling constantly tired, or being unable to visit friends as often as usual are typical, and possibly inevitable, aspects of being a new mother. In other contexts these are common symptoms of depression and as such are included in most depression rating scales.[7] One widely used and well validated rating scale, the General Health Questionnaire, which does include such somatic questions, when given to a sample of recent mothers scored 45 per cent of them as having a probable psychiatric illness, though an independent psychiatric interview found that the proportion was only 13 per cent.[8]

Comparisons of the EPDS with an interview diagnosis made according to strict criteria have been carried out in three community samples in Britain.[9] These have demonstrated its validity both for identifying women who are depressed and for ruling out depression. Since our study was completed a validation study has also been published from Australia.[10] The EPDS has been used in North America,[11] and is increasingly used in translation (for example, in Icelandic,[12] Dutch,[13] and Greek[14]).

Although it was devised to be used face-to-face in community settings by health professionals such as health visitors or community nurses, we included the questions in our postal questionnaire, and have since discovered that, at much the same time, others, including the scale's originator, were doing the same.[15] The EPDS has been used with mothers of older infants and toddlers,[16] with fathers of toddlers,[17] and with a 'control' group of women who were not recent mothers.[18] In all these instances it was highly acceptable.

Possible scores on the EPDS range from nought to 30. The score at which women are categorised as probably depressed was above twelve in our study. We selected this conservative cut-off point as it identifies a group of women who are all depressed or on the borderline of depression.[19] In doing so we know we will have missed some women who are depressed. A cut-off point at nine, with women whose scores are above nine being categorised as probably depressed, has been recommended for use in clinical settings where the scale will be followed up by an interview, since this will miss fewer women with depression.[20] However, using the lower cut-off means that the group of women then classified as probably depressed would be diluted by the inclusion of more women who are not depressed.

As our study was anonymous and confidential we were not able to confirm whether women were clinically depressed at the time the questionnaires were returned. We relied on the categorisation provided by the EPDS and accepted that there would be some misclassification. We preferred that misclassification to be in the direction of missing some women with depression rather than including more women without depression. This also gave us the greatest possible contrast in comparing the two groups.

DEPRESSION AT EIGHT TO NINE MONTHS

One hundred and nineteen of 771 recent mothers in the sample (15.4 per cent, 95 per cent confidence interval 12.8-18.0 per cent) were found to be depressed on the EPDS, having a score above twelve. The nineteen women excluded from this calculation and the subsequent analysis did not complete all the items and had total scores in the range where a missing item score might or might not have resulted in categorisation as depressed. The mean score on the EPDS was 7.6 (SD=4.8) and the median was seven. In our culturally and ethnically diverse population the EPDS proved to be highly acceptable with only 2.4 per cent (19/790) of the women who returned the questionnaires unable to be categorised.

Some of the women commented on this section of the questionnaire, often in order to put their answers into a wider context:

> I think some of the questions are misleading as the way I have felt (Q 54) has been due to problems with my estranged husband, not the baby.

> Some of my struggles afterwards are because when [the baby] was 5 months my husband and I moved to another state — away from both our families, our church family and therefore our support systems.

I also left a *very good* health centre sister, plus my childhood doctor. [emphasis in original]

Because I have 2 other children aged 9 and 11 years, everyone presumed I would be just fine but in fact it was like starting all over again as things have changed so much and I was out of touch and couldn't remember a lot of things I had done with the other two. Also emotionally I was feeling shaky but I had to pretend everything was just fine.

Answers to Q54 are not due to postnatal depression. My baby, now 8 months, has been operated on at 11 weeks and suffers from asthma and apnoea attacks so I have had a hectic few months though I get a lot of support from all family members.

At present I feel worthless in my job as a mother, because my husband is always saying how easy it is to look after children, therefore what I do, and in turn I, am taken for granted. Motherhood is rewarding but emotionally and physically draining and a thankless job. I love my kids but I am always tired and often depressed.

I had to return to work when my baby was 3 months old because of financial restraints — my partner is a student, this I feel has made it extremely difficult for me to cope at times, especially as I'd rather be at home with her. This strain prolongs the tiredness and frustration of early motherhood. As for the past week — well I've got a cold and feel much worse then usual!

I feel caesarean patients are expected to recover a little too quick ... I think women who have caesareans also need a lot of psychological support afterwards.

I found it difficult to rest during the first few months. My husband works long hours and I had many minor problems after the birth e.g. milk fever, sore episiotomy, severe haemorrhoids, gastro. It would have been helpful if I had had some child care for the older children [3 and 4 years] just for a few hours here and there. The rest of the family are all busy with their own children or jobs and I felt it would be imposing if I asked for help.

I usually cope well after the children are born but the third child has spent some 4 months being continually sick with croup, colds, a hospital visit, subsequent weight loss etc. and is just recovering now...

These themes of concern over the child's health, poor health of the mother, need for physical recovery, isolation, lack of support, marital problems and physical exhaustion will come up again in the follow-up study (see Chapters 9 to 13).

DEPRESSION OR 'POSTNATAL DEPRESSION'?

Many of the factors women mentioned in their comments on the survey form are not specific to early motherhood, and this raises the question posed at the beginning of the chapter as to whether depression is in fact any more common in the year after birth than it is at other times. One problem in answering the question has been the very real possibility that the number of 'new' depressive illnesses (incidence) identified in longitudinal studies through pregnancy and the postnatal period may under-estimate the true incidence since participation in a research study involving a series of interviews with skilled mental-health professionals might well have a preventive or therapeutic effect in its own right.[21] Studies that tried to answer this question by carrying out a parallel longitudinal study with a control group have encountered problems in identifying, recruiting or following up an appropriate group of women for comparison. Finding a representative group of women similar in all respects — except for not having had a child in the previous year — who agree to participate in a longitudinal study has proved virtually impossible.[22]

The other approach has been to compare the prevalence of depression in women after birth with the prevalence over one year reported from a similar community study of the general population.[23] All three of these comparisons have suggested that there is no significant difference in the prevalence of depression between women in the postnatal period and other women, though the third comparison detected a higher incidence of depression in the first three months after birth.

A recent study in Britain assessed depression in a population sample of women six months after birth and a group of women from the same community — matched for age, marital status, social class and number of children — who were not pregnant and had not had a child in the previous year.[24] Women who scored nine or more on the EPDS and a random sample of women with low scores received a standardised psychiatric interview with particular attention to the onset and duration of depression. This carefully controlled study confirmed that the prevalence was similar in recent mothers and matched controls, but it also confirmed that there was an increased risk of depression beginning shortly after birth:

> A finding which suggested that childbirth and its immediate psychosocial sequelae were likely to be important causal factors for the non-psychotic depressions ... [25]

The apparent discrepancy (higher incidence but no difference in prevalence) could be accounted for by the long duration of depression among women in the control group who also had young children and by the women in the control group whose depression had followed a previous birth. The findings in that study on the timing of depression with respect to birth are very similar to those from our follow-up study, which are discussed in Chapter 9.

The debate around this question has often seemed to miss the point that the impact of the birth of a child or the presence of a baby brings with it highly positive rewards likely to promote well-being, as well as highly negative experiences or losses. Thus there may be depressions averted by motherhood just as there are depressions initiated by it. Counting new cases of depression in recent mothers and in a comparison group of women is only part of the answer.

ASSOCIATIONS OF DEPRESSION AT EIGHT TO NINE MONTHS

There are very few consistent findings about factors associated with depression after birth, and no consistent findings about associations with the birth experience itself.[26] The explanation usually given for this — that it reflects different ways of assessing depression and different points in time after birth at which studies have been completed — may play a part, but a more likely reason is that most studies have been too small. More than half of the published studies include fewer than twenty women with depression.[27] In studies of that size, comparing the rates of depression in sub-groups of women with and without partners or comparing depression after a caesarean birth with depression after a spontaneous birth, is likely to miss even large differences of clinical and practical importance. It is a major reason why the findings in earlier studies have been so inconsistent. Our study was more powerful since it included 119 women with depression and six times as many women without depression. Yet there were still sub-groups in our present study that were not large enough for a sensible comparison to be made.

Table 6.1 summarises the significant associations of depression with social differences, pregnancy and birth events, and the subjective experiences of birth.

Although age and parity were not by themselves associated with depression, when they were examined together it became clear that for women 35 years and over there was a marked difference between women having a first child and those having later children, with the former group much more likely to be depressed (5/18, 27.8 per cent compared with 5/67, 7.5 per cent). This highly significant difference was not found in other age groups.

For comparison, the events, experiences and social factors that were *not* associated with depression are listed in table 6.2.

In evaluating the associations with later depression there are a few obvious examples of variables that the study was not large enough to assess: very small numbers of women gave birth outside a hospital labour ward; only eight women had twins; only 18 had a general anaesthetic. There was insufficient statistical power to detect differences between these sub-groups and other women.

Table 6.1 The associations of depression

Depression was less likely for women:
  living outside the metropolitan area
  who breastfed from birth
  breastfeeding at three months

Depression was more likely for women:
  living without a partner
  born overseas and of NESB
  with a prior caesarean delivery
  who rated their antenatal care as mixed or poor
  who had two or more antenatal procedures
  given pethidine or an epidural
  having a caesarean birth
  whose birth was assisted by forceps
  with an obstetric procedure score[28] >4
  who had unwanted people present at the birth
  who were unable to hold the baby after birth
  who did not have an 'active say' all the time
  who rated care in labour as only fair or not very kind
  who did not get enough sleep and rest in hospital
  who rated advice/support for breastfeeding as fair or poor
  who found it difficult to get information about themselves or their babies after birth
  who rated postnatal care as only fair or not very kind
  who felt their hospital stay had been too short
  who felt fairly confident or definitely anxious about looking after the baby when they left hospital
  who were uncertain about having further children or had decided not to have more

Questions about the experience of labour were not asked of women who had an elective caesarean birth, so the associations related to labour, summarised in tables 6.1 and 6.2, exclude those women except for operative delivery itself.

Table 6.2 Events and experiences not associated with depression

- maternal age
- number of previous births
- maternal education
- family income
- health insurance status
- mother's birth in Australia or overseas
- paid employment or otherwise in pregnancy
- time of ceasing paid employment in pregnancy
- paid or unpaid maternity leave
- prior pre-term birth or infant of low birthweight
- prior stillbirth, spontaneous abortion (miscarriage), or induced abortion (termination of pregnancy)
- prior breech, forceps or vacuum birth
- prior postpartum haemorrhage
- attitude to becoming pregnant
- provider of antenatal care
- attendance at childbirth-preparation classes
- hospital admission during pregnancy
- cigarette-smoking or alcohol consumption in pregnancy
- length of labour
- rating of pain in labour
- prior discussion of pain relief
- use of gas and oxygen for pain relief
- success of pain relief
- insufficient information provided by doctors or midwives
- whether or not labour was managed as liked
- place of birth (hospital labour ward, birth centre, home)
- doctor or midwife care at birth
- sex of the infant
- the extent of separation from the baby after birth
- actual length of hospital stay after birth

THE CONTRIBUTION OF BIRTH EVENTS, BIRTH EXPERIENCES AND SOCIAL FACTORS TO DEPRESSION

Some of the significant factors identified in this analysis have already been shown in earlier chapters to be linked to one another: dissatisfaction with antenatal care is associated with dissatisfaction with care in labour and postnatally; women living outside the metropolitan area have lower obstetric intervention scores and are less satisfied with the management of labour; women 35 years and over have more antenatal procedures; women with high obstetric intervention scores have slightly lower rates of breastfeeding. The next step was to carry out an analysis that took all the significant factors into account together. This process was described in Chapter 3 in relation to dissatisfaction with the management of labour.

The exclusion of cases with any missing values from the data file before statistical modelling resulted in a final sample of 698 women (88 per cent of the original respondents). The characteristics of those excluded were compared with those retained for all the variables in the analysis. The proportion of women who were depressed was 15.2 per cent, compared with 15.4 per cent in the full sample ($\chi^2=0.06$, $p=0.8$). The only statistically significant difference was the loss of women of NESB, who made up almost one-quarter of those excluded (23.9 per cent). The reduced sample size of the final file meant that the power of the study to detect differences was also reduced. The final file included all the variables that had a significant association with depression in the original univariate analysis, together with maternal age and parity. Stepwise logistic regression was carried out and the results are shown in table 6.3.

Once the factors listed in table 6.3 had been incorporated into the model, the other measures of satisfaction with care in labour and after birth and the significant social factors from table 6.1 (being unmarried or of NESB) did not make an additional contribution to depression.

SOCIAL DIFFERENCES AND SOCIAL ADVERSITY

The much *lower* odds of depression in women living outside the metropolitan area of Victoria was wholly unexpected. A New Zealand regional study of women's mental health could not detect significant differences between rural and urban areas,[29] but the city included in the study (Dunedin), and its surrounding country region (Otago), would both have been regarded as rural within our study, which contrasted the Melbourne metropolitan area with the rest of Victoria. A large population-based study of mental illness in the United States carried out in a number of different areas confirmed a decreased rate of major depression in younger rural residents (those aged 24 to 44), with this being more protective for women than men.[30] The rural recession was well under way at the time of the survey and we had evidence of other problems for country women, so we were left wondering what processes contributed to the lower prevalence. Were local community networks stronger outside the metropolitan area? Were local communities more supportive? Are there aspects of the natural environment in rural areas that can promote human well-being?

The interaction between parity and maternal age was a particularly interesting finding. It was not unexpected that the very small group of women having a first child over the age of 34 years might have a much higher odds of depression, since this is a common perception of those providing clinical services, but the very low rate among multiparous women of the same age was unexpected. Women over 34 years having a first child are a very small proportion of women giving birth (2.3 per cent) so this factor explains a relatively small proportion of depression in the community.

Table 6.3 Factors associated with depression in the model

Variable	Adjusted odds ratio	[95% CI]	p
Parity (previous births)			
1 none			
2 ≥1	0.36	[0.09-1.52]	0.16
Age			
1 <25			
2 25-34	1.19	[0.08-17.2]	0.90
3 >34	0.02	[0.0005-0.72]	0.03
Parity x age 25-34	0.65	[0.14-2.92]	0.57
Parity x age >34	9.47	[1.07-84.1]	0.04
Residence			
1 Melbourne			
2 Country	0.56	[0.32-0.98]	0.04
Birth			
1 Spontaneous			
2 Assisted	2.03	[1.17-3.56]	0.01
Antenatal care			
1 Very good, good			
2 Mixed, poor	2.12	[1.21-3.71]	0.01
Unwanted people at birth			
1 No			
2 Yes	2.98	[1.29-6.85]	0.01
3 Elective caesarean*	0.90	[0.43-1.91]	0.78
Feeding method from birth			
1 Breast			
2 Bottle	1.86	[1.01-3.43]	0.05
Confidence when leaving hospital			
1 Very confident			
2 Fairly confident	3.05	[1.80-5.19]	<0.001
3 Anxious	9.04	[4.07-20.1]	<0.001

All factors mutually adjusted
* Not asked of women who had an elective caesarean birth

Women without a partner and those of NESB born overseas had a significantly increased odds of depression in the univariate analysis (table 6.1). Both these groups of women had a low response rate to the questionnaire (see Chapter 1), so it is difficult to know whether these factors can be regarded as risk factors for depression. However, lack of a supportive relationship with a partner is one of the most consistent associations of depression in other studies.[31]

Both groups, but especially women of NESB, had reduced representation in the final sample for the logistic regression analysis and this reduced the study's power to assess associations with depression. Women of NESB constitute a very heterogeneous group including refugees, recent migrants speaking very little or no English, and women who have lived in Australia since childhood. Their susceptibility to depression is also likely to be heterogeneous and the postal survey was not large enough to analyse differences within this group. Any future studies of depression would need to explore cultural beliefs and practices about the postnatal and infancy periods, to examine the appropriate use of standard questionnaires in translation, to include interviews in community languages as well as in English, and to look at these issues within specific communities. A study in inner-urban Melbourne some years ago identified language problems and lack of family support as important mediating factors in depression among immigrant mothers of small children.[32] That study, and the findings from the postal survey, suggest that this might be an important area for future research and action.

Although it may seem surprising that there were no associations of depression with income or education, it is another consistent finding about depression after birth that low socio-economic status itself is not a risk factor.[33] More severe measures of social adversity, such as lack of housing tenure[34] or extremely low family income,[35] have shown an association. We did find that having a pension as the main family income was a risk factor, but this was accounted for by the almost total overlap with being a single parent.

OBSTETRIC COMPLICATIONS AND OBSTETRIC INTERVENTION

Five recent studies confirm the links between caesarean birth and depression found in our study. Green et al., using a modification of the EPDS, reported lower emotional well-being six weeks after birth in women who had a caesarean section.[36] The same association with operative delivery was found in two hospital-based follow-up studies using the EPDS.[37] In the light of two prospective Australian studies showing mood disorders *after*, but not before, caesarean delivery,[38] it seems very probable that the association is causal. It reinforces concerns about high and rising rates of operative delivery and other interventions when these are found to be associated with subsequent psychological morbidity. Almost one-third of women in the study had an assisted delivery, so this risk factor is potentially very important in terms of its contribution to depression in the population (its attributable risk). The study finding that the obstetric procedure score and the antenatal procedure score were associated with subsequent depression in univariate analyses, while none of the indicators of perinatal complications (antenatal hospital admission, low birthweight, length of labour, or prior reproductive complications other than caesarean delivery) were associated, lends weight to the view that it is obstetric practice that is relevant.

The other event linked with depression in the final model was having unwanted people present at the birth. It was notable that the unwanted people mentioned included family members as well as staff and students.

BREASTFEEDING, HORMONES AND DEPRESSION

One of the more surprising findings was that women who were depressed at eight to nine months had been less likely to breastfeed their infants. Almost one in five (19 per cent) had bottle-fed from the start, compared with 11 per cent of the group who were not depressed. There was also a significant difference between the two groups of women at three months after birth: 51 per cent of the women who were depressed were bottle-feeding, compared with 37 per cent of the others. Breastfeeding is often believed to be a contributing factor to depression; a belief reinforced by theories about the hormonal basis of depression after birth. The rationale for hypotheses that link mood changes after birth with 'hormones' lies in the dramatic changes that occur in steroid hormones through pregnancy, birth, lactation and the re-establishment of the menstrual cycle.[39] The concentration of some hormones in the blood changes a hundred-fold in the few days after birth. If there were a hormonal basis for postnatal depression, it would have to be a hormonal pattern characteristic of the period following birth. This unique pattern is maintained by breastfeeding, only to be replaced by the usual cyclic hormonal pattern once suckling is reduced in intensity and frequency, and menstruation resumes.

There are of course many other ways in which breastfeeding might contribute to depression: it might increase women's social isolation in places where breastfeeding is something to be carried out in private; it might reduce a mother's 'time out' if no one else can care for her baby for any length of time; it might be physically exhausting and demanding, allowing the mother even less sleep and rest. The latter has been documented in a large postal survey of women's health after childbirth in Britain.[40] Breastfeeding might also contribute to depression in women who have feeding problems or are unable to feed for as long as they planned to. If a mother was very keen to feed and problems such as cracked nipples, mastitis, or a hungry, dissatisfied baby developed or recurred then weaning or supplementary feeding might well be associated with a sense of failure or a feeling of loss, contributing to depression.

Whatever the proposed mechanism might be, the findings are quite consistent: there is no association of breastfeeding with depression after birth (see table 6.4), though most individual studies are too small to draw conclusions with any confidence. Table 6.4 also shows dramatic differences between studies in the proportion of women breastfeeding around three months after birth. One might expect to see these reflected in inter-country differences in depression if breastfeeding were indeed an important determinant of depression.

Table 6.4 Depression and infant feeding

Study	Proportion (%) breastfeeding	No.[#]	Proportion depressed (%) Breast	Bottle	p
England[41]	71.4	35	50	50	ns
England[42]	36.5	14	12	5	ns
England[43]	88.5	33	13	31	*
Wales[44]	18.6	27	19	23	ns
Scotland[45]	70.5	29	31	39	ns
Scotland[46]	55.2	8	13	15	ns
Scotland[47]	62.1	2	5	17	ns
Scotland[48]	69.0	4	7	0	ns
Finland[49]	51.0	4	11	19	ns
Australia[50]	77.8	20	10	18	ns
Current study	62.9	119	10	22	*

[#] number of women in the study who were depressed
p (probability):
ns no significant difference between breast and bottle feeding
* significantly lower rate of depression in women breastfeeding

In our survey, the difference in infant feeding was apparent at birth and became greater, but not significantly so, by three months of age. A recent longitudinal study in two English towns has clarified this relationship by demonstrating that depressed mood precedes weaning. In addition to the established social factors of young maternal age, low socio-economic status, and lower levels of formal education, this study showed depression to be a significant factor associated with bottle-feeding or early termination of breast-feeding.[51] The authors went on to say:

> This finding calls into question the alleged role of hormonal changes consequent upon breast feeding or its cessation in the genesis of depression.

The opinion that hormones play an essential role in the development of depression after birth masks profound disagreements about which hormones or mixtures of hormones are relevant. Low levels of progesterone,[52] low levels of oestrogen and progesterone, possibly high levels of prolactin (in breastfeeding women),[53] high levels of oestrogen and progesterone (combined contraceptive 'pill' in breastfeeding or bottle-feeding women),[54] low levels of prolactin (in breastfeeding women), low levels of progesterone (in breast-feeding women), high levels of progesterone (in bottle-feeding women), not taking the oral contraceptive 'pill' (in bottle-feeding women),[55] low levels of oestrogen (unsupplemented breastfeeding)[56] have all been blamed. Only one of the studies listed above included any measurements of hormone levels or changes in activity[57] and the methodology of hormonal studies in the postpartum period has received substantial criticism.[58]

Given both the lack of agreement on which hormones are relevant and the lack of evidence it is puzzling that opinions about the link between hormones and depression remain so strong. A recent review of research on this topic exemplifies both the lack of evidence and the continuing nature of the belief in hormonal factors:

> The results of endocrine research in puerperal mental illness are not encouraging. Despite a feeling that hormones 'have something to do with it' there are few positive data.[59]

DISSATISFACTION WITH MATERNITY CARE

One measure of dissatisfaction (the rating of antenatal care) remained in the final model, as did having unwanted people present at the birth. The other satisfaction variables did not make an additional contribution to the model. It can be argued that because the study was retrospective, its findings are not as strong as those from a prospective study would be. On the other hand, there are certain advantages to retrospectivity in so far as it is able to elicit from participants, directly and overtly, their subjective interpretation of the link between past events and current feelings, which is psychologically significant in its own right. What may be viewed from one perspective as retrospective bias may be seen by the women concerned as salient components of their life history. Further, the psychosocial consequences of current depression are likely to be strongly related to the woman's own view of its causes. Her retrospective construction of meaning will powerfully inform her current and future behaviour, including, as we have seen, her plans for subsequent pregnancies, her attitudes regarding her own competence, confidence in looking after her infant, and her sense of emotional well-being.

It is, of course, debatable whether the dissatisfaction characteristic of depressed women in our study followed the development of depression or was equally present at the time the events actually occurred. This cannot be elucidated in a cross-sectional study. However, if the dissatisfaction reported by women exists more strongly at one point than another, when an important mediating process like depression occurs, it should not automatically be seen as an artefact of that mediating process (the distortion of perceptions by depression). An alternative view is that perception of an event can legitimately change after time and considered reflection.[60]

As time passes and the physical and psychological 'danger' associated with the birth recedes, especially a birth with a high level of intervention, it may become possible to explore and revise one's views of and the events associated with the birth. Thus while the management of labour and birth might need to be considered satisfactory at the time, some months later this management may be questioned and feelings of anger, dissatisfaction, sadness and depression may surface. Shearer has commented on the importance for women who have just given birth to believe about interventions like caesarean section that 'the right thing had been done'.[61] These self-delivered explanations serve a beneficial function 'forming the fulcrum around which the experience is revised and made palatable'.

CONCLUSIONS
The events and experiences of pregnancy, birth and the early postnatal period have significant associations, both positive and negative, with depression after birth. These leave a great deal unexplored and unexplained. It was for this reason that we conducted the follow-up study described in the second half of the book.

Judith Lumley, Jill Astbury, Stephanie Brown

The Follow-Up Study

Introduction

In the last five decades profound social and economic changes have transformed women's lives. Whereas in 1947, 6 per cent of married women in Australia were in the paid workforce, by 1990 this figure had risen to more than 50 per cent.[1] The introduction of the principle of equal pay for work of equal value in 1972, and the introduction of government-funded child care have made it both easier and more financially rewarding for women to combine paid employment with motherhood. On the other hand, women's average weekly earnings remain only a fraction of male average earnings; in 1992 the median full-time wage for women was still only 83.7 per cent of male full-time weekly earnings.[2]

The steady growth in the proportion of women in paid work has been just one of a number of transformations in the areas of work, population, and social and economic policy that have altered the lives of Australian families in the post-war period. After the Second World War Australia experienced an economic boom. The growth of manufacturing and service industries not only drew women into the paid workforce, but also prompted a major wave of immigration to Australia from all parts of the globe, especially from Southern Europe and, more recently, from Latin America and Asia. Between 1947 and 1980 the Australian population doubled in size, with more than half of this growth accounted for by migrants and their families.[3] In 1989, 15 per cent of all births in Victoria were to women born overseas in countries where English is not the first language.[4]

Social and economic policies in Australia have also changed dramatically in the post-war period, reflecting the rapid pace of change in other areas. Of particular relevance to families have been the introduction of the *Family Law Act* (1975) allowing 'no fault' divorce, a Supporting Parents Benefit for sole parents, and Medicare which provides universal health insurance. While these and other policy changes have had positive effects for women, many continue to be at risk of violence (either domestic violence or sexual assault), and female-headed families remain one of the most impoverished groups in Australian society.

Although comparatively wealthy, Australia is still marked by social divisions. Phil Raskall has documented a growing divide between the wealthiest members of Australian society and an expanding group with limited financial security or economic opportunities.[5] Australia has also become a society in which two incomes are often no longer a luxury, but an economic 'necessity'. In 1989, 44 per cent of women with children in the newborn to four-year age range were in the paid workforce or were actively looking for work.[6] As the economic recession of the late 1980s and early 1990s deepened, many families lost one or both incomes. Job losses in manufacturing and the public sector placed substantial stresses on families, particularly those who had lost jobs or whose jobs were threatened. In 1991, 9 per cent of couples with children did not have either parent employed.[7]

What does it mean to be a mother in this environment? The follow-up interviews took place in the latter part of 1990 and the first half of 1991, before the worst impact of the recession was felt in Victoria. At the time of the interviews all of the women had a child who was between eighteen months and two-and-a-half-years of age, and 48 percent were in the paid workforce, the majority working part-time. Of the 90 women in the sample, only four were not living with a partner. In four cases fathers were at home full time; two of these had recently been retrenched. Fifteen of the women interviewed were born overseas; eight of these were of NESB. There were also a number of second generation migrants in the sample. None of the women in the follow-up study were under twenty years of age. This reflects both the under-representation of younger women in the original survey, and the relatively small proportion of women under twenty having babies in Victoria — in 1992 only 3.8 per cent of women giving birth were under twenty years of age.[8]

During interviews of around one-and-a-half to two hours, we talked with women who lived all over Victoria about their experience of the time since the birth of their child. In the second half of the book we draw on these interviews to describe what being a mother meant to these women. A question we asked all women in the study was how they would describe a 'good' mother. The conversations this prompted form the basis for Chapter 7. Chapter 8 draws on responses to the Experience of Motherhood Questionnaire, and continues a focus on the experience of being a mother. In Chapter 9 we concentrate on the 60 women in the sample who had experienced depression at some stage since the birth of their child, in particular what women said about what it was like to be depressed and what factors they saw as contributing to their experiences. Chapters 10 and 11 look at aspects of the social context of motherhood for women who had been depressed and those who had not, focusing on important differences between the two groups in terms of social support, negative life events, and involvement in domestic labour and paid work outside the home. Chapter 12 contains edited excerpts from the transcripts of interviews with three different women, all of whom scored as depressed at the time of the original survey. Chapter 13 explores women's accounts of how they had tried to cope with being depressed, and what advice they would have for other women going through the same experience.

Stephanie Brown

SEVEN

Troubled Thoughts on Being a 'Good' Mother

Reflecting on her experience of being the mother of three sons during the 1950s and 1960s, Adrienne Rich recalls that she was haunted by the belief that a mother's love should be both unconditional and available 'at call':

> I remember a cycle. It began when I had picked up a book or began trying to write a letter, or even found myself on the telephone with someone toward whom my voice betrayed eagerness, a rush of sympathetic energy. The child (or children) might be absorbed in busyness, in his own dreamworld; but as soon as he felt me gliding into a world which did not include him, he would come to pull at my hand, ask for help, punch at the typewriter keys. And I would feel his wants at such a moment as fraudulent, as an attempt moreover to defraud me of living even for fifteen minutes as myself. My anger would rise; I would feel the futility of any attempt to salvage myself, and also the inequality between us: my needs always balanced against those of a child, and always losing.[1]

Being the mother of a small child is both physically and emotionally demanding. Adrienne Rich's memory of the tension she felt between simultaneously wanting to meet the needs of her son and wanting to grab some small spaces in the day for herself was echoed in the conversations we had with women about motherhood. As one woman commented, a good mother is someone 'who's patient, always there ... caring, loving, can do ten things at once, that knows how to put two kids on one lap'. Her assessment of the qualities required to be a 'good' mother, and her acknowledgment of the balancing acts this requires on a daily and constant basis, were very familiar themes in the interviews.

In this chapter, we explore women's ideas about motherhood drawing on a section of the interviews where we asked women the question *How would you describe a 'good' mother?* Occasionally, when we asked this question, women faltered at the idea of categorising mothers in this way.

Collete Prout Really, I don't believe there is any such thing as a really good mother. I think every mother is just — they do their best to each situation.

Amanda Joseph I think it's each to their own. I don't think you can criticise anybody else, and every child is different.

These women were not prepared to think of mothers as either good or bad, and explicitly rejected the idea that they could pass judge-

Table 7.1 Descriptions of 'good' mothers*

	%
Attributes	
caring and loving	38
patient	25
calm and relaxed	11
listens to and talks to children	8
understanding and sensitive	7
responsible	7
able to juggle competing demands	7
non-judgemental	6
consistent	5
does their best	5
able to handle children in any situation	4
is there any such thing?	4
never loses temper	4
not perfect	4
children respect her	2
fair	1
creative	1
energetic	1
Tasks	
spends time with children	26
fosters children's emotional development	16
does the basics/attends to feeding, hygiene	11
disciplines children	8
always there for children	8
keeps children under control	5
Sense of self	
good mothers are good at what I'm not good at	15
children come first	8
confident about being oneself	5
keeps a sense of own interests and needs	2

*Most women gave more than one response

ment on other women. However, this resistance to our question was not characteristic. Most women readily listed attributes they associated with being a 'good' mother. Even the occasional mother who commented that it was a 'hard question', usually went on without further hesitation to give an account of the characteristics she believed were necessary to be a 'good' mother.

We analysed their comments in a series of steps that employed both qualitative and quantitative approaches (described in detail in Appendix 1). The list of attributes women associated with being a 'good' mother is a somewhat daunting job description. If all these attributes were prerequisites for the 'job' of being a mother, we wondered if anyone would ever, even momentarily, contemplate applying. Giving preference to the qualities women mentioned most frequently (see table 7.1), the 'good' mother is required to be loving and caring, to have 'never-ending' supplies of patience, to willingly and regularly spend time with her children, and in this time provide her children with the right sort of attention, stimulation and guidance. She is required to remain calm and relaxed at all times, to be a good listener and communicator, and to be understanding and sensitive to children's needs. Amongst the tasks she must competently perform are the disciplining of her children, teaching of appropriate behaviour, and everyday basic care tasks of feeding and keeping children clean. In order to manage all this she must have highly developed skills in juggling competing demands; she must be responsible, consistent, fair, able to handle (control?) her children in any situation, never lose her temper — and it would help also if she was energetic, creative, and had a sense of humour. Of course most women mentioned only a few of these and the heterogeneity of women's responses is one thing that is striking about the list in table 7.1.

RECOLLECTING THE PAST: 'THE OLD STYLE GOOD MOTHER'

It is interesting to compare these ideas about being a 'good mother' with the reports Lyn Richards and Jan Harper give of a study they conducted in the 1970s, in which 60 Australian-born women who had recently had a first child were asked to answer a very similar question. Richards and her colleagues used long, open-ended interviews to probe the feelings and beliefs of 60 couples regarding marriage, family life and parenthood. In *Having Families*, Richards argues that women generally adhered to one or other of two overlapping discourses about 'good' mothers. She distinguishes between these by labelling them the 'old style good mother' and the 'new good mother'. The 'old good mother' discourse stresses the importance of love and security, and what Richards describes as 'passive qualities — patience, reliability and willingness to spend time'.² The 'new good mother', according to Harper and Richards, is more interested in retaining her own independence and individuality, and in providing a stimulating environment for her child's development, rather than the 'loving presence of a patient mother'.³ We will return to Harper and Richards' concept of the 'new good mother' later in the chapter. Below we consider the concepts associated with the 'old good mother'.

Patience, love and the giving of time to children featured often in the accounts of 'good' mothers given by the women in our study. Patience, of all the qualities associated with being a 'good' mother, was the most likely to be mentioned first.

> A good mum, I think is never-ending patience (laughs); spending a lot of time with them; loving, all that sort of thing. I don't know even hygienic and that sort of thing.
>
> *Tessa Smith* Someone with a lot of patience, and can organise themselves, which I can't do. I'm terrible, I get sidetracked.
>
> *Sylvia Greenwood* A good mother ... try and think of one looking at the TV or something. One who has a lot of patience.

Spending time with children and patience were often linked together.

> *Fiona Neilson* A good mother is one who has time and patience for her children. Patience I think is the big key for children.
>
> *Lilian Roth* [A good mother] Somebody who spends a lot of time with their kids, has a lot of patience.

Consistency and reliability, central to many womens' accounts in Lyn Richards' earlier study, were mentioned only infrequently by women in our study.

> *Sharlene Dawson* Patience is one of the things I aim for and consistency. Well, I do my best, you can't do better than your best.
>
> Someone that views it as a responsibility. I hate seeing children just left and nobody can much care about them. Responsibility, and I suppose that gives them the love and care that they need. As long as they do that I think you give the child a really good start.
>
> [Another woman] I don't know. Somebody who's affectionate, calm, energetic. ... Somebody who can put themselves aside for their child, takes their child's needs into consideration before worrying about whether they can afford to buy cigarettes for themselves this week, or going to the pub or whatever.

For some women who described 'good' mothers consistent with the Richards' 'old style good mother', our question seemed relatively straightforward. They gave brief responses that had an almost matter-of-fact quality to them, and there was little indication that being a 'good' mother posed any more than everyday difficulties. Other women were very open about how they tried to be 'good' mothers, but often felt they lacked the necessary patience and capacity to make time for their children.

Wendy Elliot   Oh, you have to be more patient, I think. You have to learn to be more patient. I don't know. I'd say you should put your kids before anything else; before your housework and everything — although I don't always, but I think you should.

Caitlin Adamson   I always admire those women who've got all the patience in the world, that can sit down and play and be really creative, yeah. I'd like to be like that, but I'm not. [Caitlin was in our case group and was also depressed at follow-up. She is one of three women whose accounts of being a mother are included in Chapter 13.]

Jacinta Campbell   [A good mother] One that never loses her temper; always got patience; nothing's ever too much trouble: they do the baking for the school fetes and all this, all that sort of thing. I mean I don't do any of that, but I look at some mothers I know, and they do all of that and I think, 'I can't, I can't, I can't do it ' (laughs). It's beyond me that part. These are getting tough questions!

Women who spoke candidly about their own attempts to be 'good' mothers often seemed to think other mothers managed better than they did. While some compared themselves to friends and mothers on television, several made comparisons with their own mother or mother-in law, or someone else from an earlier generation of mothers.

Stephanie   How would you describe a good mother?
Lucy Barden   I don't know. Maybe that's part of my problem, that I'm ... I think someone who can really listen to the child. I suppose I sort of think a good mum is someone who has their children under control all the time, too whereas I don't. You know ...
Stephanie   They do exactly what you tell them?
Lucy   Mmm. And I suppose I think a good mother is someone who's a lot fussier than me, 'cos I'm not over fussy with them.
Stephanie   Fussy in what way?
Lucy   Oh, probably I suppose I think of my mother-in-law all the time. Like just to be careful with things, and the ornaments and things, and also things that are dangerous.

> *Stephanie* So you seem to be saying you don't really see yourself in that way?
> *Lucy* I suppose I'm looking maybe more at other people's ideas of a good mother.
> *Stephanie* I'm really interested in what you think.
> *Lucy* But I sort of get confused between the two ... It's hard really 'cos sometimes I mean I'm fairly patient, but sometimes it just gets too much.

It might have been a relief to many of the women who took part in the study to hear *each other* talk about how often they found it all got 'too much'. Most had found motherhood harder than they expected. The realities of having one, two or more children who begin their day at 5.30 or 6.00 a.m.; who are on the go almost constantly all day, wanting to go to the park, wanting to be read a story, not wanting to have nappies changed, hair brushed or faces wiped; who have tantrums in the supermarket when they are not allowed to take home the toys and lollies strategically located near the check-out counter; who follow their parents everywhere, even to the toilet; and who even after they have been settled in bed for the evening wake at 2.00 or 3.00 a.m. needing a cuddle before they will settle back to sleep, are enough to test the patience of even the most saintly parent.

But women were often extremely critical of their own efforts at motherhood. They imagined not only that other mothers managed a lot better, but that other mothers did not share their sense of frustration at dealing with the constant trail of children's demands. For example, Bronwyn Meier, who had two children, described a 'good' mother as one who

> seems to have more kids. They let a lot of stuff roll off their back, sort of thing. They don't let it affect them. Don't get mad by different things that happen. So [an] easy going person.

Asked whether she saw herself as a 'good' mother she replied,

> Yeah, pretty good. Probably not a natural mother. They have more kids, and sort of ... natural mothers ... . I think a lot of that's got to do with when you have your kids older. You've been used to working for ten years before you have kids, and it turns your life upside down now. I might have been a more natural mother at twenty than at thirty sort of thing. It's a different kettle of fish.

Bronwyn's ambivalence about her own skills as a mother and judgement that she is not what she calls a 'natural' mother reflect an assumption that only women who embark on motherhood with no other life experiences can be 'good' mothers; that somehow once you have other experiences, such as 'working for ten years', you lose the apparently innate capacity to offer children what they need. Motherhood is seen here as unlike other life tasks for which greater experience is an advantage. While becoming a mother in our society does often involve a series of losses for women — giving up paid work, never or rarely having time to oneself, never or rarely seeing friends without the company of little children — why is it that having no other experiences in life (less to lose) is seen as the best route to being a 'good' mother? In reality, being able to respond to children around a 24-hour clock whenever they want or require attention, and at the same time deal with the consequences of this for one's own life is something which arguably demands a great many skills. The recurring themes in women's accounts of 'good' mothers — patience, the capacity to switch off other things and focus on the children for at least part of each day, seeing children as a responsibility — are attributes which require a great deal of commitment and the preparedness to accept everything going wrong one day, and still be able to get up and start again the next.

Not all women who took part in the study subscribed to the view that the generations of mothers who stayed at home with the kids while Dad went out to work did a better job of being a mother than the current generation:

Judith Do you see yourself as a good mother?
Amanda Joseph I feel I am a good mother to Emma, yeah.
I try to — a lot of things that I feel maybe that I missed out on in childhood — I give her. Like, we were never a huggy, kissy, cuddly family, and I don't know whether that's because my Mum virtually brought us up 'cos Dad was working quite a lot and never had time, and then if you were sort of the younger children, the older ones tend to play with you and that sort of thing. So I try and really give her lots of hugs and kisses and tell her I love her and that sort of thing which I feel that I never had.

Amanda's account flags the realities for women of running a household before the advent of washing machines, pre-packaged foods and microwave ovens. Smaller families and new household technologies have lifted a considerable burden of domestic drudgery from women's shoulders. At the same time they have made possible a different kind of relationship between mothers and children.

Cathy Urwin argues that women in Britain spend more of their time playing with children, reading to them, and being involved in their activities than women at any other time in the nineteenth and twentieth centuries.[4] Her evidence for this is based on work by

Hilary Land, which suggests that although women's involvement in paid work has increased, the number of hours of domestic work and child care women undertake has remained fairly constant. Land argues that as family sizes have gradually decreased and labour-saving devices have been introduced into the home, women have spent an increasing amount of time on child care as opposed to cooking and cleaning. Urwin's own interview-based study of 40 women in London, all of whom had children under two, although not representative, provides further evidence of the extent and nature of women's involvement in child-related activities. Women in her sample themselves emphasised that mothers spend 'more time with the baby nowadays'; 'we want to be more involved in our children's development'; 'It's what they need at this stage, lots of one-to-one attention' and 'the more you put in the more you get out — I feel I'll reap the benefits later'.[5] These ideas of what it means to be a mother suggest a very different emphasis to the 'old style good mother' qualities of patience, reliability and willingness to spend time. The women Urwin interviewed expressed a very active engagement in their children's lives. In this context, 'having lots of time to spend' takes on a very different meaning related to what mothers do together with their children, rather than the question of whether or not they are at home all or most of the time.

EMBRACING 'QUALITY TIME'

What did the women in our study mean when they said 'good' mothers have 'time to spend with their children'? Although there were six women who stated unequivocally that it was important for mothers to be 'always available' or 'full-time at home', most women did not say this. The women who identified spending time with children (but not all one's time) as important elaborated on this in a variety of ways. In some cases what women said appeared to be an extension of the qualities Richards associated with the 'old style good mother'.

> *Sandra Richards*   I think I am a good mother. One that can cope. Just a good mother is someone who can just tune off other things and devote her time to her children, and not rush them around and expect them to keep up ... mothers that sort of keep the same speed as their children, not rush them, and being frazzled which I have done from time to time too. That's when I don't feel a good mother.

Although in this account Sandra does not use the word 'patience', the capacity to keep the same speed as one's children that she describes clearly builds on the idea that patience is a quality of 'good' mothers. But Sandra's account also stresses that a 'good' mother is someone who can switch off other things and devote her attention entirely to her children. This suggests a different concept of motherhood, in which the time mothers spend with their children has an important purpose.

Several other women reiterated this view. Elena Long was most explicit.

> [A good mother] One that's very patient and thinks of the child before themself. Like sometimes I want to finish what I'm doing but I know she wants me to do something, and that's a bit frustrating. But now sometimes I just leave — like when I first brought her home I would just worry about if the house wasn't clean and this and that, but now I worry about her more than making sure the house is alright. *So when the child comes first I think, mainly, and taking time to play with them and read to them.* [emphasis added]

The importance of playing with children, 'reading to them', and helping older children with homework was brought up by several women. Listening to children and providing them with an immediate response when they wanted attention were also recurring themes.

> *Sophia Hegazi*   Good mother (laughs). Gee whizz. A good mother, … I suppose one that is kind and understanding, willing to spend time and listen, but still with a firm hand — a little bit strict.

> *Bettina Copley*   I really hate going to visit other mums when their child comes up to talk to you and they don't actually listen, and they don't give them any attention 'cos it must be very hard for the kids to work out when it's alright for them to be noticed and not noticed.

> *Kristen Watson*   Good mother, good mother (laughs). Someone who's patient. Someone who will listen to their children. Someone who will discipline their children, as well. Someone who'll also let them have time to themselves. Quite often if one of them wants to go off the deep end, they are allowed to, but they are in their own — in their room. Nobody else has to put up with it. They can do, they can have their space too. And someone who'll respect their opinion too I suppose … It might not always be something you like, but the fact is they do have opinions too … And someone who's willing to give quality time, time to sit down and play with them, and teach 'em things, and things like that.

Some women clearly worried a great deal about whether or not they were doing enough in this regard. For example, Charlotte Williams reflected at length on the time she had been able to spend with her son, Joseph, in the week just prior to the interview:

[A good mother] One that's got a lot of time one on one, for their children, which is what I was saying to a girlfriend the other day, Monday. It's been a few days since I've spent that one on one time with Joseph 'cos we've just been really busy. We've had outings, like I've gone out with him and we haven't left him, oh except for Monday, but just with one thing and another happening I've just sort of been really social wise busy, and I've been minding other children and I found that he was starting to get niggly. Normally at least once a day I try and sit down, whether it be half an hour or an hour, just take the phone off the hook and play puzzles or play dough or something, read him stories or something like that. And I've just found like — and with yesterday working — he got it with Tim [child's father] all day, 'cos Tim didn't do a scrap of housework — washed the dishes that was about it — but even today, we've been to playgroup and he's gone down for a sleep, and this afternoon I spent some time with him. But I was starting to feel guilty because I hadn't spent that one on one time with him, but nearly every day I try to do that.

The focus of Charlotte's concern is on what implications there will be for Joseph if she fails to provide some 'one on one time' to him on a regular basis, but she also notes that there are repercussions for herself here too. Even though her partner has spent the whole of the previous day with Joseph apparently giving him his sole attention (since he 'didn't do a scrap of housework'), she comments that she feels guilty about not having spent enough 'one on one' time with him herself.

Another recurring theme in women's beliefs about 'good' mothers was that it is important for mothers to understand children's feelings. Sometimes this was linked to the idea that all children are different, and require individualised responses catering to their particular character and personality.

Liza Rogers [A good mother] someone to talk to, someone that would understand how you feel, if you don't feel like talking, but knows what to do to make things better. Just to be there when you need someone.

Ursula Redman A good mother would be someone who spends quality time with her children and knows their personality traits well enough to cater to their need, not just their general care, I guess is what I'm trying to say. That you know them well enough to be able to turn each situation to suit them, 'cos each child is so different.

[Another woman] I don't know, [a good mother] one that can sort of handle their child in any situation, sort of like letting the child not do what they want, but sort of still showing them what they want to say without just squashing their feelings, by the same time, still letting them know who's the boss.

These accounts add yet another layer to spending time with children. They describe mothers who are skilled at reading their children's behaviour and feelings, and who make use of this knowledge to 'turn each situation to suit them'. The idea of 'quality time' is merged here with the belief that mothers have a responsibility to provide children with guidance, but in subtle ways linked to children's individual personalities.

Mothers in these accounts are very powerful people who are responsible for their children's present and future happiness. But to some extent this is a two-edged sword. The idea that mothers are the major influence on children's futures gives meaning and purpose to the many hours women spend caring for young children, but it has a downside. The possibilities if one is aiming to provide children with 'quality time' are endless. And since children are never 'good' (happy, inquiring, engaged, not bored, tired or frustrated) all of their waking hours, how can a mother ever know if she is providing the *right sort* of inputs, or *enough* of her undivided attention?

THE POSSIBILITY OF PERFECTION

The idea that mothers should provide their children with a stimulating environment (opportunities for play, time to listen, etc.), and that they should actively engage in the child's world of discovery, reflects a major shift in the child-care literature in the post-war period. Whereas in the immediate aftermath of the Second World War mothers were advised to stay at home full time with their children in order to avoid the damaging effects of 'maternal deprivation', from the 1970s onwards mothers were encouraged to maximise opportunities in their daily interactions with children for fostering children's social and intellectual development.[6] Post-Freudian psychology, which informs most of the child-care literature currently available to mothers, assumes that mother–infant interaction is pivotal to the psychological, emotional and relational life of the child, and that it is the quality of the interactions between mother and child that determines future psychological development. Mother and child in this framework are, or have the potential to be, the perfect unit. Penelope Leach, for example, gives the following advice to new mothers in her book, *Baby and Child*,[7]

> The more you can understand her [the child] and recognise her present position on the developmental map that directs her towards being a person, the more interesting you will find her. The more

interesting she is to you the more attention she will get from you and the more attention she gets the more she will give you back.

Leach outlines the perfect symmetrical relationship between mother and child where understanding and meeting the baby's needs contributes to the mother's sense of purpose and self, and the baby's response in turn fuels the mother's interest and capacity to give appropriate care and attention to her child.

For a very occasional woman in our sample, motherhood did seem to be like this.

> *Annette Flynn* A good mother is one who cares for her children and her family, provides a happy environment for them, also feels fulfilled and satisfied in some senses in what she is achieving.
> *Stephanie* Most of the time would you see yourself as a good mother?
> *Annette* Yes, yes. I'm always here for the children, and I do things for them, love them.

Others had found a workable way of relating to their children that accommodated the times when they felt their responses were less than perfect.

> *Gayle Lazzaro* [A good mother] Someone who's tolerant, consistent, I suppose natural in the sense that they can express all their feelings ... this is all hypothetical, it doesn't really happen like this.
> *Stephanie* Do you see yourself as a good mother?
> *Gayle* Oh, I'm on the better end of each of those things (laughs). I mean sometimes you're not, sometimes it's easy to fly off the handle, things like that, but if the kids see you do that, then I think you have to accept that they're going to do that too. I mean it's all part of life, isn't it, it's real life. You can't create an artificial environment for them.
> *Stephanie* So most of the time you would see yourself as a good mother?
> *Gayle* Yeah, I think I do a reasonable job.

But several women were far less sanguine about what it is like to try to be a 'good' mother on a constant basis.

> I don't know how to word it, but [a good mother] remains calm around their children. Like if they're really het up about something, go somewhere else and express their concern. You know, go out in the back paddock and scream and yell. I've been guilty of spinning it with —— [child] a couple of times, or near him, and I've seen what it's done to him, so if I'm getting uptight about something I try to get away from him before I show it.

> *Rhonda Do you see yourself as a good mother?*
> No. (laughs)
> *Rhonda Do you want to say a bit more about that?*
> I don't know. I desperately want to be good mother, and I like being a mother. But, yeah, I seem to be full of failures, and I think a lot of that stems from receiving a lot of criticism, but also you know, I think I am fairly insecure as a person, too.

Although the focus on mother–infant interaction in post-Freudian psychology renders it *de facto* a theory of motherhood, the implications for mothers of, in theory at least, shouldering the responsibility for children's social and intellectual development, have rarely been researched or described. What are the effects for women when they find themselves unable to be consistently patient, understanding, loving and attentive? It is clearly impossible to be these things all the time, but how do women determine what is enough patience, or under what conditions it is okay for them not to remain patient, loving, calm, etc.? Dawn Harrison summed up this dilemma as she experienced it in her relationship to her four children. Her conclusion was that a 'good' mother would have to be a superwoman.

> A superwoman! A good mother. I don't know. Anybody that could discipline their children and be able to turn around and feel all motherly toward her child must be able to work miracles, because I certainly can't do it. If I'm angry because I'm disciplining, I certainly can't go up and give them a cuddle. I just can't do that. It would be nice to be able to get over the emotions I suppose. Or to be able to relax and enjoy them without all the pressures of running a household and that as well.

When we first began the interviews all of us felt some unease about asking women how they would describe a good mother. The notion of 'good' mother and even the qualified 'good enough' mother popularised by object relations theory[8] carries the implicit assumption that some women do not make 'good' or even 'good enough' mothers. It is almost axiomatic given the tradition within western rationalist thought of thinking in dualities, that these other mothers — the ones who are not 'good' mothers — must logically be bad mothers. The dichotomy good/bad belies the possibility of being both good and bad or sometimes the one/sometimes the other.[9] As we have seen, few women challenged the good/bad dichotomy. The attributes they described as being the qualities of good mothers, in the main, also fitted within an either/or framework. When women found themselves unable to remain patient, calm, understanding, loving and attentive to their children's needs, they felt they were not good (and therefore bad) mothers.

GETTING THE HOUSEWORK DONE

One of the stumbling blocks women described coming up against in attempting to be 'good' mothers was housework. Research by the Office of the Status of Women shows that new mothers spend an average of 56 hours per week doing unpaid work.[10] This includes doing household cooking, laundry, cleaning and shopping as well as tasks associated with the care of children. The effort involved in trying to juggle these competing responsibilities was a topic that came up often in the interviews. The comments of Josephine Cucinotta below illustrate a tension that several women described between being a 'good' mother and managing to get housework done.

> *Judith*   *Do you see yourself as a good mother?*
> *Josephine*   Yes and no. Yes, when I don't yell and scream. Depends like if I'm really busy that day and I'm not — like if I'm not that busy, it's fine — like I don't mind; but if I, like now and then you can't let go of the housework and let go of all the things you have to do around the house because it's gonna put you back behind. That's the only thing I find really hard.

The kind of work that women do when they are at home with small children remains, despite all the efforts that have been made to draw attention to it, a socially hidden form of labour. The census does not count hours of unpaid caring and household work; time spent taking children to kinder, school and visits to the local doctor or health centre; or the number of hours involved in doing the household shopping. When new mothers are depicted in television commercials and 'soapies', they are usually relaxed with a freshly bathed, smiling, and obviously thriving baby. Sick babies, babies with feeding problems, mothers with mastitis, mothers who are chronically tired from long-term sleep deprivation and the physically demanding nature of motherhood with its routine of domestic labour are rarely seen.

In the descriptions women gave of 'good' mothers we also saw only part of this picture. No one in this section of the interviews talked about how difficult it is for mothers to remain patient and calm when they are themselves physically exhausted or unwell. Nor was there any mention of babies that cry for several hours a day no matter what strategies are tried to console them; babies who never sleep during the day, and want to be constantly in someone's arms; or that wake several times a night until they are five years old. Women talked at length about what it is like to manage under these and other stressful circumstances in other parts of the interviews, but they were silent about these stresses when we asked them about 'good' mothers.

Why did women talk about housework intruding upon their capacity to be good mothers, and not these experiences? One plausible explanation is that domestic labour has a legitimacy as a demand on women's time that being tired, physically exhausted or having a baby that cries a lot does not. The perfect mother–baby unit described by Leach excludes these realities, except as the consequences of mothers being poorly adjusted to their role. Implicit in Penelope Leach's description of the strategies parents might use to calm a crying baby, for example, is the assumption that if these strategies are tried a 'good' mother will succeed in allaying her baby's cries. If she does not succeed it is imputed to be a failure of her mothering style; she either needs to become less anxious or more attentive and receptive to her particular baby's needs.[11] Housework, on the other hand, is something with which all mothers must contend. The child-care books counsel that a lowering of standards may be necessary in the short term, but there is no debate regarding the necessity of basic housework getting done some time.[12]

'IT'S NOT USUALLY ANYTHING FOR YOURSELF'

In the following extract, Camilla Jackson describes vividly the things that make her lose patience and feel she is not being a 'good' mother. In her case, it is not the domestic workload associated with caring for her three children, but all the commitments she has to doing things for school and kindergarten, that intrude upon her time.

Rhonda How would you describe a good mother?
Camilla (Sighs) Someone who can say no. That's my big fault. I'm everything to everybody: 'I can do that', 'Yes, I'll help you out there', 'I'll do that', 'I'll do that'. And in the end you have to look back and say my family's really suffered this week because I've been anywhere but here, and my patience hasn't been wonderful because I've had to do so many things, either for kinder or school or whatever. It's not usually anything for yourself, it's always for somebody else.

So I admire a mother that can say no. I've got an older sister like that. She'll say 'No, that's detrimental to my family, I'm not doing that', and she's so organised and always on the ball ... If someone asks me, I'll say yes. I try. Originally, this last time I thought I was getting really good. I filled in the fete form and I said no, I'd only help out on Monday to clean up, and I'll do all the cakes and the chutneys and the sauces, all that sort of thing, but I wouldn't help out on the day 'cos I wanted to go away for the weekend. But they rang up and said, 'Camilla we're desperate, you always help out with the fete. Why can't you do it this year?' I said okay what time do you want me? So I cut the weekend short and came back for it. And although I'd done well and truly what I considered to be — but that's the sort of person I am.

But it gets me down, 'cos I think when my in-laws come they say 'Camilla, what are you doing, what are all these people coming in to your house for?' They get really agitated about it and say 'You're not thinking of my son, you're not thinking of your children, you're thinking of everyone else instead'. So I get fairly negative about myself after they've been here ... They don't mean to, and I think they realise that that's life these days. It's not like it was years ago, but they still don't understand someone who can't say no. [Camilla was in the case group, and was also depressed at follow up. She is one of the three women whose stories are told in Chapter 12.]

Although Camilla feels judged by her parents-in-law for her preparedness to help out with activities outside her immediate family, the point she makes about these activities 'rarely being something for herself' is an important counter to this. The activities she talks about are all for the local kindergarten or school, and so indirectly for the benefit of her own children. Even though these involvements take her away from home and add extra burdens to her already busy domestic workload, the fact that they centre on her children indirectly means that she can still at one level feel they are a legitimate part of the role of a 'good' mother. If it had been something for herself that was occupying her time and taking her away from her children, it would have been very much harder for her to equate with being a 'good' mother.

The desire to maintain involvements that predate a woman's entry into motherhood — the life she had had before — was rarely mentioned in the context of talking about 'good' mothers. It was as if 'good' mothers did not have partners with whom they liked to spend time alone; or ever play tennis, read a book, or have lunch with friends; or go to work and enjoy it. Elsewhere in the interviews women talked about how they missed doing the sorts of things they had done in their spare time before they had children, and a proportion of women described how they had tried to keep up at least some of these activities (see the discussion of 'timeout' in Chapter 11). But when it came to the question of 'good' mothers, the idea that mothers might do things for themselves, even occasionally, was rarely raised.

The following extracts come from two women who were exceptions to this general rule. Both talked in a fairly abstract and rational way about 'good' mothers who take time for themselves.

Frances Heringslake spoke about mothers needing to look after themselves in order to stay in good health for their children.

> I suppose overall [a good mother] one who really does love her children and listens to them and tries to cater to their needs. I suppose if you look after yourself and stay healthy too, so you're able to be around.

The second extract is from a woman who gave an expansive commentary on what she described as the global and specific aspects of being a 'good' mother. It is reproduced here in full, although it is only in one small section (italicised in the text) that she talks about mothers having to recognise their own needs as well as their children's. In the range of issues she discusses, and the perspectives on motherhood she presents, this mother was most unusual among the women who took part in our study. We were unable to contact her to ask permission to use a pseudonym for her interview as she had moved without leaving a forwarding address.

> *Stephanie How would you describe a good mother?*
> Oooh that's a tricky one. Do you want it in sort of general terms? There are lots of specifics that I think are important.
> *Stephanie Do you want to go through them?*
> I might just get global first. I think a good mother is somebody who recognises that her child is an individual and needs the space to be one, so you'd basically let the kid be just what they are, and who they are, don't try and push them and direct them all the time. *And I think it's really important that you recognise your own needs, in terms of being a parent and in terms of being in a relationship — which is a separate issue I suppose.* [emphasis added]
> I suppose a good parent also has to recognise that if they can't provide the care that a child deserves, then they can get somebody else responsible to do it, and make sure it's being done by someone. You don't have to be a good parent yourself all the time, I don't think, as long as there's somebody else doing it, and that doesn't even have to be their partner.
> *Stephanie And the specifics?*
> I think there are lots. I think breastfeeding is really, really important. I think having the baby sleep with you is really important. I think not saying 'don't!' is really important, letting them take risks for themselves, like not stopping — I don't stop her — well — there's not a lot of things I actually stop her doing — I mean potentially harmful things like falling off stairs and all that sort of stuff. I let her do those things, and fall off or whatever if she's going to — and she doesn't

very often — and I think that's the way it works. Not giving her junk food. (Laughs) I mean those things are actually — I think they're really important and I think they're quite hard to implement — all these ideals. You have to be quite determined to keep them in place, to make sure that your kid's getting a good diet all the time. It's harder than I thought it would be, to do that, and I think it's really important.

This account of what is required in order to be a 'good' mother is exceptional in a number of ways. It is one of only a handful of responses women gave to our question about 'good' mothers where women's own needs are acknowledged as being both important, and separate from the needs of their children. This mother was also the only one among all the women we interviewed who transposed the notion of 'good' mother into 'good' parent, and one of only four women who mentioned their partner at all in this section of the interview. The length and breadth of issues she covers without any prompting by the interviewer also distinguishes her comments. Although most women had a ready answer for our question, there were many for whom it seemed the interview was the first time they had put into words their thoughts on motherhood. The extract above, on the other hand, is striking because of the sense that the woman had clearly worked through her ideas about motherhood before the interview and appeared to be more resolved and confident about her beliefs than was characteristic of most other women.

Yet her comments remain a fairly abstract commentary on what it is like to be a mother. There is much less lived experience in this long exposition of the attributes of a 'good' mother than in the comments women made about how they juggled housework and child care alongside more active involvement in their children's lives. What it actually meant for Frances or the woman quoted above to try to negotiate the emotional space and time to pursue their own interests and needs in a way that is compatible with their lives as mothers and their beliefs about motherhood, we are not privy to or at least not in this section of the interview. Perhaps it is too hard to put into words in a culture where the idea of mothers having needs of their own is not acknowledged or accepted. Counter to the sense conveyed by Harper and Richards that the qualities of independence and individuality are associated with an emerging concept of the 'new good mother', we could find no evidence that the notion that mothers may have lives that extend beyond their children's lives was any more common in 1990–91 than when Harper and Richards interviewed couples in the mid-1970s.

FATHERS AND OTHERS — WHAT HAVE THEY GOT TO DO WITH BEING A 'GOOD' MOTHER?

In women's accounts of 'good' mothers we rarely heard about fathers or about other people (family members, friends, day-care staff, etc.). Why? The isolation of the mother–child dyad is, of course, a physical reality for a majority of women. Over 70 per cent of partners were absent from the home for more than ten hours a day, or for more than five days a week. Although some men contributed a great deal in the time they were at home, and four fathers were at home full time, the reality for most women was that they did the majority of the work of caring for their children during both day-time and night-time hours (see Chapter 11).

But the isolation of mother and child in women's accounts of 'good' mothers was about more than women's greater responsibility for the physical workload of child care, and about more than the amount of time women spent 'alone' in the company of their children. It also had a potent psychological dimension.[13] The sense that 'good' mothers offer their children a very special commitment, and have a very deep-rooted emotional bond with them that is non-transferable to others came across strongly in some women's comments. For example, Collete Prout stated that a mother's relationship to her child had to take precedence over all others:

> *Rhonda   How would you describe a good mother?*
> *Collete*   Well ... just to be a friend of them, and always take care of them, not to leave that role to any fathers or other relatives. It has to be — I mean mother has to be first, of education, of everything! Even if you're planning to buy something for them, just mother has to think about it first, what they really need.

Liza Rogers also conveyed in her response a sense of the special psychological bonds between mothers and children:

> Well, I'd say a good mother is someone to talk to, someone that would understand how you feel if you don't feel like talking, but know what to do to make things better. Just to be there when you need someone. Someone to help you with things, do things with you, and all those sorts of things, be a friend.

And Henrietta Woodhouse explained how she chose not to employ a live-in nanny in order to develop a strong relationship with her daughter.

> *Jill   How would you describe a good mother?*
> *Henrietta*   Loving, guiding, responsible ... I don't think it's a mother who has to be on duty and around 24 hours a day, and

obviously that's to clear my conscience about the number of times I leave my children, but I have also made the conscious decision not to have a live-in nanny 'cos I want to be a mother ... I choose to do a fair amount myself, because I feel that's important. Next year in London I will have a live-in nanny ... because I will want to have more free time to enjoy London, and Jane will be old enough that I think that *the bonding will be strong enough* there to go through with it. But for this twelve months, two years I'm choosing not to have it. It's a conscious choice. [emphasis added]

Fathers were only rarely brought into the constellation of women's thought about 'good' mothers. The following extracts, particularly Judy Gower's reference to mothers and fathers working as a team, were unusual.

Judy A good mother is one that's ... as a team you have to work, as a husband and wife. As long as they're happy. I want them to be happy throughout their life, and doing what they're happy doing. It's really difficult to answer that. I just want my children to be happy and have a good life, and go to the beach, and things like that.

Rhonda Do you see yourself as a good mum?
Eliza Ross Yes, but not everyday.
Rhonda But overall?
Eliza No, I flip my lid quite regularly. But even that's not a bad thing. I think your children have to see you ... I think it's through watching Graham [partner] and myself that they pick up problem-solving strategies and so on. It can't all be rosy — that's unrealistic. I don't think it hurts anyone to be exposed to a raised voice, or as I say, to see you lose your cool a bit, so long as the overall effect is a positive one.

Rhonda How would you describe a good mother?
Katrina Peterson One who's not perfect but is just there for her children, I think. I think for me it's coming down to an issue of being able to feel and express love for them very openly.
Rhonda And do you see yourself as a good mum?
Katrina I feel like I'm learning. I don't know, it's hard to know — things like where you set boundaries and where don't you. We're not disciplinarians. We have trouble with that sort of thing, so it's hard from that sort of respect. But yes — no I think I give them a lot. We're managing. We've learned a lot.

A DEPRESSING VIEW?
This chapter was written 'blind' to the case/control status of the women whose reflections on motherhood are described above. As

we ourselves reflected on what women's beliefs about 'good' mothers tell us about what it is like to be a mother, we did not know whether certain of the ideas women expressed about 'good' mothers were linked in any way to having experienced depression or being depressed currently, or to the social background of the women themselves. Only after we had written this chapter did we make a computer file that enabled us to look at these questions. What we found was that there was no association between any of the most common beliefs expressed — good mothers are patient, loving, give their time freely to their children, stimulate and encourage children's emotional development — and depression at eight to nine months after birth, or at the time of the interview. Nor were any of these beliefs associated with any social background factors (including parity), with the exception of encouraging children's emotional development, which was more often expressed by women who had done some tertiary level studies (25 per cent compared to 6 per cent non-tertiary educated women).

Given the variety of ideas about 'good' mothers conveyed in the interviews, which meant in some categories we had very few responses, we grouped together a number of the categories to make one variable that we call 'the perfect mother'. We included in this variable all the attributes of 'good' mothers that fitted within a dichotomous either/or framework (patient, loving and caring, consistent, fair, non-judgemental, responsible, calm and relaxed, able to handle children in any situation, listening attentively/talking with children, showing sensitivity to children's needs, never losing one's temper). Our hypothesis was that women who experience depression might be more likely to adhere to an either/or construct of the 'good' mother; that the sense of failure inevitable within this construction of motherhood may contribute to depression. In fact, we found this was not the case. Women who had been depressed at eight months postpartum or were depressed currently were not more or less likely to adhere to this conception of the 'good' mother. The beliefs women expressed concerning 'good' mothers were shared beliefs — culturally pervasive and therefore normative in our society. Depression was not explained by them, although the picture of motherhood they evoke is in some ways depressing. After analysing this section of the interviews, we were left with a powerful sense of how impossible it is to be a 'good' mother in the terms women had described. Women's voices on this question reiterated a conversation recorded by the American author Phyllis Chesler in her diary in 1978:

I asked a Mother what she thinks a 'good mother' is.
   'A good mother is nothing like me,' she said. 'A good mother

always knows what to do, and does it well, without complaining, without yelling, without manipulating anyone. A good mother uses her power to protect her children from all harm. A good mother has healthy, happy, wonderful children. A good mother is nothing like my mother, or like my grandmother ...'

'You're describing a faery goddess and a machine,' I interrupt.

'Yes, maybe I am. But I think that's what a good mother *should* be.' [emphasis added][14]

To be both 'faery goddess' and 'machine' is more than is asked of any human being in any other role in life, yet it is expected of women in their relationships with young children.

Stephanie Brown, Rhonda Small, Judith Lumley

EIGHT

The Experience of Motherhood

The 'invisibility' of the stresses involved in the work of mothering goes a long way towards explaining why past researchers have focused on looking for a hormonal cause for postnatal depression.[1] The invisibility of the work of mothering is partly due to the fact that it is literally unseen. Taking place within the privacy of the home, the unpaid physical and emotional work of mothering is idealised, on the one hand, as the most important and fulfilling work a woman can do, but on the other hand goes unremarked, uncounted and unpaid.

In the nineteenth century, the home and all that went on within it was deemed to be private, a 'separate sphere', quite distinct from the public world of paid work and exempt from all outside scrutiny. Even today the division between home and work, while not so rigid, still remains. Ignoring the work of mothering and the other work carried out in the home because it counts for nothing in official statistics of economic productivity is one reason why this work and its emotional consequences for women is ignored by researchers and health professionals.

Another reason that this work and its stresses has not received the attention it deserves stems, Elliott argues, from a reluctance by women themselves to discuss the emotional impact of motherhood.[2] To disclose feelings of stress and inability to cope to others, when these feelings are believed to be 'unnatural', is to experience them as stigmatising. Such a disclosure can feel like an expression of personal failure as a woman and as a mother, which reinforces the view that if other people knew about these unmotherly, unfeminine feelings, they would react with disapproval and rejection. Anticipating a reaction of this kind is a potent incentive for remaining silent.

Another motive stems from the belief that no one else feels the same way.

Cassandra Lightfoot I think a lot of it was personalising it and not sharing it, and realising that other women felt like that.

Some women had attempted to share their feelings with either partners or health professionals, but the reaction they received — disbelief, avoidance, anger, rejection, dismissal and trivialisation — caused them to keep their feelings to themselves.

Very often the cumulative effect of this self-censorship was to deepen and extend the distress already being experienced. Another reason to 'silence the self'[3] probably stems from accepting as real, and attempting to live up to, what are really unattainable ideals of motherhood (see Chapter 7). Other research on the experiences of motherhood has also commented upon a pervasive ideology of maternal sacrifice, whereby women always place the needs of others in the family above their own and accept that mothers should be endlessly patient, giving, nurturing and unselfish.[4]

> *Eliza Ross* You look at the ads on TV and so on, and Mums are superwomen: the house is spotless, the children are in beautiful designer gear, and there's this immaculate dinner put on the table, and you're really made to feel that's how you're meant to be. So I think that those advertising images are very harmful, and to have an honest friend who can say, 'I got two hours sleep, I feel lousy', just occasionally to have someone say that. But I find a lot of my girlfriends and the girls I listen to at Playgroup and so on, talk about how their kids go to bed at seven and they eat broccoli.

Thus the qualities a good mother is supposed to have tell us a great deal about the way in which socially constructed and sanctioned ideals are translated into self-imposed demands that women tell themselves they must meet if they are to live up to the ideals of good motherhood. All the women we interviewed valued the work of mothering highly and felt responsible for its successful outcome by fostering the development of a happy, healthy child. At the same time, women were aware that in becoming mothers they experienced irreversible changes in their own lives and their sense of themselves.

Becoming a parent is known to affect women and men differently and to have a more marked effect on a woman's sense of identity. This differential effect on identity has been found to derive from palpable differences in the amount of personal change that occurs in women's lives on becoming mothers compared with changes in men's lives when they become fathers. As well as experiencing more personal change than men, women feel more responsibility for the health and well-being of children.[5]

This difference in how parenthood is experienced and its lived consequences for women compared with men can begin in pregnancy:

> *Lucy Barden* [mother of three small children] I was really devastated [when she found out she was pregnant for the third time]

and he sort of didn't see that it was so devastating 'cos he wanted to have three children anyway, and he couldn't understand why I was so upset and got so worked up. And by the time Sam had been born, in the morning all three of them would be crying and I'd just be crying and feeling ... 'cos they were very young, and I had three of them to feed.

Even when men and women carry out the same tasks they tend to be differently construed in social terms. When a man looks after a child he may be seen by others or see himself as babysitting. The time has not yet arrived for child care to be viewed as an equal responsibility of fathers and mothers. This distinction struck some women as unfair.

The worst thing is the responsibility, always having to be there. Even if you go out and he falls over, everybody's screaming out: 'Where's your mother? Where's your mother?' And you think: 'Why don't you say, Where's your father, Where's your sister?'

Georgia Trembath That's the one thing I hate, it really pisses me off — if you go out, or if you stay home, you're looking after the child, because you're the Mum, right? But if you go out and the father stays home to look after the child, he's babysitting. You know, as if it's not his job. I mean he put it there in the first place. You know, it wasn't an immaculate conception; he has some responsibility for it .

Another woman was annoyed by the adulation a man received if he did some ordinary household task:

If somewhere in passing I mention that he cooked tea last night, it's the mass hysteria, 'Oh, haven't you got a wonderful husband, isn't it just fabulous, and does he do the washing too?' ... Oh yeah, sometimes ... I don't think people have to fall on their knees and worship a guy because he cooks the food and changes a baby's nappy every now and then. You know. I mean I certainly appreciate the fact that he does it, but I don't really think I need to be continually thanking him, and I don't think other people need to see him as being God's gift.

To find out about the nature and extent of the changes that took place in women's lives as they took on responsibility for a new baby, we asked women to complete a specially designed questionnaire focusing on these changes and a woman's reaction to them. We decided to use a specific measure, rather than one of the more general measures of stress and life events, for a number of reasons. General measures do not focus on the particular changes and events that contribute to the experience of motherhood. General measures also tend to be phrased in a way that suggests they are gender neutral and apply equally well to both men and women. Very often, however, the content of the individual items which make up the questionnaires, is more applicable to the events that occur in men's lives than in women's. For this reason, it is doubtful whether findings from studies employing questionnaires that primarily reflect men's interests and experiences and overlook women's can be valid for women.

Researchers interested in representing women's experiences accurately have found it necessary either to modify existing questionnaires or to devise questionnaires specifically addressing crucial aspects of women's lives. An example of the first approach is found in Jane Norbeck's Life Experiences Questionnaire for use with women,[6] which we used in our study. Norbeck devised this questionnaire because she found that traditional assessment measures of life events actually left out questions and issues that were centrally important to women. So she added new items under existing headings. For example, under the heading of 'Health' she added a question concerning major difficulties with birth-control pills or devices; under 'Parenting' she added items such as a change in child-care arrangements, conflicts with spouse or partner about parenting, taking on full responsibility for parenting as a single parent, and custody battles with former spouse or partner; and for the section on 'Crime and legal matters' she included being a victim of violence, such as rape or assault.

In our study we also adopted the second approach of devising a questionnaire that specifically addressed a crucial aspect of women's lives — motherhood. The twenty-item questionnaire, which covered a wide range of changes and experience related to motherhood, was called 'The Experience of Motherhood Questionnaire' (EMQ).[7] A high score on the questionnaire indicates a high level of stress and dissatisfaction with motherhood, while a low score indicates a low level of stress and a high level of enjoyment and satisfaction. As previously noted, becoming a parent is typically a very different experience for women than for men. We wanted to focus on the changes associated with motherhood that disproportionately affect women; their satisfaction and enjoyment of various facets of their lives and their sense of themselves.

Responses to the questionnaire revealed far-reaching changes in women's lives consequent on becoming a mother. This chapter will consider first those that affected more than 50 per cent of the women we interviewed.

HOW LIFE CHANGES ON BECOMING A MOTHER
There were five areas of women's lives that changed for most

women on becoming mothers:
- 59 per cent of women reported not having time to pursue their own interests
- 57 per cent did not have an active social life
- 55 per cent needed a break from the demands of the child
- 55 per cent had less confidence since becoming a mother
- 53 per cent did not enjoy mealtimes with the child.

The biggest area of change concerned having, or rather not having, time to pursue one's own interests. As we have seen, almost 60 per cent of women in our study stated that their ability to do this had changed quite dramatically as a result of becoming a mother.

Confinement: 'The Tied Down Feeling'

The term confinement, when applied to childbearing women, usually describes the period of restricted physical activity following the birth. For women in our study, this confinement was simply the start of a longer and more complete physical, emotional and social confinement that was inextricably bound up with the mothering role.

At a physical level, the ability to come and go at will was severely constrained. For a number of women, this was quite an unexpected and distressing part of becoming a mother.

> The tied down feeling was what I wasn't expecting. You sort of can't just go and do what you want to do.

It was a shock for women to find that things that could be done freely and easily before children arrived became difficult or impossible afterwards. This confinement severely affected where they could go and what they could do outside the home, but also constrained behaviour and activities inside the home. Having children was frequently at odds with having any uninterrupted time, space or privacy to do things previously taken for granted as an unremarkable part of adult life.

At an emotional level women could feel cramped and intruded upon:

> *Melissa Dean* They're both fighting and they're both jealous of each other; both always on top of me, fighting for me. Like I said, I can never do anything without them. I can't go anywhere without them. It's not that I don't want them, it's just that I need a bit of space sometimes; even going to the toilet.

The changes that take place extend from the level of lacking time and personal freedom to pursue sporting, cultural or intellectual interests or hobbies — an enjoyable and important part of adult life — to changes and adaptations in basic living, right down to no longer being able to go to the toilet alone.

Social Confinement
Given the inroads motherhood makes into a woman's ability to pursue her own interests, it is not surprising to find that the second most commonly mentioned negative effect of motherhood related to its impact on being able to have an active social life. This effect was mentioned by 57 per cent of women. To some extent, not having an active social life meant the loss of a sense of self as a social being and the loss of affirmation by others as a person. This loss linked into profound emotional role changes whereby women sought to redefine themselves and reorganise their lives around a very different set of circumstances and responsibilities.

> *Cassandra Lightfoot* And a lot of it was just going through those emotional role changes. You know, being a rager who goes out drinking and having a great time, to being someone who is pregnant and can't drink, and so, who am I? Working out a new life.

The world the woman inhabits shrinks and at the same time she and her baby are alone within it, occupying all the available space.

> *Sally Osler* I find after I've had the children that I sort of lack a lot of self-esteem too. You feel like, really there's nothing else in the world except you and the baby and it just — it's all there is. All of a sudden you think, 'Oh, there's gotta be more to — there was more to life than me and a baby, and now there's not. It's me and the baby. So I think you lost a lot of self respect.

Often the way in which life changed was difficult to explain for someone who had not experienced it before.

> *Georgia Trembath* Some things you just can't explain. And also, like they say it's a 24 hour job but — you know, a 24 hour job is going to work, clocking on — so it's not a job, it's a lifestyle. It's just suddenly everything changes.

Further evidence of the contraction of one's world and interests is found in the fact that 31 per cent of women said that they had 'little to talk about besides the baby'.

Needing a Break
The emotional toll of trying to respond almost single-handedly to the child's ongoing needs for physical and emotional care and attention was apparent in the wish, expressed by more than half of

the women interviewed (55 per cent), for a break from their child's demands, some personal time and space.

> *Dawn Harrison* [who had five children]   I just wish everybody would leave me alone. I'd like some peace and quiet. It's very demanding.

> *Katrina Peterson*   If I come in tired from work, I can't there's no way I can back out of emotionally still giving to them — they still need me; or if you just want space to be quiet for a while, it's just not there; or time to talk together. But they give us back a lot.

Use and Control Over Time
Becoming a mother meant the inability to be able to control or define the use of time, amounting to a personality change, and for some women this was the major psychological effect of motherhood.

> *Camilla Jackson*   You don't expect it to affect your personality as much, I don't think. I think that's the major change. Your time's not your own.

Loss of Confidence
More than half the women interviewed believed that their confidence had been adversely affected since becoming a mother, for a variety of reasons.

> *Katrina Peterson*   Having worked out that I don't like the parenting styles of either of my parents leaves me in limbo as to where I actually go.

> [Another woman]   I mean socially I went into my shell a bit, and it was very difficult. Just in terms of working out who I was and what I was and feeling really unsure about what a good mother should be and wanting desperately to be a good mother.

For some women, this uncertainty could never be laid to rest.

> *Clare Thornton*   You can do as many courses as you like, it's not going to fix your personal ... the questions in my mind are always, 'Am I doing it right? Am I going to give her a good life?'.

Camilla Jackson was clear about her maternal instincts, but still lacked the inner conviction that allowed her to act on them.

> I know the right thing, but I'm not confident enough to follow my instincts and do it, do what I know to be right, at the time, 'cos I keep thinking, 'oh, maybe I'm not right'.

Sometimes the loss of confidence came from a feeling of profound inadequacy at not knowing how to cope or come to terms with some aspect of the child's behaviour.

> *Lucy Barden* Sam at the moment — he's the terrible twos where he's throwing tantrums and you really get embarrassed when you go out, and that really destroys your confidence.

Stressful Mealtimes
Mealtimes with the child also proved to be a source of stress, with 53 per cent of women indicating that they did not find this activity enjoyable. Although the majority of women responded in this way on the questionnaire, the topic of mealtimes was not included as a specific question in the interview. Other difficult aspects of life with children such as problems with sleeping, eating, crying, battles of will or temper tantrums were more frequently mentioned in response to a question about the child's temperament. Thus one mother who commented on how her son had no regular patterns of sleeping also mentioned his irregular eating habits.

> *Ann Marie Burke* Sometimes he will eat it, sometimes he doesn't. Even to get cereals into him I try to put some fruit, or just a bit of sugar, he sees me put sugar on mine, so I put a bit of sugar on his, to help him. Sometimes it works, sometimes it doesn't. Just depends on whether he wants it or not. He's not a regular, cereal every morning, or toast every morning. It's whatever he wants. Froot Loops, anything, it could be just cheese, or even just a juice. He's not a regular ... like some kids have their slice of toast and their cereal, there's no way.

Taking these five separate but connected domains of life as a mother together, it is apparent that becoming a mother imposes great demands for adaptation, change and re-organisation in a woman's life. For more than half of the women in our study, motherhood involved the loss of significant aspects of their 'old self' and changes to their sense of identity. Becoming a mother diminished the sense of being an individual with time to oneself, unstressed by the needs and demands of a child; someone who could and did pursue personal interests and was able to have an 'adult' social life, to say nothing of uninterrupted sleep and enjoyable mealtimes. For the majority of women the multiple changes and adjustment in their lives had an adverse effect on the confidence they felt in themselves.

More than one-quarter of the women in our study also reported stresses or lack of satisfaction with six other areas of their lives. Sheer physical and emotional fatigue was the most important of these, with 44 per cent of mothers agreeing they felt 'run down'. More than one-third (39 per cent) found the trouble of arranging a baby-sitter took away the pleasure of going out, suggesting that there are potent practical or possibly financial difficulties related to the falling away of one's social life on becoming a mother. A similar proportion wished that those close to them 'would share the work of baby care with me', another likely reason for feeling run down.

In view of the multiple sources of stress in their lives it is not surprising that more than one-quarter of the women (28 per cent) reported that they had not enjoyed sex since their baby was born and did not like their lives as they were at the time of the interview (26 per cent).

GAINS AND REWARDS OF MOTHERHOOD

It would be inaccurate and misleading, however, for the weight of these negative changes and difficulties to hide the very real pleasures and satisfactions also inherent in the experience of motherhood. If the responses to the Experience of Motherhood Questionnaire are looked at from a positive rather than a negative perspective, then more than 80 per cent of women felt they were coping well with these stresses (81 per cent), were not concerned about their child's progress (81 per cent), felt relaxed whenever they thought about their child (82 per cent), did not feel cut off from friends (83 per cent), and felt fulfilment in looking after their child (82 per cent). Very few did not have easy access to transport (15 per cent), felt anxious when they remembered their baby's start in life (13 per cent), believed relatives undermined their confidence in looking after the baby (12 per cent), or got so much different advice it was hard to know what was best for the baby (12 per cent).

In the interviews we were particularly interested in exploring which aspects of being a mother brought with them the most joy and satisfaction. Consequently we asked all women: 'How would you describe your overall experience of being a mother this time around?' In keeping with the responses on the Experience of Motherhood Questionnaire we found that three-quarters of the women in our study rated their overall experience as either very positive (43 per cent) or mostly positive (32 per cent). Just over 22 per cent of women rated their experience as 'mixed', with some positive and some negative elements, and only one woman described her experience of motherhood as mostly negative.

We then asked 'Thinking about being a mother, what are the best things?' All the women, even the one who reported having a mostly negative experience of motherhood, were able to nominate something that was good about being a mother and usually women nominated several. The best things, in order of how often they were mentioned included: watching a child's development (47 per cent), the love you receive from children (43 per cent), being needed and responsible for the child (27 per cent), giving love to the child (21 per cent), helping to shape the child's life (20 per cent), having the child's company (13 per cent), and feeling contented (10 per cent). One-third of the mothers we spoke to also mentioned a variety of other enjoyable, satisfying things about motherhood.

Answers to this question were similar whether or not women were currently depressed, had been depressed at eight months, or had no experience of depression at any time over the two years since giving birth.

> *Amanda Joseph* Oh, just seeing her learn new things all the time and — not that I force her to do the alphabet. I mean she learnt all that on her own. Just seeing her growing and experiencing new things and coming back and showing me a flower or different things like that.

Marcia Goldie, who had experienced depression, encapsulated in her comments the way in which the positive and negative aspects of motherhood were part and parcel of one another.

> The best thing — is just really watching them and the feedback from them; and although I talk about the restrictions on me and that, there are times when you have lovely days when you are just free to enjoy the day and go out and go to the park or catch a bus into the city. I mean, yeah, it's all there, it's just a matter of getting out there and enjoying it.

Many women were aware of the co-existence of ambivalent or mixed feelings about motherhood: needing a break from the needs and demands of their child, but at the same time enjoying being needed and gaining enormous satisfaction from being with their child.

> *Camilla Jackson* The best thing I 'spose is always having someone beside you, either in your arms, or clinging on to your leg, or pulling at your skirt, dirtying up your clothes, whatever.

> *Carlotta Gould* Even though you are on call 24 hours a day, it's a nice feeling, knowing that when they want something they'll always want you to do it for them. And teach them things and watching them doing what you taught them.

For Clare Thornton being with her small daughter was sheer good fun:

> Well, it's company, if that makes sense. Like we're friends. Even though she's so little. I like sharing with her. I like playing with her toys with her. Feed times, we have good fun at mealtimes. Bathtime, splashing you know. Sometimes I'll jump in the bath with her and we'll have a splash game. Play peek-a-boo, and we run round the house playing hide and seek. Besides she brings out my childhood for me, it's good fun. And as far as all the cleaning and all that goes, that's just part of the game. I just accept it. [Clare is one of the three mothers whose stories are told in Chapter 12].

Besides watching and being responsible for the development of another human being, giving and receiving love and enjoying the company of a son or daughter, mothers also mentioned a range of other pleasures.

> *Mary Sainsbury* It's a very sensual experience as far as I'm concerned, being a mother. I mean I just love watching them: the perfect flesh, and ... and I still do with the other children too, especially in summer, just watching them.

> *Cassandra Lightfoot* It's also a very nice experience to share with Ben. Just being able to drool over them.

What another mother liked best was the openness of her children towards her.

> They accept you as you are, and they're open — like they'll say, 'I don't like that dress on you' — so they're honest.

A number of the mothers we interviewed also saw motherhood as an experience that was crucial in fostering their own emotional growth and maturity and that changed them irrevocably from the people they had been before.

> *Annette Flynn* I think it can be very rewarding and it can also strengthen your character; it makes you more mature, more aware of life. We have lots of friends who don't have children, and sometimes I feel really different from them — not superior in any way, but just as though I've experienced a lot more of life than they have. I mean you make many sacrifices when you're a parent and I think that it's all part of expanding your knowledge of life.

Perhaps the feelings of the majority of the women who spoke to us, could be summarised in these sentiments:

Fiona Neilson I don't think I could go through life without — not having children. My brother and his wife are going to do that, I think and I think they're crazy. Even though it's not easy having children around at times, I don't think I could go through life without. They do bring a fulfilment to your life.

Jill Astbury, Rhonda Small, Judith Lumley, Stephanie Brown

NINE

Depression: Women's Voices

Perhaps the most striking inadequacy of the postnatal depression literature is the almost total lack of reference to women's experiences. One could be forgiven for thinking that this phenomenon renders mothers speechless, so rarely are their voices to be heard. It is as if the only way one could gather knowledge about depression in recent mothers was through the case histories written by doctors and psychiatrists or the results of standardised tests and questionnaires administered by researchers looking for causes or associated factors. It should be said, of course, that such questionnaires are painstakingly completed by women — women who nevertheless are rarely asked to tell their own story.

In one sense it is true that the experience renders women speechless. In societies where motherhood is held up as the ideal of womanhood and having a baby a matter of unbounded joy, women literally cannot speak about any distress they may feel following the birth of a baby. If they do speak, they are admitting to being less than a 'good' mother. If they do speak, there is the risk of having their baby taken from them. If they do speak, few will want to listen. Many women in our study had actually had these experiences, or felt fearful of the consequences of making their distress public in any way. Clare Thornton, for example, whose story is told in Chapter 12, was concerned not to tell her Maternal and Child Health nurse about the distress caused by her husband leaving her when she was five months pregnant, because of the fear that she 'was going to try to take my baby off me'. But this does not explain why researchers who seek to understand the phenomenon of depression after childbirth so rarely do the obvious and talk to mothers about the experience.

In conducting the follow-up study of mothers depressed at eight to nine months after birth our express purpose was to fill in some of the gaps in knowledge about depression in recent mothers, gaps which have arisen precisely because of the lack of attention paid to women's experiences. We wanted to ask women what it had felt like to be depressed, what they thought were the contributing factors, if they had done anything about being depressed, whether they had sought help, what had speeded recovery, and finally what advice they would offer other women having similar experiences.

These are areas where the research literature on depression in recent mothers has been largely silent. In fact, when we began the research we could find no other study that had posed such questions to women. By 1993 just one similar study — of 60 first-time mothers in Glasgow, Scotland — had been reported in the literature.[1]

It is also worth emphasising at this point that our study was not designed to answer questions about the aetiology of depression after childbirth, but rather to document the salient factors of the experience as women themselves perceived and described them. We have taken women's beliefs about their experience at face value because we believe their understandings have important implications both for how women themselves deal with the experience, and also for how health professionals seek to help women recover from depression.

In this chapter, we present women's accounts of what the experience of depression was like. When had women begun feeling depressed, how long did it last, and what changed to improve women's emotional well-being by the time their children were two years old? In Chapter 13 we document women's responses to depression; whether and from whom they sought help; and women's advice to other mothers about how to deal with being depressed.

WOMEN'S RECALL OF EMOTIONAL WELL-BEING

We talked to women about their emotional well-being in the latter part of the interviews, after we had talked at length about their experiences of motherhood. Sometimes well before we asked women directly about whether they had been depressed, they offered this information themselves. In reply to a question about whether looking after her daughter had been easier or harder than she expected, Amanda Joseph commented that 'initially it was a lot harder':

> I think I cried every day for the first six months. ... Sometimes I look back and I think I actually had postnatal depression probably for a lot longer. 'Cos I also haemorrhaged for ten weeks after she was born, so that didn't really impress me a lot. Then I had the mastitis the three times, and she was a constant feeder every two hours, and you think 'Goodness, what's happened to my life? I used to be so organised' and sort of also that independence, of losing work — that played a big thing in it.

When women in the case group did not comment spontaneously on their emotional well-being, we began the final section of the interviews by feeding back to them that their answers to some of the questions on the original survey form indicated they may have been depressed at that time, and asking if this was how they remembered it. We were interested in checking whether their recall of this time matched with their scores on the EPDS. We also wanted to know whether describing their state as 'depressed' was something women would find accurate or acceptable.

Only one woman disagreed with the assessment of her emotional well-being given by her score on the EPDS. Sally Osler said that looking back on it she thought she had been 'more tired than depressed', though she also said that she probably would have viewed it differently at the time. Forty of the 45 women agreed that they had felt depressed, three said perhaps, and one could not remember. Women's recall of their feelings eight to nine months after the birth were thus well matched to the assessment made on the basis of their EPDS scores, and there seemed to be no reluctance to naming their state at the time as depression. We also asked women in the control group whether they had felt depressed for more than a week at any stage since the birth and fifteen replied that they had. Twelve of these fifteen had in fact felt depressed for four weeks or more.

Interestingly, however, when we asked women whether they would call their experience 'postnatal depression', over one third of all the women who had felt depressed since the birth did not agree with this label of their experience. There were no differences in this regard between women in the case group and the fifteen women in the control group who had felt depressed at some stage. For these women, feeling depressed often had 'nothing to do with the baby'.

Georgia Trembath People were saying I had postnatal depression ... I was suffering from post marriage depression!

Jacinta Campbell No! (laughs) I mean I know ladies that have had that [postnatal depression] and nah I can honestly say no, I've never had anything like that ... Well it's not actually to do with Heather.

The importance of the finding that over one-third of the women did not wish to call their experience of depression 'postnatal depression' lies not in whether women are more or less likely to be depressed in the first postnatal year than at other times, but rather in the implications of this finding for how a woman feeling depressed at this time might be helped and supported. If the focus from helping professionals is on 'postnatal depression', or centres primarily on improving the mother– infant relationship (as help for depressed mothers often does), then a considerable proportion of the women who may be feeling depressed and in need of support are unlikely to view such 'help' as relevant to them. Jacinta Campbell, who is quoted above as saying she did not have postnatal depression, for example, had talked to her Maternal and Child Health nurse about her daughter's constant crying, which was eventually diagnosed as lactose intolerance, but had never talked to her about her own feelings and level of stress related to her marriage and her adolescent stepson.

'THEY'RE DOING A WONDERFUL JOB. WHY CAN'T I?'

Women's descriptions of feeling depressed commonly included statements about feeling alone — both in terms of feeling unsupported or isolated at home, but also in feeling that they were the only ones not coping. They rarely knew other mothers who openly acknowledged feelings of depression; women's silence acting to reinforce the belief that there must be something the matter with them, rather than something the matter with the circumstances of their lives. One woman who spent a lot of time 'alone' with her two children on an isolated farm commented,

> You sort of look at them [other mothers with young children] and think, they're doing a wonderful job. Why can't I?

This woman's partner was away from the farm five days a week working in his own business. He left at 7.30 a.m. and returned after 5.00 p.m., often spending the remaining daylight hours and considerable time at the weekend doing farm work. He made hardly any contribution to the work of running the household (scoring one for this question in the interview), never changed nappies, and never got up at night although their two children woke frequently. There was no one else on whom this woman could rely to assist her in running the household or looking after the children. These are difficult circumstances in which to care for young children, especially when one or other of them is sick or you are sick yourself. Despite this, when this woman had tried to talk to her husband about how overwhelmed she felt, his response was to say

> I was crazy (laughs). He thought I was just nuts, I think. You know, I'd flipped my lid — which didn't help.

The physical isolation experienced by this woman was thus compounded by psychological isolation from her partner. Yet, he was the only person she felt confident enough to talk to about her feelings until her general practitioner registered the stress she was under, and broached the subject during a consultation for one of the children. At no stage did she mention how she was feeling to her Maternal and Child Health nurse, laughing at this suggestion because of the social stigma she felt would be attached to any admission that she was not coping. Nor did she talk to friends about it, although in hindsight she felt it would have been useful to do so.

As mothers ourselves, we frequently identified with women's accounts of what motherhood had been like for them. We too had experiences of the whole family coming down with vomiting and diarrhoea all at the same time; of what it is like at mealtimes with a boisterous, loud toddler; of having repeated bouts of mastitis; of feeling isolated from adult company; of running out of ideas for what game to play next before nine o'clock in the morning, having been up since five-thirty. We fed back to women that they were not alone in these and other experiences; that the stories they told were familiar to us from other women's accounts and sometimes from our own experiences as well; that other mothers did not always manage better or cope with the stresses of motherhood without becoming stressed themselves.

FEELING DEPRESSED

Feeling that everything was too much, that there was no light at the end of the tunnel and that no one really understood her feelings featured often in women's descriptions of feeling depressed.

> *Elena Lang* I thought she'd never grow, she'd never be able to respond. I thought she'd never get easier to look after, and I felt that I was always tied to her. I was just there for her ... Probably because I couldn't get out of the house either [because she didn't have a car] — I was here with her all the time.

> [Another woman] I did go through a pretty bad patch with her. I just felt very — not lonely but isolated. As to how I was feeling — my husband and I were also having a bad time together, not over the children but through them as well. We couldn't agree on anything with them, so that was causing conflict in other areas. And I couldn't communicate with anyone as to how I was feeling, 'cos I didn't want to say to my friends this is how I am feeling in case they sort of said well, is she cracking up a bit? ... it wasn't just any one thing. [This woman was in our case group and was also depressed at the time of the follow-up interview.]

> *Joanna Douglas* It was a nightmare. I'd wake up in the morning and think — well I was hoping I'd go to bed and I didn't want to wake up in the morning — just couldn't go through another day like that one. The next day came and went and it went on and on. Some days she was better than the day before and I thought oh well wouldn't you know, and I would feel better and then the next day would come ...

Joanna was included in the control group, but described herself as having been depressed for a couple of months beginning around six weeks after the birth. She attributed her depression to her daughter 'screaming all day' for the first few months after birth. Joanna had been hospitalised for a short period in a mother and baby hospital to enable her to get some rest.

Not surprisingly, many women talked about feeling depressed in the context of the overwhelming physical exhaustion that characterised much of the first half year (or more) of life with their baby, and made them feel less than human a great deal of the time.

> *Jacinta Campbell* I was just so tired that I just got depressed ... you try, like one part there, she went into hospital, I think I had two hours sleep in 75 hours and I couldn't work out why when I came home I actually ran into the door.
>
> *Katrina Peterson* I think it was more that you weren't — that you had to keep on coping, even when things were tough, so you tended to just deny how you were feeling more than anything. It was more that you didn't feel the 'happys' as well as the lows; that you had to get tough. I think earlier in my life I would have cried a lot more, but I stopped doing that and I sort of survived from day to day ... I was very, very tired.
> *Rhonda* *That was from waking up every two hours?*
> *Katrina* Breastfeeding every two hours, yes. He was six feeds a night up until he was seven months old.

Another common theme was feeling inadequate. Sometimes women talked about feeling depressed in the face of criticism from family about how they were tackling the job of mothering.

> *Freda Holding* It was a very depressing time, with Karl being sick and I was getting sick, and very tired, and emotionally drained. Plus with him being sick, my husband's parents turned around and sort of blamed me that he was sick — I got depressed at that stage too.

Freda's baby had been hospitalised with bronchiolitis and gastroenteritis. Freda herself was hospitalised for depression some months after these events, and although she described herself as feeling 'good now' she scored as depressed at the time of the interview.

Some women talked about losing confidence in themselves like the woman quoted below,

> [I felt] a real failure, that's for sure, very concerned to do the right thing for [the baby], guilt ridden in case I wasn't. And yet wanting to

follow not only how we felt she should be read, but intuition I suppose, mother's intuition to a certain extent, but that seemed to be in conflict with what I was being told.

Others blamed themselves for their own or their baby's difficulties.

Joy Freeman   I somehow think that I've failed her, like her illnesses must be a reflection — I know realistically it's not, but I somehow think that her illnesses are something that I've done wrong. You know right from the word go, perhaps if I'd done something else.

Lucy Barden who had three children very close together in age blamed herself for having a third child so soon after the other two.

Lucy   I suppose it had to do with having the three kids, yelling and screaming at them, getting really frustrated. I'd get really annoyed, I suppose and feel like it wasn't fair, because I didn't seem to have the kids under control, and blame myself.
Stephanie   Would you see yourself as having postnatal depression?
Lucy   No, I don't. I think it was more related just to having kids that small ... I felt really guilty.

Reflecting on the sorts of symptoms they experienced when they were depressed, women most commonly talked about feeling exhausted, lacking in energy, feeling overwhelmed by tasks they normally had no problems completing, being easily upset and irritable, and crying readily.

I can remember going in one night, going in when she was in the middle of colic [and saying] 'Take this baby before I throw it through the window.' And that shocked me that I could feel like that, and it scared me ... I suppose it's all intertwined because I was tired, I wasn't doing those things to make me happy ... But it was mainly the tiredness. Once I got a few nights sleep I was a different person. [This woman was in the control group, but described herself as 'frequently depressed in the first twelve months'.]

Margit Gunn   You felt as if you were not in control of your life or your emotions, and what you did and when you did them. You know, you could just burst into tears for no apparent reason — fairly regularly. And it doesn't matter where you were or who you were with, you just didn't have any control.

[Another woman]   I've never known a kind of tiredness that I had, and it's very hard to explain. I mean even looking at it now, it just sounds pathetic, but yeah I was just completely overwhelmed with it ... just couldn't get going in the morning I think too; impossible to get out before midday with organising this one, and then you see other Mums who can do it with three or four of them (laughs) ... I mean look at Felix [Rhonda's baby] you can take him out and you can do this sort of thing and he's quite contented. —— [daughter] would have been very impatient with that because she wanted my attention all the time.

Women's descriptions of being depressed were not, however, simply stories of despair and negativity. Not everything about their lives was viewed through the bleak eyes of depression and it was not uncommon for women to tell their stories with a large measure of humour and courage in the face of considerable adversity. Georgia Trembath, whose husband began using illegal drugs soon after their baby was born, described how determined she was not to let this get in the way of the responsibility she felt for the baby.

Georgia ... when we first met, he was on it, and we both — he wanted to get off it — and we both worked and got him off it. But this time I said 'Well, you're on your own. I helped you once. I've got a baby to look after. I've got a house to look after. You wanna do it, you do it on your own'.

For some women, the experience of depression marked a turning point in their lives which, however painful, had led to special insights and changes that left them with a view of the experience as something both important and ultimately positive. The woman quoted earlier who lived on an isolated farm described how she felt her partner not understanding her feelings had contributed to her depression, but concluded towards the end of the interview that things had significantly improved as a result of her seeking help from her general practitioner, and her partner then taking more notice of the way she was feeling.

Stephanie You mentioned when you were thinking about going to a counsellor that things changed at that time.
Yes, I think they did, because we were both so — I mean you hit rock bottom is all I can say. And because we were both so awakened by that fact, that we made a big effort to change it, and it did change dramatically. [This woman was in the case group and was also depressed at the time of the interview.]

Jacinta Campbell also described herself as having learnt a lot about herself through managing to cope during the period her daughter was not sleeping, and with other things that had happened since.

> I didn't go in there [Maternal and Child Health Centre] and say I'm not coping please help me. I'd just sort of go in there and say look she's not sleeping, she's crying all the time, I don't know what's the matter with her. So I sort of transferred it all onto the baby. It came back to the old cliche, you know, if she got better, I'd be alright ... well, since then I've learnt a hell of a lot more just with different other things that's happened, but I'm not ashamed now to go and get help, which I have done just recently and it's the best thing. Really once you've got someone to listen to you and talk to you, whether they advise you or what, but you come out — even if they didn't say a word — you come out thinking that was good.

ONSET AND DURATION OF DEPRESSION

For some women depression came within days of the birth.

> It was sort of euphoria for the first day, a lot of visitors the second day so I didn't have a chance to think about it, and then sort of downhill from there. Crying every day, not wanting to go home from hospital, I wanted to stay there. I was in there for nine days. The specialist said 'When are you going home?' and I said 'When he's five!' (laughs). 'When I feel qualified to look after him.'

For others the onset of depression was more gradual coming over a period of weeks or months.

> I can't sort of put any time on that. It was probably just a gradual slide down I would say. I sort of can't say like suddenly at four months I felt terrible. Yeah, I would just say over a period of time.

> *Caitlin Adamson*   Well, it was really bad in hospital and I was crying and whatnot and the sweats and everything else, and then I got home and I was really buoyed up and pleased to be home, and then about two months I got mastitis, and from then on it's been slowly downhill. [Caitlin's story is included in Chapter 12]

> [Another woman]   Well, there was just the normal baby-blues thing I think. No, I was just overjoyed in so many ways. I think as the tiredness got to me — I think certainly after getting home, when ——-[child] wasn't having much sleep, and then when, as I saw it my milk failed, and we were having problems with the breastfeeding, and then the problems with the marriage came along with that. So, yes, certainly it was weeks, maybe even months later — three months, something like that.

A few women described feelings of depression that began in pregnancy, and a small number of women said they felt depressed on and off over a long time.

Ann Lamb   I wasn't real happy throughout the pregnancy, but probably I think on the second day when he [boyfriend] wasn't coming to visit at the hospital, that's when I really started.

Marcia Goldie   It's very much something that comes and goes. In some ways I wouldn't even say that it's — like that it's postnatal — I would say that it's something I have all the time, not just through the children.

Camilla Jackson   Usually in the first few months you feel pretty down about things. It's just trying to cope with less sleep and feeling like a zombie, and not being able to speak to people properly because you're too tired to think ... You teeter on the edge and come back a bit, and then back to the edge and think, oh, will you jump or not? [Camilla had three children and was depressed at the time of the follow-up interview. Her account of her experiences as a mother is included in Chapter 12.]

Figure 9.1 gives a picture of the onset of depression for both women in the case group and the fifteen women in the control group who had also felt depressed at some stage since the birth. The timing of the onset of depression is very similar in both groups with the most common point at which women became depressed being somewhere between one week and three months after birth. Five women in the case group and one in the control group described feeling depressed from some time during pregnancy, and the same number of women in both groups felt depressed off and on, but were unable to identify a starting point. Almost half of the women who had experienced depression began feeling depressed within three months of the birth (45 per cent). About one-third (35 per cent) had a later onset.

Many studies of postnatal depression have concentrated on depression in the first three months after birth, which tends to lend *de facto* support to the common assumption that this is when the onset of depression occurs.[2] The fact that one-third of the mothers in our study began feeling depressed after the first three months suggests that more attention needs to be paid to depression in recent mothers throughout the first postnatal year.[3] Those who began feeling depressed later were also more likely to say that they did not view their depression as postnatal depression, something that confirms the view that knowing how women themselves view their experience is critical in providing appropriate support and assistance.

Figure 9.2 presents women's assessments of the duration of their depression. There were significant differences between women in the case group and women in the control group who had felt depressed. Women in the case group were more likely to have felt depressed for nine weeks or longer, with almost one-third (14/45) depressed for more than a year, compared with only one-fifth of the women in the control group who had at some stage felt depressed (3/15).

Figure 9.1 **When did women start feeling depressed? Cases (n=45) versus controls depressed (n=15)**

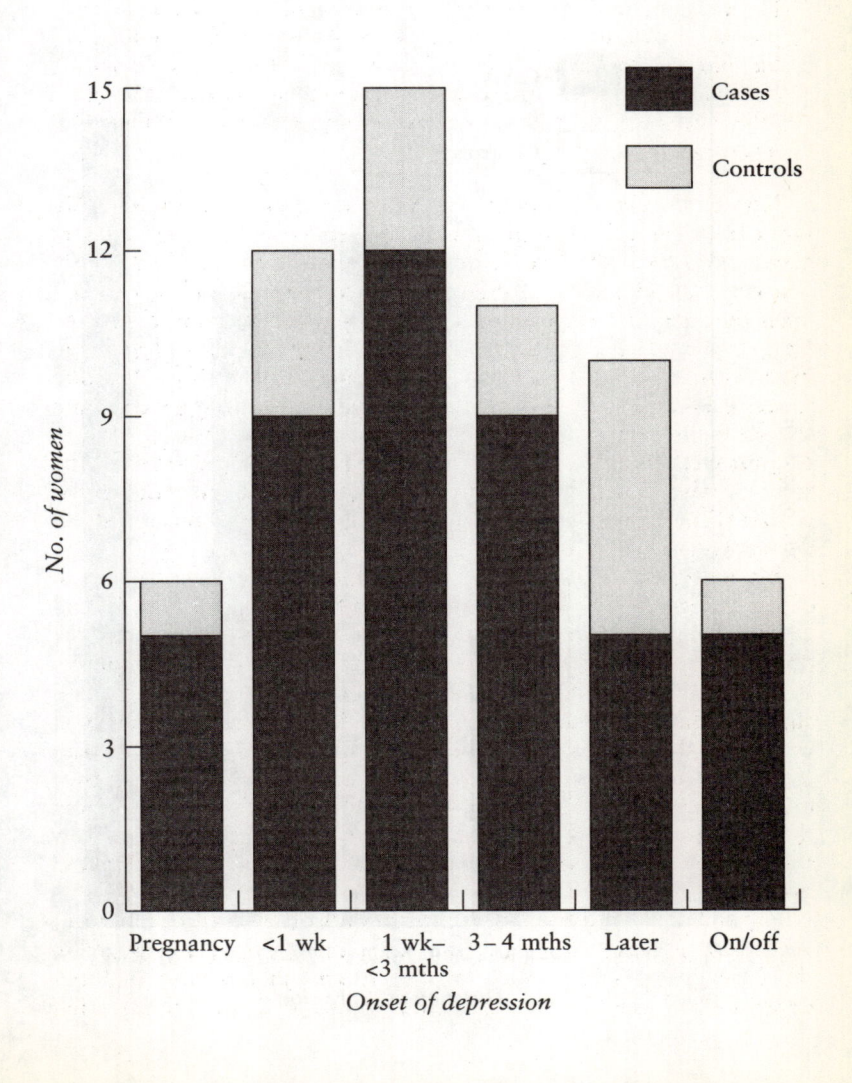

For a significant minority of the women in our study, then, the experience of depression had pervaded their lives throughout much of their child's infancy. And for the majority feeling depressed was by no means a fleeting experience, even for the fifteen women in the control group who experienced shorter periods of depression.

Figure 9.2 Length of time women had felt depressed: cases (n=45) versus controls depressed (n=15)

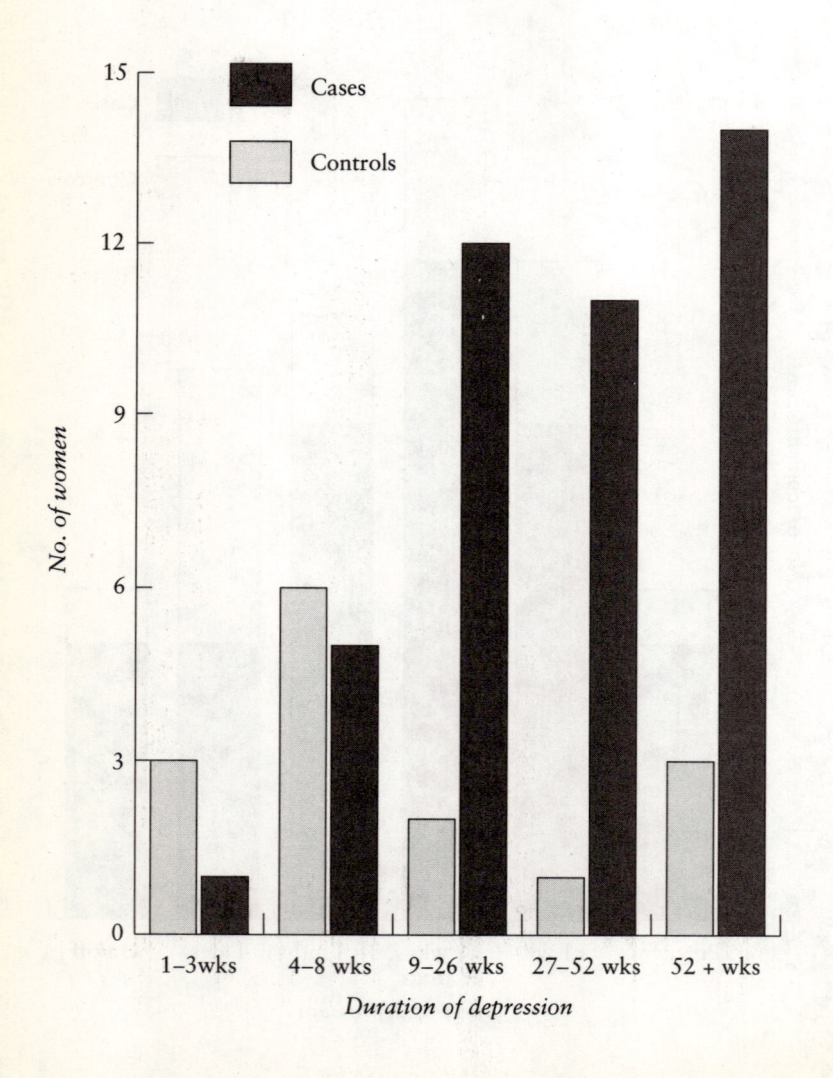

EMOTIONAL WELL-BEING AT FOLLOW-UP

We asked women in the follow-up interview whether they felt more or less depressed than they had done at the time of the original survey. Of the 60 women who had experienced depression, four said they felt about the same at the time of follow-up as they had at the time of the survey, and four felt worse. A majority had more good days than bad, although 12 per cent said that it was about fifty-fifty. The main reasons women gave for feeling worse at the time of the follow-up interview were financial problems, relationship difficulties, their children being sick, and feeling that they were less supported.

Figure 9.3 Distribution of EPDS scores at follow-up: cases (n=44) versus controls (n=44)

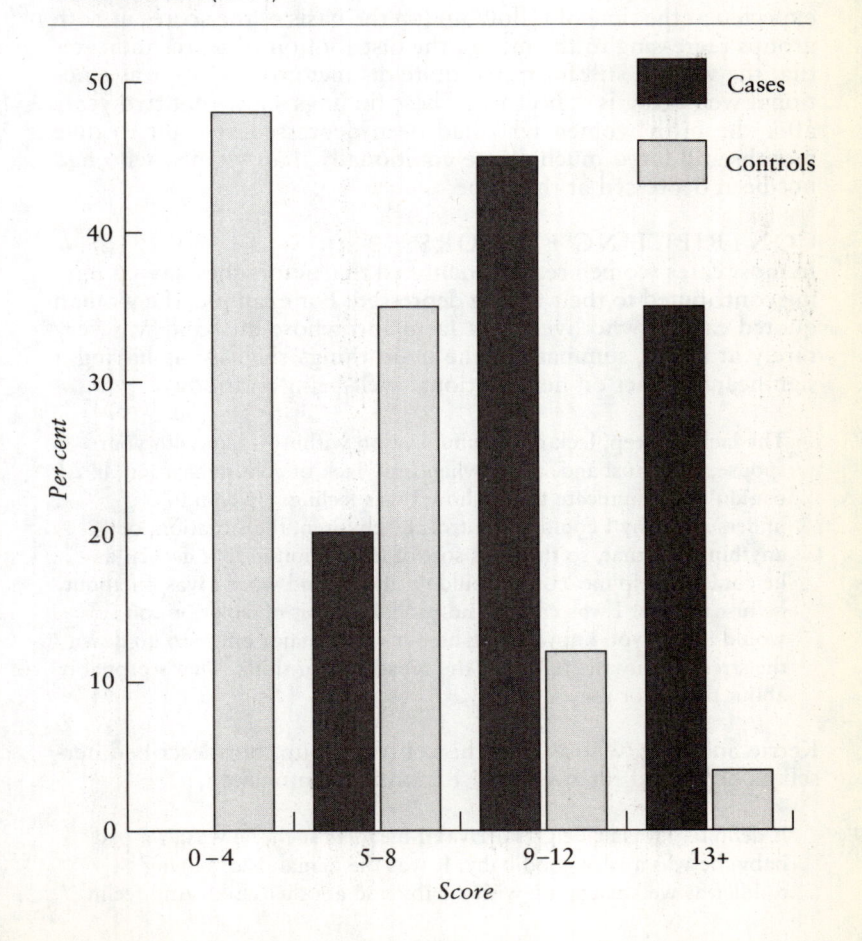

All of the women in the study were sent a copy of the EPDS to complete again just before we visited to interview them at home. Figure 9.3 gives the distribution of scores on the EPDS at follow-up for women in the case and control groups. Women in the case group were significantly more likely to be depressed (that is, scored greater than twelve) at follow-up than women in the control group. Although two-thirds of women in the case group no longer scored greater than twelve on the EPDS at the time of follow-up, they were clustered on scores of nine or more, with only 20 per cent (9/44) scoring less than nine. This means that most of them were still scoring in the region where they might be considered borderline for depression. In comparison, 83 per cent of women (37/44) in the control group scored less than nine at follow-up. Thus, while greater similarity in the scores of cases and controls might well be expected at the time of follow-up (on the basis of the scores in both groups regressing to the mean), the distribution of scores indicates that the women still form two quite distinct groups as far as emotional well-being is concerned. These findings show that two years after the birth women who had been depressed at eight to nine months still fared much worse emotionally than women who had not been depressed at that time.

CONTRIBUTING FACTORS

In most cases women readily identified the factors they saw as having contributed to their feeling depressed. For example, the woman quoted earlier, who lived on a farm and whose husband was very rarely at home, summarised the main things she saw as having a significant impact on her emotional well-being as follows:

> The lack of sleep, lack of communication within — like with your spouse, your husband, as to, when I say lack of communication, like I couldn't communicate to him how I was feeling. He couldn't understand why I couldn't control the children, the situation, or anything like that, so that was sort of frustration in that aspect, and he couldn't help me 'cos he couldn't understand what I was on about, he just thought I was crazy. And probably a bit of isolation too I would say — you know, being here it was a major effort to go down the street to buy the milk and the bread sort of thing. That's probably about the major issues.

Kerrie Sneddon, who was in the control group, but described herself as depressed for over twelve months, commented,

> It definitely wasn't Leigh's arrival. I mean as such, he wasn't a bad baby, he was a very good baby. It was the demands of having a toddler as well as coping with a baby and another child. And feeling,

I just felt hemmed in. I mean I've got the car, but I felt it wasn't so easy to just jump in the car and go somewhere.

It was not unusual for women to blame a number of different factors.

Ann Marie Burke I think because of the colic, and not having my family here to help me, and being new in the area. Even though everybody made me feel welcome, because they're very friendly round here, and people are very helpful. But just moving to this area, I really wanted, I needed my mother and my sister-in-law.

Amanda Joseph ... as I said, I think it's due to the birth, the bleeding, the mastitis, the colic — those sorts of things.

These comments were made in reply to an open-ended question in which we asked women to explain what had contributed to their becoming depressed. Women's replies to this question are recorded in the 'Initial responses' column in table 9.1. Of the 60 women who had been depressed, 22 said that lack of emotional support was a factor, and nineteen blamed isolation, tiredness and/or their own ill health. Lack of time to oneself, material circumstances (such as financial difficulties, housing problems)

Table 9.1 Women's views about what factors contributed to their depression (n = 60)

What women said	Initial responses	Most significant factor	Other factors after prompting	Totals
Feeling unsupported	22	10	15	37
Being isolated	19	9	18	37
Tiredness	19	8	*	19
Physical health factors	19	4	8	27
Lack of time/space for self	14	2	26	40
Material circumstances	15	2	18	33
Illness/death of loved one	12	7	4	16
Baby temperament	9	4	11	20
Hormones/biology	9	1	10	19
Tendency to depression	3	1	6	9
Other factors	31	12		31

* Tiredness was not prompted as the questionnaire asked about physical health factors and tiredness together. However, women's responses in fact distinguished these so they are listed separately in the 'Initial responses' column.

and the death or illness of a loved one were also commonly listed factors. A number of factors mentioned were particular to individual women (accounting for the 31 factors categorised under 'Other factors' in Table 9.1). For example, one woman was unhappy because she was living with her parents-in-law; another woman was living with her father (whom she did not like) as a way of feeling safe in the context of her ex-partner's threats of violence; and three women described conflicts over naming the baby arising from their partners' wish to have the baby called after their own fathers.

> *Helen Bakoula* It's a long story, but I'll try to make it brief. Greeks usually name their children after the father's parents. So, usually it's the son that has number one. When Anna was born I thought I could sneak out of it and call her after my family because she was a girl. But Peter's mother insisted ... Then when Nick was born, I felt that I had just lost my father, his sister had a son called Nick anyway ... so I wanted to name him after my father. [In hospital] I was bawling my eyes out. I thought he would say okay we'll do it your way. But he just kept going home and that was it.

Twelve women identified a factor we listed in the 'Other factors' row as the primary factor contributing to their depression.

Any factors on the list *not* mentioned in a woman's initial reply to our question were then prompted to check whether when asked directly about these factors women perceived them as contributing to depression. The same factors continue to rate highly, but more women said that lack of time and space to oneself and material circumstances had influenced their emotional well-being when they were asked about these factors directly. It seemed that these things were in a way taken for granted; that having young children necessarily means never having time alone, and a period of financial insecurity. Women laughed when we asked about these issues, or replied with comments like 'I suppose money is always a worry'; 'I don't have time to recharge the batteries'; or 'definitely, yes that was a part of it'.

The factors women identified as playing the most significant role in their particular case are also of interest. Of the 60 women who had been depressed, ten identified lack of support as the most important contributing factor, nine said it was being isolated, eight said it was tiredness, and seven felt that the illness or death of a loved one had been the most important factor. None of the other factors was seen as the most significant influence on their emotional well-being by more than four women, and in the light of the controversy surrounding the role of biological and hormonal factors it is of particular interest that only one woman linked her depression primarily to hormonal changes.

Despite some major recurring themes there was also much diversity in women's accounts of the factors contributing to their feelings of depression. It was also clear from the ease with which women pointed to relevant factors, that depression was not something they saw as having descended upon them quite inexplicably after the birth of their child, as implied in some literature on this subject.

For the most part women's own explanations of their depression lay firmly within the context of their lives as mothers: feeling unsupported or isolated, being exhausted, or physically unwell, having no time or space to oneself. Perhaps not surprisingly, what women believe about this experience actually matches well with those factors most firmly established as important by postnatal depression research to date, particularly lack of social and emotional support.[4] There is also a striking similarity in what women said about the reasons for their depression in this study and the views of a sample of 60 working-class mothers in Glasgow.[5] But women's perspectives on contributing factors also raise issues which to date have been given little attention in studies of depression after childbirth; the study powerfully demonstrates the relevance of women's physical health after childbirth, the instrumental support they receive from partners in the areas of household work and child care, and the responsiveness of health care providers as factors contributing to women's emotional well-being.

RECOVERY

The majority of women who had been depressed (87 per cent) said their emotional well-being had improved by the time of the interview. The most frequently mentioned reasons for their improved emotional well-being were: their child getting older (52 per cent), having more support from their partners (31 per cent), going back to work (27 per cent), and not feeling so tired (25 per cent). Just under one-fifth of women said they had adjusted their expectations of themselves or their children. Very few women (less than 4 per cent) said that professional intervention (either counselling or medication) had been a major factor in their recovery. An equally small number mentioned making new friends or simply the passage of time.

Although most women in the case group stated they felt better at the time of the interview than they had done when their children were eight months old, there were, as we noted earlier, fifteen women for whom depression was either continuing or had recurred by the time of the interview. For them recovery from depression was either elusive or fleeting.

Rhonda Small, Stephanie Brown, Judith Lumley

TEN

The Social Context of Motherhood

In this study we wanted to explore the social context and the social arrangements in which mothering occurs and how differences in these can impart quite a different emotional flavour to how women experience motherhood. In particular, we were interested in how the lives of women who were depressed differed from those who were not.

One source of information for considering these differences in women's lives comes from the richness of the interview material. Using this material the previous chapter recounted women's experiences of depression including their views of the contributing factors. It drew attention to the finding that women who had been depressed at eight to nine months were much more likely to be depressed two years after the birth than other women. This chapter will focus on some key elements in the lives of women which made the experience of motherhood more difficult, stressful and depressing for some mothers. These key elements are the role of partner support, the impact of negative life events, and the influence of the temperament of the child.

The psychometric measures used were the Experience of Motherhood Questionnaire (EMQ),[1] already described in Chapter 8; the Life Experiences Questionnaire (LEQ),[2] the Toddler Temperament Scale (TTS),[3] the Social Support Questionnaire (SSQ),[4] and the Edinburgh Postnatal Depression Scale (EPDS).[5] Each of these is described in more detail in Appendix 3.

DEPRESSION AND THE EXPERIENCE OF MOTHERHOOD

Two years after the birth women who had been depressed at eight to nine months had a significantly higher mean score on the EMQ than women in the control group (43.30 versus 37.00, t= −3.77, p=0.001). The higher the score on the EMQ the greater the stress, negative life change and dissatisfaction a woman is experiencing as a mother. Women who were depressed at the time of the interview also had much higher scores on the EMQ than other women suggesting that feelings of depression are intimately connected with the emotional experience of motherhood.

The particular areas of experience found more stressful by women who had experienced depression were different depending on whether they had been depressed at eight months or were depressed at interview. The original case group, for example, compared with the original control group, were much more likely to feel cut off from friends (27 per cent versus 7 per cent), not to like their lives just as they were (36 per cent versus 16 per cent), and almost one-third (compared with 7 per cent) did not feel they were coping with the stresses of parenthood. They were more likely to feel 'run down' (54 per cent versus 32 per cent), and 73 per cent (compared with 43 per cent) said they did not have an active social life.

By contrast, the much smaller number who were depressed when their children were two years of age had marked concerns and anxieties over mothering their children. Over 40 per cent of these women did not feel relaxed when they thought about their babies, compared with 13 per cent of those who were not depressed at this time. The same percentage felt concerned about their baby's progress and 41 per cent (compared with 11 per cent) did not feel great fulfilment in looking after their children. Another area of distress and dissatisfaction that characterised them was that they were far less likely to have enjoyed sex since the birth of their baby (47 per cent versus 23 per cent).

There were two areas in which women who were, or had been, depressed differed from those who had not. The two commonalities were not liking their lives as they were (36 per cent of women who were depressed at eight months felt like this and 47 per cent of those depressed at interview) and feeling that they were unable to cope with the stresses of parenthood (32 per cent and 47 per cent respectively).

These findings provide insights into which of the changes that accompany motherhood happen to most women and should therefore be considered 'normal' and which are disproportionately associated with depression. For example, not having time to pursue one's own interests affected the greatest number of women in the study, nearly 60 per cent, but it did not affect mothers who were depressed more than those who were not. On the other hand, the second most commonly agreed-with statement — not having an active social life — did differentiate between mothers who had been depressed at eight months and those who had not. Other views about life as a mother that occurred to the majority of women, but no more frequently to women with past or current depression, were needing a break from the demands of the baby, losing confidence since becoming a mother, and not finding mealtimes with the baby enjoyable.

PARTNER SUPPORT

We, like a number of other researchers, found that women were more likely to be depressed two years after birth if they felt unsupported, especially by their partners. For example only four of the fifteen women who were depressed on both occasions described their partners' reactions as supportive or very supportive. Women from the case group had a significantly lower mean score for partner support, less support overall, and lower satisfaction with the support they did receive, than women from the control group. However, women who were depressed did not differ from other women in the degree of support they saw themselves getting from other family members or friends.

During our interviews we asked women who had scored as depressed on the EPDS at eight months whether their partner had noticed or commented on how they were feeling at this time. Ignoring what was happening, escaping from the situation or just not being around at times of greatest need were commonly reported partner responses.

> *Nina Cooper*   No, he didn't [react to her being depressed]. He doesn't notice anything like that. He didn't even notice when I was in labour; he went to work, didn't he?
>
> [Another woman]   He took up playing footy again. He tried to walk away from the situation and let me deal with it too much of the time.
>
> [Another woman]   I'd be in tears, and he would say, 'You'll be all right', and off he'd go to the back shed.
>
> *Ann Marie Burke*   He's very hard to talk to. Because of the long hours he works he feels he's done ten hours at work … that I'm a mother, I'm home, it's my responsibility. That's his viewpoint.

Other partner reactions included anger, criticism and defining women as crazy.

> *Kaylene Shaw*   He may notice [how I was feeling] I guess. He's more likely to get annoyed with me and say, 'wake up to yourself', you know, rather than try and solve the problem. So I guess I don't talk to him a lot about why I'm feeling depressed.
>
> *Charlotte Williams*   He probably even got angry with me because I was still neglecting him and that as well.
>
> *Amanda Joseph*   Yeah he sometimes thought I was going crazy, because if he was five minutes late, I used to just really crack it because, you know, if he said he was going to be at home at six-thirty, he should have been home at six-thirty to take her from me

and help with the dinner and that sort of thing. And he thought I was going off the deep end.

Georgia Trembath recounted how her husband had started using drugs again and she noticed how a large sum of money came out of their bank account whenever they visited certain friends. Initially, he accused her of spending too much money but when she confronted him with spending the money on drugs he told her 'Oh, you're suffering from postnatal depression'. She retorted:

'Well, bullshit, I know what I'm suffering from and that's not it'.

Angelina Razos A lot of it is lack of self confidence ... I think the woman could be feeling down slightly — which won't actually be postnatal depression — and somebody'll turn round and say 'snap out of it, don't be so stupid'; just being treated with contempt, putting you down; your self-being gets stamped into the ground and trod on real hard, and I think that probably could be a big start of it, because I mean the assistance for mums just isn't there, that is needed. I mean you can't ring somewhere at ten o'clock at night when you're feeling really rank, and you can't wake your husband 'cos he needs his sleep to go — 'bloody kids are up all through the night and then you've gotta get me up as well'.

The inability of some men to listen empathically to their depressed partners or even to know what spending a day with a fractious infant was like and to react with anger or ultimatums to women's accounts of what they were experiencing, significantly deepened the distress. Ann Marie Burke's partner told her: 'Don't complain'. And she said,

I'm not complaining, I'm just saying what happened today, what I had to go through. You think 'cos I'm home that I can rest. I was feeding every two to three hours, I'd be breastfeeding, so I never got a big break in that time. You might sit down and cook your lunch and have your lunch and you just get your dishes done and he's up again and he wouldn't sleep very often. So you couldn't ... he didn't have a sleep pattern, so you couldn't plan your day.

Deborah Tannen suggests that much of the distress generated in women by their partners' response to their emotional states is due to differences between men and women in the style of their verbal communication, its goals and the values that inform it. Women, Tannen writes, are more likely to engage in 'rapport talk' in which they want to attain intimacy through connection with others and for whom 'conversations are negotiations for closeness in which people try to seek and give confirmation and support, and to reach consensus'.[6]

Men, however, are more likely to engage in 'report talk' — to deliver a report, complete with 'facts' and a 'solution' to the problem at hand. Tannen writes that this style of communication is fuelled emotionally by a desire to maintain a sense of independence and defend one's position in a hierarchy. She goes on to suggest that these differences begin in early childhood, when research on how boys talk and play has found they often give orders and try to get others to follow them in order to achieve and maintain status in a hierarchical world.[7]

When women are troubled emotionally they are likely to feel comfortable in and gain comfort from talking about how they feel. An important part of such conversations is to confirm the authenticity and legitimacy of their feelings through interaction with their listener, to receive support and to feel properly 'heard'. They are unlikely to build the rapport they wish with male partners who are concerned with maintaining a dominant position by showing that they know more, who foreclose on the conversation by presenting immediate solutions or answers, who issue ultimatums and who interrupt or challenge what is said rather than listen in an accepting way. Listening may be particularly difficult for men who equate talking with the giving of information and the occupation of a higher status role, and perceive listening, albeit unconsciously, as the function of one in a lower status or subordinate position. Men may feel uncomfortable in the role of listener because this is a role women have typically occupied and it may be experienced as 'feminine', passive and unmanly. Conversely, being told what to do by a woman who in this way is doing 'report' talking like a man by delivering orders, can be seen as threatening and evoke feelings of hostility.[8]

A woman who sets out to establish rapport and intimacy by expressing her feelings, but finds her partner won't or can't listen to what she is saying without interrupting, telling her what to do or judging her, may decide there is not much point in attempting to communicate with him. What then happens is a process of self-censoring in which the woman decides to be silent about what she is experiencing because she knows how her partner is likely to respond.

Freda Holding He didn't know that I was keeping all this — like he knew I was upset, but I thought I was keeping such a big burden and not saying anything about it. Like if I said anything he probably wouldn't listen, so I wouldn't say anything.

The response of professional care-providers could also play a big part in a woman deciding to stay silent about her depressed feelings. Dawn Harrison told her doctor she was feeling 'not right' about things when she went for her postnatal check-up six weeks after the birth.

> He then asked me if I was abusing my children. And I said no, and he said 'Don't worry'. Which I just could not believe. So after that of course I just didn't mention it to many people. Then I found I was getting very depressed all the time. I was isolating myself from my friends, my family, I was staying home a lot, crying a lot. Just getting totally frustrated.

The issues of practical support by partners, and partners' involvement in household work and the care of children are taken up in Chapter 11.

NEGATIVE LIFE EVENTS AND EXPERIENCES

It came as little surprise to find that women who were depressed eight months following the birth of their infant were more likely, at the follow-up interview, to report a greater number of negative events in their lives since the birth than those who had not been depressed at this time. Of greater note, because it is contrary to the view that depression causes both current and past events to be perceived in the same distorted, depressing way, was the finding that women in our study did not see all aspects of their lives in a pervasively negative light. We found they reported just as many positive life events occurring in the two years since the birth as women who had not been depressed.

The kind of negative life events and experiences reported by women who had been depressed ranged across the whole gamut of such things covered in the LEQ. Women had experienced problems in their relationships, including separation and divorce; the stress and disruption of moving house; legal and financial difficulties associated with the recession, unemployment or the failure of a business; problems in parenting; illness or sometimes even death of significant people in their lives; their own ill health, and upsetting disagreements with family or friends. Women who were depressed were particularly likely to have experienced negative events in the areas of health, love and marriage, parenting, family and in the personal/social sphere where their scores were significantly higher than those of women in the control group.

Some health events that bear crucially on the emotional well-being of women as mothers in the year after the birth, such as breastfeeding and weaning, prolonged bleeding or episiotomy pain and associated sexual difficulties, are not included in the health section of the LEQ. The only items relating to women in this measure, even after its modification to make it more relevant to women, are 'pregnancy, miscarriage and abortion, menopause and major difficulties with birth control'.

It was not these health events that were important for Nina Cooper's feelings of depression eight months after her baby was born, but the multiple and intermeshing effects of trying to give up breastfeeding.

> I had a lot of trouble getting rid of my milk at that stage; I couldn't get rid of it, it just kept coming and coming, and I didn't want to, I didn't want to breastfeed any more 'cos it was coming up the hot weather, and that was really depressing me. I was sick 'cos I was filling up so much. The doctor couldn't get rid of it that I went to, but finally I went to another one who got rid of it. So that's basically why I wasn't very happy at that stage.

She recalled how her decision to give up breastfeeding set in train multiple, unforeseen negative consequences which affected her physical and mental health.

> I was pretty tired; 'cos that was also when she was waking up a lot in the middle of the night and we were trying to — she'd fallen into a bad habit of falling to sleep with the bottle and then she would have this habit of waking up and expecting the bottle to be there still and we had to get her out of that routine. I went to the paediatrician and we had to go through controlled crying technique and giving her a substitute for the bottle — like a teddy bear or something like that and that took ages — you'd still be waking two or three times of a night. So I was pretty worn out then too.

Despite the lack of relevant items on the LEQ concerning the specific difficulties of early motherhood we found that women who had been depressed eight months following the birth of their baby had significantly higher scores regarding the impact of negative health events than women who had not been depressed at this time. This suggests that whatever influences the physical well-being of new mothers has an indirect but critical effect on their emotional well-being. So far, the relationship of physical health to emotional well-being following birth has been under-researched. This oversight probably derives from the bias in older psychological research, which places primacy on the impact of the mind on the body — the psychosomatic model. The privileging of the psychosomatic model within research has meant that the possibility that the reverse might be true — the body exerting a significant effect on the mind — has been largely overlooked.

It became apparent that the negative events women experienced often came in clusters. Adverse psychological effects seemed to be partly a function of the cumulative physical and emotional exhaustion of attempting to cope with too many things at once. Women would comment on coping with a difficult situation for a while or being able to cope with a few stressful events, but then becoming worn down by the chronic nature of the stress or overwhelmed by the sheer number of things that were going wrong.

Good social and emotional support, especially from their partner, could ameliorate the difficulty of the negative events and experiences women faced, and make the difference between feeling that stress could be coped with and feeling emotionally overwhelmed.

Kaylene Shaw recounted having a large number of stressful things occurring in her life at the time of the eight month survey, when she scored as depressed on the EPDS, but thought that a small amount of practical and emotional support from her husband would have made all the difference. She was the mother of five children and lived on a farm where there was always a lot for her to do, in addition to her already heavy workload as a mother. She saw herself as having to respond to her husband's need for assistance, but felt she had little control or autonomy over how she spent her time. She could trace the course of her depressed feelings according to the demands of her workload as well as more obviously emotional triggers.

> If it's cropping or if it's harvest, then it's usually a pretty low time because so much is expected of you and instead of one body, you need two bodies to be helping out on the farm, sometimes three ... the other children are at school, there might be something on at the school that they'd really like you to come to, but you can't. So that's pretty depressing, not being able to do things.

For Kaylene, too, physical health factors were extremely salient in determining her emotional well-being. After the birth of her last child, she had been hospitalised at a place some 80 kilometres away from where she lived, making it difficult for her husband to visit her.

> Every now and then you mightn't feel real crisp and it's easy to get depressed when you're not feeling ... And also after that I had my appendix out, I had the kidney infection and after that I had a miscarriage — in the January — and then in the July I was pregnant again, and everything was fine, and by the October it died — I don't know why — and that was another time, you know? And it was a worry, too, because you know, 'God, six kids, how are we gonna cope, we've got three bedrooms and five kids now'.

As well as her physical workload at home and on the farm, and her poor health, Kaylene's cluster of negative life experiences included a strong sense of personal and social isolation, little autonomy and no time out, as well as a lack of emotional and practical support.

Conversely, women whose partners were able to understand the difference their support could make in buffering the stresses of mothering, told us how much this helped in lifting their sense of despondency. For Freda Holding who was so depressed she had to be hospitalised, having a more emotionally responsive partner following this episode made an enormous difference to her well-being.

> That's how he's changed, and he's helping me a lot more — even before he helped me, but I think if this hadn't happened — which I don't want to happen again — but if this hadn't happened, well I don't think he would have woken up to himself.

TODDLER TEMPERAMENT

The final factor to make a significant contribution to the likelihood of a woman experiencing depression was the temperament of her infant. While women who had been depressed at the time of the postal survey were just as likely to have a child categorised as 'easy' on the TTS (40 per cent) as those in the control group (40 per cent), they were somewhat more likely to have a child rated as having a 'difficult' temperament (24 per cent versus 9 per cent) though this difference just failed to reach statistical significance. Just over 24 per cent of the toddlers of women who were depressed were classified as having a 'difficult' temperament and this is almost double the rate reported as the Australian population norm for the TTS (13 per cent).[9]

Despite the fact that the TTS was designed to give an objective rating of a child's behaviour there has been considerable controversy over the extent to which this is possible.[10] In particular, it has been asked how far the responses of mothers to questionnaires on the temperament of infants or children reflect a biological or constitutional predisposition of the child and how far they reflect parental characteristics and expectations.

The issue for our study was whether mothers who are depressed rate their toddlers as having a 'difficult' temperament because they are depressed or whether the rating is an objective estimate of the child's behaviour unmediated and unaffected by a mother's emotional state. That is, does the rating of temperament by mothers who are depressed say more about them than it does about the behavioural style of their children? In fact the fifteen mothers whose toddlers had a 'difficult' rating did not necessarily perceive them in that way: six of them were described by their mothers during the home interview as 'easier than expected' or 'pretty much as expected'.

As we had no other assessment of the children's behaviour in this study we are not in a position to compare mothers' ratings with those of other people and ascertain whether differences exist and, if so, in what form. However, it seems likely from previous research on infant temperament that mothers' rating of temperament (like fathers') have both objective and subjective determinants.[11] Nevertheless, the comments women made during the interviews about how their infants' behaviour and temperament affected their emotional well-being left us in no doubt that women themselves felt having a child with a difficult temperament could make the difference between coping pleasurably and coping miserably with motherhood.

Rosemary McLean was convinced that the difficulty of her son's temperament was paramount in the development of her depressed feelings.

> His temperament had a lot to do with it, yeah. When he was awake he was screaming, when he wasn't awake he was — his sleep times and feed times didn't coincide, and you were stuck — it was the isolation and the continual crying, just wore you down.

The crying, unsoothable baby can arouse powerful feelings of anxiety, stress, failure and depression in its mother.

> *Jacinta Campbell*   It just seemed to be getting on top of me, that this baby was just crying non stop — an hour's sleep if I was lucky, but two hours at the most — and going down to 7 stone 8lbs doesn't do you the world of good, and of course you start thinking all these whacko things: why did I have the child?'

Sometimes mothers felt they were unequally matched temperamentally with infants who had more energy, less need for uninterrupted sleep, and greater determination than they did.

Faith Thompson felt she was engaged in this kind of unequal relationship with her child who she saw as 'very strong willed'. Faith believed that her ability to cope with her daughter could be described as 'sometimes in very small doses'. She freely acknowledged 'it gets very frustrating for me' and laughingly said that one of the things she liked best about looking after her daughter was her sleep time.

Antisocial, aggressive or embarrassing behaviour by the child was another aspect of temperament that distressed mothers, who often felt uncertain how to respond because they did not want to reciprocate with similar behaviour themselves, such as hitting a child who was hitting smaller children, but could not find any workable alternative.

Sometimes it was not until the issue of how the child's temperament might relate to the mother's depression that the difficultness of temperament was considered by mothers as a possible cause.

> *Cassandra Lightfoot* That's an interesting question. I suppose it must have. You tend not to think like that. You tend to think that it was all things you're doing. I'd say it must have, but I've never really thought about it in terms of that.

This response suggests the potency of the discourse on motherhood, which attributes all difficulties to the personality and psychological functioning of the mother.

As with the other factors that contribute to a woman becoming depressed after she has become a mother, the emotional impact of having a difficult toddler is lessened if the woman's partner has an empathic and preferably first-hand experience of what she is going through.

> *Rhonda* *And did your husband react at that time — did he notice or comment on how you were or you felt?*
> Oh he was nearly as bad as I was, and then of course he wasn't getting — he wasn't sleeping either. I think he was on the raw edge emotionally — we both were — and I think our time in [a mother and baby] hospital really confused him, but in a way he let me go there because he knew I was at the end of my rope physically and there wasn't support coming — I think if there'd been support coming from elsewhere we wouldn't have found ourselves in that situation.

> *Elena Lang* I know since he's had her that it's — when I did start work and he had her for the afternoon, he said he never realised how difficult it was, looking after a child. I said, 'well it's easier now than it used to be'. Maybe he's understood a little bit more.

PUTTING IT ALL TOGETHER

The final step in the analysis of the standardised questionnaires employed a statistical technique called discriminant function analysis. The purpose of this was to discover which factors best discriminated between mothers who were depressed and those who were not, and to see what contribution the social factors we had investigated with standard measures made to depression. We found it was possible to correctly classify 85 per cent of all the women in our study as to whether their EPDS scores would be less than nine, or nine and over, two years after having a baby, on the basis of the following factors: a high score (above twelve) on the EPDS at eight months, high scores on the EMQ, a high total number of life events on the LEQ, and a low level of satisfaction with the support available from other people. The prediction and classification was almost equally good when the original EPDS score was omitted from the analysis. Birth events, summarised in terms of the obstetric intervention score (see Appendix 3), made no additional contribution to explaining depression in this analysis two years after birth. This was in contrast to depression eight months after birth (see Chapter 6). The analysis confirmed the importance of the social context of the mother in looking at depression.

'SO MANY THINGS HAPPEN AT THE SAME TIME'

This chapter has shown how several different factors can contribute to the experience of depression. One of the problems with looking at things like negative life events, lack of social support or difficult toddler temperament separately is that this separation is largely artificial. Unfortunately, as one of the mothers in this study remarked, 'so many things happen at the same time'. Life, unlike the scientific tradition that informs research practice and breaks problems down into small, separate, manageable bits, is indivisible.

In reality, women cannot neatly compartmentalise difficult aspects of their lives as mothers and set them aside for coping with one by one in an orderly sequence. On one level, it is clear that each of the separate parts that make up motherhood contribute to the whole emotional flavour of the experience, as the quotes from women we interviewed about the support of their partner or the temperament of their infant, show. What this approach cannot provide is a holistic, integrated understanding of how each part can be differently weighted within the psychic economy of an individual woman. It is for this reason that we have included longer extracts from the 'stories' of three different mothers in Chapter 12.

Jill Astbury, Rhonda Small, Judith Lumley, Stephanie Brown

ELEVEN

Balancing Acts: Work and Family

'A woman's work is never done' is a phrase embedded in our language and our cultural consciousness. In spite of this, motherhood is rarely seen in terms of the work involved. Becoming a mother is so often represented as a 'taken for granted' part of being a woman that the work women do in the name of motherhood, their 'labours of love' — child rearing and domestic work — remain invisible. There are some major problems with this that the women in our study were grappling with on a daily basis, not least of which was that caring for children was much harder than most women would ever have imagined prior to starting their own families. Yet once they did have children, the work of motherhood was very real for women. It took up practically all their waking hours — if they were not also employed outside the home — and often some of their sleeping hours as well, yet it so often went unacknowledged by their partners or anybody else. Often, women's work at home — and many women readers are likely to identify with this — was only noticed when it did not get done.

In this chapter we are interested in all the work that mothers and fathers do and how work in its different forms, namely paid work outside the home and unpaid work inside the home, has an impact on women's emotional well-being in the early phases of motherhood. Today, most mothers and fathers are in fact engaged in both types of work, albeit to very different degrees.

Over the past two decades a considerable amount of social and psychological research has been undertaken on women's role in the paid workforce, the division of domestic labour between men and women, and changing roles within the family. There have been numerous studies of motherhood with a particular focus on the combination of motherhood and employment for women. These have such telling titles as: 'Balancing Acts', 'Double Identity', 'Managing Mothers' and 'Double Shift'.[1] There has also been an upsurge of writing in the 1980s about the 'new fatherhood'.[2]

What this tells us about the lives of mothers and fathers is that in the 1990s, as in the 1970s, most women in Australia, and elsewhere in the western industrialised world, continue to do most of the domestic labour and most of the caring and rearing of children. Furthermore, although more women than ever before now combine these jobs with paid work,[3] there is little evidence to date that men's participation in household tasks and child care has increased to an equivalent extent as their partners have moved into paid employment.[4] Few men spend much time caring for their children: most are likely to be working long hours outside the home precisely when their children are very young.[5] There is little evidence yet of a new cultural norm that men should spend less time at work and more time working at home, thereby sharing with women the burdens and rewards of combining employment with domestic labour and the care of children.

To date, the mental-health consequences of different patterns of work within the family have been the subject of only limited research. Research on the 'double shift' worked by many women, outside and inside the home, concludes that despite the extra burdens this imposes, which may have some effects on physical health,[6] mothers who are also employed tend to fare better in terms of mental health than mothers who work solely at home.[7] On the other hand, men's participation in domestic labour and child rearing, and the effects of different rates of participation on women's emotional well-being, has received little attention. Only two small studies of postnatal depression in mothers have considered this question, the findings indicating that mothers who were depressed received less help from partners in relation to housework and child care than mothers not depressed.[8]

We were interested in exploring the consequences of current patterns of work within the family on the emotional well-being of women. What are the consequences of a partner's absence from home for long periods on most days of the week for women's experience of mothering new babies? Does the level of a father's participation in child caring and household duties have any bearing on a mother's emotional well-being in the early years of motherhood? And for mothers of young children, what effect does going 'out' to work (or not doing so) have on their emotional well-being and on their experience of motherhood? Another question we asked was how women thought their partners had coped with the changes brought about by having children, a question that so often prompted the comment, 'his life hasn't really changed that much', that we post-coded all the interview transcripts to ascertain the number of times in which this was a theme in women's responses. We also asked whether women had done any paid work since the birth of their two-year-old and, if so, how it affected their experience of motherhood.

Exploring these issues with women during the interviews was fascinating. There were repeated themes in the answers to these questions, as well as much diversity. There was also a great deal of laughter and rolling of eyes: 'he wouldn't know where the vacuum cleaner was kept!' Yet, at the same time, women empathised with the demands of their partner's breadwinning role: 'He's been working all day and he's tired when he gets home, so I can't expect much.'

THE MALE BREADWINNER: WORK, WORK, WORK

Only four women in the study were not living with a partner. Just over 70 per cent of all the women's partners were out of the house engaged in paid work for more than ten hours each day or were working more than five days a week at the time of our interview. This is consistent with other findings in Australia and overseas.[9] Men worked long hours during the week and some worked or studied at night or on weekends. Others travelled for work and were away for days at a time on a regular basis. In the extreme, some men were hardly ever home and women often found coping in these circumstances very trying.

> *Liza Rogers* With his work, we can't have a normal life. Everything centres around his job sort of thing. You can't go out late, never have holidays. We have weekends here and there, that's about it. Just not able to function as a family with normal family pleasure activities, with things to do together. I don't like coping on my own, with three kids it's too much.

There were no differences between the case and control groups in whether partners were away from home for more or less than ten hours a day or worked more than five days a week. What turned out to be significant here was how fathers contributed when they were at home: it was this that had a major impact on women's emotional well-being. We return to this shortly when considering partners' involvement in child care and domestic labour.

Men who worked longer hours were, nevertheless, less likely to be judged by their partners as having coped very well with the changes brought about by having children, than the men who were away from home less (38 per cent versus 63 per cent), and their lives were more often seen as not having changed appreciably since they had children (43 per cent versus 5 per cent).

Some women at first commented that their partners had coped better than they had, but then acknowledged that in a sense this was precisely because their partners, unlike themselves, had not been required to deal with major changes to their own lives.

> *Christine Mathews* He's coped all right. I think he's probably coped better than I have, but then again, he hasn't had to give up any sport or what he did. But I had to give up a job and sport and stay home.

Eliza Ross He's coped extremely well. Better than me I think. But I mean it's easy to say that. I'm here for every day of it. I'm sure if Peter was home with them all day and I walked in the door from work, I'd be fresh and bubble too, so ... (laughs)

Employment outside the home took up an enormous part of men's lives, and men's role as breadwinners was rarely questioned. Even the women whose partners were home full time often saw this as temporary or as a product of circumstances, such as being retrenched, or staying home while building their house.

DOMESTIC LABOUR AND THE CARE OF CHILDREN: 'EVEN WHEN YOU GO TO BED YOUR WORK ISN'T DONE'

Women in our sample did most of the domestic labour and most of the caring for children. How did women experience this work and what effect did it have on their emotional well-being?

One of the things that domestic labour and child care have in common is their never-ending nature: the task is literally never done. No wonder, then, that the commonest responses women had about their lives as mothers related to the continuous nature of the demands made on them. Caring for children was seen by two-thirds of women as more difficult than had been expected. This related to the 24-hour nature of the demands children made on them, as well as the need to manage domestic duties.

Angelina Razos I don't think you appreciate how demanding they can be till you've got them. That's the biggest problem, you don't — you know, like you're told you bring home little babies and they sleep and they're only awake for two hours during the whole day: 'Terrific, I'll get heaps done, that'll be great. I'll sit here and watch the soapies and ... ' You don't realise you're up every three or four hours feeding them or something or other though. And it takes them two hours to go back to sleep again 'cos they're screaming ... You're still sitting there at four o'clock in the afternoon in your bloody dressing gown. You haven't had lunch or breakfast and you've gotta cook dinner for your husband — ha! — that's the hard part. [case group]

Christine Mathews The fact that it's 24 hours a day and you just don't get a break from it. I think I had this idea that a child would be able to sit down and amuse itself for some length of time, and they just don't ... I don't think it ever occurred to me that you don't get to go to the toilet, on your own, for 5 years (laughs), those sorts of things. I wasn't expecting anything like that! [control group]

The exhaustion that results from never having a break, something largely unexpected, was also commonly mentioned.

Ursula Redman I didn't expect to be tired all the time, didn't expect that at all. And I'm really a different person because of it. So I guess I didn't expect to be a different personality. It's taken me a long time to cope with that, and think that I am normal sometimes. Some day I will be normal — when I start sleeping, getting eight hours sleep every night. Also, that was — definitely I didn't expect that — so in that respect I didn't think it would be as hard as it was. [control group, but had experienced depression]

Katrina Peterson For the first eight months we were just SO tired. At one stage we were throwing things at each other and we've never done that before, since or at any other time. We were wondering what was wrong with us (laughs)! [case group]

It was not that caring for children did not fulfil many of the positive expectations women had. There were very few women indeed who did not also speak about the positive aspects, the fun and joy of having children.

Katrina Peterson Suddenly you're faced with this enormous task, and it is an enormous task — it's constant every day. I mean there's the really good sides of it, being attached to children in ways that you haven't been attached to other people and all the rest of it, and it's really fun, but there's also just the constancy ... [case group]

May Sainsbury I don't think you can ever understand quite the difference it's gonna make to your life, quite how the demands just never cease. And I don't think you can really appreciate what joy it brings to your life either, until you've actually experienced it. And how it alters your fundamental focuses in life, all your basic priorities. [control group]

But as many women commented, it is the *work* involved that was both unexpectedly demanding and quite often tedious. This side of motherhood had rarely featured in the images women had of caring for children and many drew attention to the difficulty, almost the impossibility, of balancing the need to get housework done with the needs of children. This conflict came up also in relation to ideas of the 'good' mother (see Chapter 7).

Bronwyn Meier You can't get things done. Like this morning doing the dishes, about three times I got interrupted doing the dishes. Her coming up and stuff like that. So it's the interruptions that get me. I can't get anything done. And stuff like vacuuming, I don't even try to vacuum when she's around, cause she just tries to grab the vacuum and she wants to do it and all that sort of stuff. So you sort of wait until whenever, and then you wait and you wait and it doesn't get done. [control group]

Kaylene Shaw Now I'd say is probably a more hectic time because they're [two-year-old twins] wanting to do more, and you've gotta hold them back to a certain extent because they're — you've gotta do your housework, still gotta tidy. You've still got three other children to think about. And they get dirty every day (laughs). You know, it's harder now to go shopping, it's just chaos. [case group]

Did having realistic expectations about what it would be like to care for children protect women from becoming depressed? In fact we found no significant differences when we compared women in the two groups with regard to how their expectations about caring for children matched up with their experiences. Women in the case group were no more likely to feel that caring for children was harder then they had expected — this was expressed by two-thirds of women in both groups. Nor was there any difference between the two groups in relation to the amount of knowledge they felt they had about child rearing before having their own children. The number of women who felt they had known nothing or very little about caring for children was very similar in the case and control groups (51 per cent and 53 per cent).

What did distinguish the two groups, however, was a difference in how the reality of motherhood matched up with their expectations. Women in the control group were more likely than women in the case group to have found motherhood overall to be easier or better than they had expected. This could mean that they had much lower or less positive expectations than women in the case group, or it could mean that their experiences of being mothers had actually been easier than those of women in the case group. The previous three chapters have confirmed that there were indeed differences in the experiences of the two groups.

THE DIVISION OF LABOUR
We included in our home interview a series of questions about how often a range of household and child-care tasks were done by the woman herself and by her partner in the week prior to the interview. Had we asked the partners of women in our sample to answer the questions about the household and child-care tasks they perform, it is of course possible that we would have received different answers. Although there is some evidence of differences in perceptions between men and women about what men do, major differences have not been reported. In one study, for example, men said that they got up at night to their children somewhat more often than their wives reported that they did.[10] This was the only difference found for a range of child-care activities reported by both husbands and wives. In order to minimise any such possible differences in perceptions we asked women to report on how often

their partners performed these tasks in the week prior to the interview, rather than how often on average they performed them, a strategy also employed by Ann Oakley in her pioneering study of housework in the early 1970s.[11]

We went on to ask women whether they were happy with their partners' contributions in these areas, how involved they saw their partners as being in parenting generally, and how satisfied they were with their partners' level of involvement. Our scale for scoring participation in tasks was quite generous as far as rating men's participation was concerned: the maximum score of four on each item could be obtained by doing a task once or more every day. This meant that a man who worked full time away from home, but changed one nappy a day would receive the same maximum score for that item as a woman working at home full time who changed six a day.

Table 11.1 Domestic labour scores

	Average score for men	Average score for women
Woman at home full time	9.28	33.34
Woman employed part time	10.16	32.34
Woman employed full time	18.44	26.00

Table 11.2 Child-caring scores

	Average score for men	Average score for women
Woman at home full time	21.63	41.45
Woman employed part time	23.03	41.56
Woman employed full time	29.22	36.46

Overall, women did more than their partners in the areas of child care and domestic labour. Out of a possible total of 48, women's average score for household tasks was 32.1 and men's 10.6. For child care, women averaged 40.8 and men 22.9. The minority of women employed full time did significantly less than their counterparts at home full time. Women employed part time continued to score as highly as women at home full time. Significantly, the partners of women employed part time were not contributing any more on the home-front than partners of women at home full time.

However, in the nine two-parent families where women were employed full time, partners were doing significantly more domestic labour and child caring than partners of women at home full time (see tables 11.1 and 11.2).

In only four out of 90 families were fathers at home full time and even in these cases, their female partners did a considerable amount of child caring and housework on top of paid employment. In two other families, domestic labour and child caring were shared and both partners worked part time. Partners of women in the control group did more domestic labour (mean score: 11.93 versus 9.12, t=2.00, p=0.05) and more child caring (mean score: 25.67 versus 20.07, t=2.61, p=0.01) than partners of women in the case group.

Women's emotional well-being at follow-up was also related to their partners' contributions in both these areas. Women who felt better emotionally had partners who did more at home. Interestingly, when we divided women's partners into two groups on the basis of their scores on the social support scale using the median score as a cut-off point, it was also the partners judged by women as more emotionally supportive who were doing more domestic labour (mean score: 12.15 versus 9.00, t=2.29, p=0.02) and child care (mean score: 26.70 versus 19.38, t=3.50, p= 0.001).

Women in the case group were more likely than women in the control group to express dissatisfaction with their partners' contributions to both domestic labour and child caring and to say they wanted more help from their partners in both these areas. As discussed above, this association has received little formal attention to date.

Men's scores on child caring and household tasks were highly correlated (r=0.69): men who contributed to child caring were also likely to contribute in relation to domestic labour. This finding is somewhat different to that of Ann Oakley's study of housework in the 1970s, in which men's involvement with children proved to be no indicator of their involvement in domestic labour.[12] It may be that the men who now embrace a notion of more active fatherhood also have begun to accept a greater role in the performance of domestic labour. Partners of women with college or university education were also likely to contribute more, in line with findings of other recent studies in this area.[13] We found no association of participation with family income.

The belief that if a woman is at home full time looking after children, then her job is also seen as encompassing most, if not all, the domestic labour was rarely questioned by women. Most women at home full time had low expectations of their partner's contributions to domestic labour, largely because of the perceived demands of their breadwinning role.

> *Helen Bakoula* I suppose I wouldn't really expect him to do the cooking and make beds and stuff if I'm home. [case group]
>
> *Arlene Bell* I understand that he is the breadwinner, and he works very long hours, and is away from the house, so therefore he's not really in a position to do the housework. By the time he gets home, he's exhausted. He's done his bit for the day, so ... [control group]

Involvement in child care by partners was also seen to be precluded by partners' employment commitments.

> He's not around when these things [with the children] need to be done ... I mean it's the situation he's in. If he's working all day he can't be home with the children. [case group]
>
> It's difficult for husbands when they're at work all day. It's six o'clock — rush, bath, tea, listen to the reading and go to bed, so ... I mean he does as much as what he can, within that time limit ... [control group]

Expressed dissatisfaction with their partners' contributions to domestic labour and child caring appeared to stem not from any sense that these tasks should be shared and were not, but rather from a sense that when their partners *were* home they didn't pitch in and help.

> *Arlene Bell* Weekends I find that he just sits down and watches the cricket all weekend, and I just keep working seven days a week ... [control group]
>
> *Annette Flynn* On Saturdays he'll tend to lie in and read the paper rather than play with the children, and I get quite cranky about that. [control group, but had experienced depression]

A number of women had clearly resigned themselves to the reality of a non-contributing partner. Asked about whether she was happy with her partner's contributions to domestic labour, one woman who had been depressed said:

> Not really happy with it, but I wouldn't really expect him to do it. I've sort of accepted that he doesn't do it, so I suppose I am happy in that sense. It wasn't as if he's suddenly changed, and he used to do it and he doesn't. I mean he never has, so ... I've accepted that I suppose.
> *Stephanie* *Would you like more assistance?*
> Well I *would* like more assistance, yes.
> *Stephanie* *You can't see it happening?*
> No, that's right (laughs).

Although such expressions of resignation and discontent occurred in both the case and control groups, they were noticeably more frequent among women in the case group. This is to be expected given that there were indeed significant differences between the two groups in terms of men's contributions both to domestic labour and child caring, and significant differences in women's satisfaction with their partners' contributions. However, although partners of women in the control group were doing more at home, they were not doing a huge amount more. It may be that the differences had been greater earlier on. Certainly some women who had been depressed said that their partners were helping more by the time we interviewed them and that this had made a difference to how they were feeling. However, it would also appear that it was not just what partners did at home, but their readiness to be involved and their acknowledgment that the task of caring for children was important, often difficult and, perhaps most importantly, worthy of what little time they did have left over at night and on weekends.

Women in the control group frequently expressed considerable gratitude for the support they did receive from their partners and made it clear that this support made life happier for them. Women whose partners acknowledged the demands of their role at home, who offered assistance when they returned from work, or even just accepted that sometimes the house was not tidy or their dinner not cooked were the women who seemed to have fared better emotionally.

> *Frances Heringslake* I know that if I'm in a real pickle Paul will come in, he won't expect it to be immaculate when he gets home. He doesn't come in expecting to be waited on or anything like that. And I suppose, I'm a nurse, and I worked shift work when we were first married, so that's made it easier. I haven't been here every evening so Paul has had to get meals himself ... So if I'm in a bit of a pickle he'll start getting the meal or start tidying up, or whatever's appropriate at the time. So we don't feel pressurised during the day that it's all tidy and neat and meals are ready to go. [control group]

> *Wendy Elliott* He more or less looks after the kids for me [when he gets home from work], or he'll bath them. He baths the kids and does things like that, and he takes them outside and gets them away from me for a while. [control group]

The phrase 'looks after the kids *for me*' encapsulates a set of deep-seated beliefs and expectations about responsibilities for children.

Even when one partner was hardly ever home because of the demands of his job, the fact that he recognised his wife's need for a break when he *was* at home, was very important to her and to her satisfaction with his contribution.

> *Henrietta Woodhouse* I mean obviously I do 90 per cent of it, but if he's around, he says: 'Look, why don't I — I'll put them to bed, you sit and watch this' or 'Finish your book'. [control group]

Women in the case group, however, rather than commenting on help freely given by partners were much more likely to say that their partners never seemed to notice when things needed doing, or that they would help, but only when the women asked. This was often a source of disappointment and dissatisfaction.

> *Melissa Dean* He does help if I ask him, but he just doesn't see anything. If I tell him, he'll say: 'alright, that's all you have to do is tell me' but I wish I didn't have to tell him, yeah. [case group]

A number of women in the case group commented on what might be termed 'avoidance behaviour' by their partners; a tendency to cope with all the changes brought about by having children around by absenting themselves from the scene. They either became completely engrossed in work or sport, found it hard to spend even small amounts of time with the children and avoided doing so, or suddenly spent all their time at home in the garden!

> *Margit Gunn* I think he probably struggles [to cope] ... I think he's — he's very career conscious. I think he'd just love to spend all his time work-wise, and the children sort of distract him from his work, or I push him to be home. [case group]

> [Another woman] He always finds other things to do to get out, and they're usually things where [their son] can't be involved in them — like going and collecting firewood, and things like that. Which are things that have to be done, but I've never seen so much wood in the shed (laughs) — and I've never seen the garden look so good, and those sorts of things. So yes, there's a bit of avoidance there ... but whether he's avoiding me or [the son] or the both of us every now and again, I'm not sure! (laughs) [case group]

> *Faith Thompson* Sometimes he acts like a father, but most of the time he's just like a friend. 'Cos with umpiring, he's got training nearly every night of the week, plus also Saturdays he's umpiring, and Sundays nine times out of ten he's umpiring as well. So on average, he'll see her probably on a Monday for about an hour, and on a Wednesday for about an hour or two, and on Friday, and that's about it. [case group: partner also works more than five days a week]

For these women in particular the task of rearing children was often a very lonely one.

The importance of partners' support for women's emotional well-being was also highlighted by the sixteen women who had been depressed, but who felt that their partners' becoming more supportive over time was one of the things that contributed to their recovery. These women spoke about how their husbands had initially failed to understand how juggling the demands of a young baby (and often other children), doing housework, feeling isolated and alone could all combine to make them feel trapped and miserable. Sometimes, being responsible for caring for the child himself had helped to bring about a change in the partner's attitude.

> *Amanda Joseph* I don't think he really understood what I was going through ... So one of the best things was for me to go back to work and he had her for 24 hours — well not, you know, 8 hours — and he enjoys it. He says that's the best time because I'm not there and he learnt to feed her ... I mean that's been good for him, good for me and good for her. [case group]

Frequently, it seemed that men found it easier to be involved with children as they got a bit older.

> Earlier on he found it very hard — well like when she was first born, in the first few months, he was very frightened of holding her — like a lot of men are — and I felt that then he could have helped me a lot more than what he did. But as time's gone on and he's seen her get older and all the rest of it, he's helped more and, so it's gotten better. [case group]

As other studies in this area have found[14] men tend to be more involved in the enjoyable aspects of caring for children (playing, cuddling, going on outings), than those which require more work (changing nappies, getting up at night). In the 76 families who had children who woke at night in the week prior to the interview, 54 per cent of the men had not been up to children during the night at all. Almost one-third of men (30 per cent) whose children were still in nappies had not changed a single wet nappy, and one-third had not changed a dirty nappy in the week before the interview. There were nineteen men who had not spent any time in the past week alone with their children and over half of the men (55 per cent) had not been alone with their children on more than one occasion.

Partners of women in the control group were more likely to have got up at night to children in the week prior to the interview (57 per cent versus 29 per cent), though there was no difference in the amount of child waking between the two groups. Control partners were less likely to have had no time during the week when they were responsible for the child or children (14 per cent versus 29 per cent), though this difference did not reach statistical significance. These two areas are probably quite important in relation to mothers' emotional well-being. Sharing care at night means that women are likely to feel less tired and more able to deal with daytime demands. When partners take on looking after small children on their own, there is the potential for women to have more time for themselves. The division of labour at home can clearly be recognised as a factor contributing to, or preventing, exhaustion, distress and depression in the lives of women.

MOTHERS' EMPLOYMENT

Forty-three of the 90 women in the study were in paid work at the time of our home interviews, with eleven employed full time. Eighteen other women had been employed at some stage since the birth of their two-year-old, but were at home full time at the time of the interview; half of these had a subsequent child. Of the 47 women not employed, only six had no plans for employment; five would probably take up paid work at some time in the future; five were uncertain. Five women planned to join the workforce quite soon, nineteen women planned to work outside the home once their children had started school, and another twelve planned to return to employment, but did not have a definite time for doing so. These findings are broadly consistent with those of a recent large survey of Australian mothers:[15] 14 per cent of mothers were in the paid workforce before their child turned one, with two-thirds of mothers employed by the time their children started school.

Women who had returned to employment at the time of the follow-up were equally divided between the case group (22) and the control group (21). Resuming employment was rated by 72 per cent of the mothers who had done so as having had a positive impact on their lives, and there were no significant differences between case and control groups in this respect.

When asked how returning to employment affected how they felt as mothers the picture was more complex. Of the 59 women who had been in paid employment since the birth of their two-year-old, 29 believed it had a positive effect on how they felt as mothers, nineteen felt it had both positive and negative effects, seven reported only negative effects, and four felt it made no difference.

Employment was seen as providing a break from the constant demands of caring for children and a chance to recuperate so women had more patience and energy when they were back with their children.

Joy Freeman I enjoyed it [motherhood] far more. Yeah. Yeah, I could come home to the children and everything took on a different perspective, you know? [case group, now at home with a young baby]

Amanda Joseph Mm, I work. But I still call that time off! [case group, working one day each weekend]

This concept of paid work being a rest when compared to full time parenting was expressed most potently by one mother who job shared a full-time nursing position with her partner:

It gives you a break. Whoever needs a break goes to work (laughs). Whoever's very tired goes to work!

For one woman, however, her job as a teacher meant she felt she had somewhat less patience for her own children at the end of the day.

I guess I'm a little less tolerant. I s'pose because I have to tolerate kids all day long, you come home and it makes it difficult to tolerate your own. So I'm a little less tolerant.

Social contact and adult stimulation were also important and positive features of employment, particularly when compared to the isolation some women had experienced when at home full time.

Rosemary McLean I'm quite happy to be at work. I need the social contact. [case group, working full time]

Gayle Lazzaro It is pretty isolating being at home. I don't think you're challenged when you're around the kids. You can only do so much. You can only be happy for 70 per cent of the time, you know: painting and colouring in, all those sorts of things; making cakes and ... The rest of the time you need to yourself. You need to provide something for yourself. [control group, working full time, partner currently at home]

Amanda Joseph It's great to get dressed up, put a bit of make up on, and go and speak to adults and use your brains and things like that.

Increased confidence and self esteem were also seen as stemming from having 'a life of one's own' in work outside home.

Alice Spielvogel I find that when you're home with the children all the time, you seem to lose your self confidence, and going back to work gives it back — well it did with me. You sort of feel a bit like you've got nothing to talk to people about. When you're just home, all you know is babies and what they're doing and that sort of thing ... and going back to work seems to — having other people to talk to has helped me, anyway. [control group]

Sandra Richards I felt good being back at work, dressing up — I was in an office. It was a bit of a morale booster I think, to dress up in the morning and go out and get some money, and back here. [control group, had experienced depression, now at home with a young baby]

The value of being happier in themselves was also seen by a number of women as having positive flow-on effects for their children. As this mother expressed it:

Kristen Watson I feel like I'm doing more than just being a housewife and a mother, so I'm achieving a lot more, so therefore I feel far happier to spend time with the kids, and spend good time with the kids and that sort of thing, yeah. 'Cos I know what it was like before I did work. I don't think I did very much with the kids. I know I cooked and washed and cleaned, but I felt — I wasn't feeling good within myself, so therefore I didn't spend good time with the kids I don't think. [control group, had experienced depression, now self-employed, part time]

The positive value for children of attending child-care centres when both parents were working was also raised by one mother.

Carolyn Barker Being a mother and working doesn't clash to me at all. The children don't suffer at all. That probably does them the world of good, particularly in socialising; and they've always been so independent. [control group, mother of four children, now a full-time teacher]

Resuming employment was directly linked to improved emotional well-being by twelve of the 31 women in the case group who had been employed at some stage since the birth of their two-year-old and this was the third most commonly mentioned reason for women feeling less depressed now. This is hardly surprising given women's comments above on the benefits of employment for their self esteem, confidence and sense of identity. For many women, employment was an important and positive part of their lives, both as individuals and as mothers.

However, for just under one-third of women who had resumed employment at some stage since the birth of their two-year-old

(19/59), there was considerable ambivalence in their feelings about being employed. This was sometimes linked to missing their children, or to feeling that their children were losing out by not having their mother with them full time.

> *Nina Cooper* Oh I missed him terribly. I still did, until the last day I left; it felt so good when I finished ... I missed him, and that affected me more or less ... I mean if he was older, five, six, and he's going to school and I went out, it would have been different. [case group, had worked part time]

> *Sandra Richards* Penny was quite touchy and I hadn't put it down to me returning part time to work — and she was at Mum's — until I finished, and she improved and I realised I hadn't picked it up ... We packed up and went away in the morning, and there was never any tears about it, but when I finished I could see that she'd been trying to get more attention and I hadn't picked that up 'til I finished. [control group, but had experienced depression, now at home with a young baby]

Women often felt guilty about going out to work and about not being with their children all the time.

> *Ursula Redman* Well, I love the work. When I get there I love it. The only negative aspect of working is leaving the kids. I don't hate the work. I just worry about them: if they're alright ... You know, you think if you're doing the right thing all the time. You know, should I be there, are they suffering, are they coping? I'm sure they do. [control group]

In spite of reassuring herself that the children were okay, feelings of guilt and ambivalence persisted. This was also true for one of the women whose partner was taking major responsibility for caring for the children.

> *Katrina Peterson* I'm actually giving myself permission to enjoy my work and have space to myself, and it's just dealing with my feelings. I mean the children are fine — Peter's there for them — they're not missing out, but dealing with your own change when it's that major a role change, is quite difficult. I have to keep reminding myself that — you do get very guilty — particularly since because I'm working, there are things you have to do after work. For instance I'm going to a seminar on Saturday that I really want to go to, and I need to do that for myself for work, but it means that I don't get to see very much of them; so it's a balancing out. [case group, full-time social worker, partner at home full time]

Thus, women often spoke about enjoying being at work for themselves, but they found it difficult to reconcile this with wanting to be with their children, feeling responsible for them and feeling that they really ought to be at home all the time.

> *Melissa Dean* I think that a mother should stay at home with her children while they're young — if they can, but it is nice to get away from them. Like I didn't really think I'd enjoy going back to work — like I may only do one or two days a week. I enjoy being away from them but I do miss them. When I get home I've really missed them, so. [case group, had just begun part-time employment]

For some women the ambivalence this created meant that they returned to being home full time, foregoing the positive aspects of employment in favour of fulfilling their beliefs about what was best for their children and their own desires to spend more time with them. Of course there were also women who had not resumed employment for just this reason.

> *Bettina Copley* I think I'm happy in the role I've got, and I like to be the carer for the children, and obviously look after the house and manage things there, so I don't want to be out there in a man's job — person's job. I'm quite happy ... and I'd feel very disappointed to leave the children in a sort of permanent child care ... they miss out. [control group]

> *Josephine Cucinotta* I love staying home with the kids. Like, when I went to work with my first daughter, I sort of missed out, not too much , 'cos I only went to work for fourteen months, but it was just the time she started crawling, walking, saying her first words. I missed all that ... Where with Mark I was home to see all that, and it was really very exciting. [control group]

However, the sense of ambivalence about employment and being with the children was also felt by some women not currently employed, who recognised the benefits from previous experience.

> *Caitlin Adamson* I'm confused. I'd like to be working because I think since I've been at home I've lost a lot of confidence, but there again I'd like to be at home with the kids as well, especially when they're little; so I'm in two minds ... I worked after I had Amanda and I really enjoyed that two days working, it was great. I'd love to leave all my problems at the doorstep and then come home and pick them up eight hours later, it's really good. But I haven't been able to do that with Jack and not been willing to either, quite happy to stay at home. I daresay I'll get back there one day. [case group, Caitlin is one of three mothers whose story is included in Chapter 12]

Ambivalence also stemmed from women's sense that they were trying to juggle too much. Camilla Jackson summed up this commonly felt experience:

> When I went back to work I was a much better person for it, but now I find that work puts a lot of pressure on — I can't *be* at Michael's school mass if it occurs on that day, and I can't be everywhere at once any more — so it does put a lot more pressure on because I'm working. But I find that it's a way to get away from — sometimes it's the only time I get away from the children at all, and you do get a fresher look at things, by working. But I didn't really want to go back to work after my third child, I had enough to do at home trying to fit everything in. [case group, Camilla is another of the three mothers whose stories are included in Chapter 12]

As we have seen, one way women who worked full time coped with all the work they had to do was by doing less at home, particularly domestic labour. While their partners did contribute more to household work it seemed that a range of tasks were just not done so often in households where women were employed full time. Where women were employed part time and continued to do domestic tasks as frequently as women at home full time, it appeared that things were done by carrying out more domestic tasks on weekends or in the evenings.

Another way women coped with the different demands of home and employment was to attempt to keep the two worlds apart: a conscious switching off was employed when moving from home to job and back again. This compartmentalisation was also one of the coping strategies identified by women in a study of dual earner families in the United Kingdom.[16] It certainly appeared to make the demands more manageable for a number of women in our study.

> *Collete Prout* Well, when I return from work, I just completely change my mind, that I'm not working, I'm just at home ... that the time that I was working during today, was a break. [control group, full-time clerical worker]

> *Carolyn Barker* I'm a teacher — I love the teaching and when I get to school, I don't ever think about my children, and then when I finish, I don't ever think about the classroom. So I'm quite able to completely separate the two of them. I never worry about my kids when I'm teaching and I don't ever come home from school and worry about my teaching. And I keep all my work done — I do it all at school, the time I've spent at school. I might do a little bit, say, during the week. I won't ever do any on the weekends — I refuse — because as far as I'm concerned, I'm home with my family, and I'm not doing school work; and if they want me to do it that way, well, bad luck. [control group, full-time teacher]

It was not always possible for the two worlds to be kept separate and women then had to deal with the conflicts between home life and employment.

> *Joy Freeman* Well, realistically, I s'pose you can do both to an extent, but it's very limiting: you've got always to work around your children. I was working part time, and if Sally was sick — you know, it ends up jeopardising your position because you've gotta be away for your children, so realistically I don't think you can ... But I would like to think you were able to! I definitely am in favour of creches in the workplace. [case group, no longer employed, child often ill]

Attempts to cope with the very different experiences of employment and being at home were sometimes very unsettling, and led one woman to give up her part time job soon after resuming it, feeling that she had tried to combine motherhood and employment too soon.

> I went back to work at the start of this year, one day a week, and I lasted eight weeks and I just hated it. I couldn't seem to get the two worlds together ... I'd come home and I'd be very unsettled, and I'd find the next day I was unsettled, I didn't want to be home and I didn't want to be anywhere, so I stopped ... I think in years to come I will go back and do something, but in my own time. [control group]

For the majority of women who expressed ambivalence about combining employment and motherhood, the positive aspects of being employed seemed on balance to win out. Only three of the 43 women employed at the time of our interviews said they would rather be at home full time, and one of the mothers employed full time would have preferred to be working fewer hours outside the home. Of the ten women who said that resuming employment had a negative impact on their lives, three had stopped working by the time of our interviews. The remaining seven all felt that employment had positive as well as negative effects on how they felt as mothers. What was negative often had to do with the circumstances surrounding the resumption of employment: working full-time when part time was preferred, resuming employment earlier than was considered ideal, and in one case facing considerable opposition from friends about not being a full-time mother.

> *Ursula Redman* I've been really surprised by the response I've gotten from other mothers. I thought these days people would be pretty used to the idea of women working, but it's been a really negative response ... and just because you work everyone thinks they need to give you advice, like: 'Are you coping?', 'Do you think you should be doing

this?' 'I think you should sell the business'. Things like that where you weren't really thinking about it, but once everyone starts saying it, you're thinking: 'Oh, am I doing the wrong thing?' There wasn't any really positive support. [control group, running own business part time]

These extracts make it clear that women were often trying to grapple with accepted ideas about the 'good' mother devoting a lot of time to her children, while at the same time feeling better themselves, not to mention feeling themselves to be better mothers, when they had some time away. There was also the sense that only mothers (and not fathers or other people) can provide certain things for children; that it is mothers who are ultimately responsible for children's physical and emotional well-being. Yet, despite these ambivalent feelings about combining employment and motherhood, and the demands of 'doing it all', almost half the mothers interviewed (40/90) were, and wanted to be, employed.

One striking feature of women's comments about resuming employment is how very rarely they gave any indication that the question of balancing employment and family responsibilities might rest on anyone's shoulders but their own. They seemed to be trying to do it all. Sometimes extra 'help' came from partners or family, but it was almost always mothers who orchestrated the daily symphony, or perhaps cacophony, of family life.

There were ambivalences here, too. To some extent it represented an unwillingness to let go of the special, close relationship of mother and child. In *The Mother Knot*, Jane Lazarre describes how it was she who *wanted* to organise child care, and be the one involved in choosing it, having the contact with other parents and so on, as her 'right', and almost as an extension of her special relationship with the child.[17] This was true for many women in the study. One consequence of having been the primary care-giver from the beginning is the sense of having to give up something special when resuming paid employment means sharing the care with other people. An understandable response to this is to do all one can to give up as little as possible.

MEN AT HOME

There were six households in the sample that were rather different. In four of them it was the male partner who had the main responsibility for child care: in the other two the partners were employed part time and shared the day to day responsibilities for the children. Three of the six men were self-employed and worked from home, while another was in the process of building the family home. All six women continued to have a major involvement in both domestic work and child care, as well as being employed —

though not all of them were in full-time work — so these families had not reversed traditional roles but expanded them.

The much greater involvement of fathers from these six families in being with, and caring for, children was very apparent. Like women in the same situation, they found having the major responsibility for children and home very demanding. Katrina Peterson's partner was working from home, having lost his previous job due to the recession:

> He's been really good, but even for someone who already shared most of the housework and all the rest, it's still been a shock, just the demands that are made; and getting confidence that he could do it I suppose is the other issue.
> *Rhonda   That's the general looking after of the children, in that sort of way?*
> Katrina   Yeah, yeah. Like today he bought a pair of tights for dancing. He said 'Look, I can do that even, like a mum could, I can buy tights too'. It's just confidence that he can. Or, since I've been working the last couple of months, cooking dinner each night — not that — he always did cook dinners, but having to do it day after day was different. [case group]

Partners who were currently at home, or who had been at some stage in the past, were seen as having a much better understanding of the demands, the potential for isolation, and just the sheer hard work of being a parent at home full time, with young children.

TIMEOUT

We asked women whether they had any timeout from childrearing, apart from being in paid employment. Fifty-seven per cent had some timeout regularly, 33 per cent only occasionally or rarely, and 10 per cent never had any time away from their children. We looked further at what was meant by regularly, occasionally and rarely. Twenty per cent of women had timeout once or less per month, 36 per cent between one and four times and 34 per cent five or more times per month. For most women timeout meant an hour or two away to shop, play sport or visit friends.

Women depressed at eight to nine months were no more or less likely to be having timeout from child caring by the time of our interview than women not depressed at that stage, although it is worth noting that of the sixteen women who never had any timeout, eleven were in the case group. It is impossible to know whether differences would have been more evident at the eight to nine month period, although a number of things point to this possibility. For example, women's descriptions of their experiences of isolation and being cut off from friends when they were depressed, as well as their advice to other women to organise timeout from childrearing, do suggest that lack of timeout from child caring was an issue for them at that time. Some of the women who had felt depressed commented that they had realised they needed more time for themselves because of how they had been feeling, and some, like Ruth Murray, mentioned making special deals with their partners to ensure that they did get a break:

> I try to make it regularly, like on a Saturday morning, John is with Sarah, and I just go off and do what I feel like. But I'm not usually gone for very long — a couple of hours or something. That's been good. Sometimes I don't do it at all. It's been good on a regular basis. And John sort of knows Saturday morning if I feel like it I'll be out. So he can't plan anything. But then he's out all Saturday afternoon playing tennis. So that's fair. [Ruth was in our control group, but had felt depressed.]

Many women also commented that their partners were doing a somewhat better job of helping out with child caring as the child or children got older, so that their opportunities for getting away on their own had increased. It is therefore quite plausible that by the time of the interview women in the case group had in fact been able to organise more time away than they had earlier.

On the other hand, given the total amount of time women had away even when they did have regular timeout, it is perhaps unrealistic to expect that this would have a huge impact on their emotional well-being. One or two hours a week may not be enough to provide real emotional relief from the constancy of the demands women described their children making on them. This may of course depend on what is done by women when they have time away.

It is important to note that timeout for mothers was not always leisure time or time strictly for themselves. Women often used what little time they had to attend appointments, do family shopping in peace, or tackle household tasks that were difficult to do with children around.

Amanda Joseph I do my hair, or come home and clean out cupboards, or — things I can't do while she's around. [Amanda's daughter went to occasional child care one morning a week.]

Annette Flynn A lot of time[out] is spent in running the house than in time to myself.

Leila Schmidt Well I just do a bit of shopping, do the shopping in peace ...

In other words, timeout allowed women some extra leeway to get things done that would otherwise have been much more onerous with children around. Perhaps this contributed to better emotional well-being or perhaps it just helped to keep the lid on the pot.

There was one striking difference between women in the two study groups regarding what they did when they had time away from child caring. Women in the control group were twice as likely to play sport (20/45) when they had timeout than women in the case group (10/45). This is an interesting finding in that of all the things women commonly did when they had timeout — visiting friends, shopping, playing sport — the latter is the most clearly identifiable as a leisure activity for the person involved. Some women also linked keeping fit directly with how they felt about themselves.

> *Fiona Neilson* I've kept fit and that makes me happy, and I'm not happy if I feel lazy and overweight. I'm not one to sit still for too long. [Fiona was in the control group and did aerobics several times a week.]

Both shopping and visiting friends can of course be purely leisure activities, but they can be, and often were, activities done *for* others as well as for the woman herself. Sporting activities usually also involve a specified and therefore predictable time on a regular basis. When women went shopping or visited friends, even when they did this regularly, it was usually fitted in when the opportunity arose, rather than women having a set time every week which they could count on. It is therefore possible that the women who played sport gained more emotional or restorative benefit from this purely 'selfish' and regular activity.

Wanting more timeout was very common, with 31/45 mothers in the case group wanting more free time and 21/45 mothers in the control group. Although this difference did not reach statistical significance, there was a significant difference between full-time mothers at home in the case group and full-time mothers at home in the control group, with more of the case group mothers wanting more time out (18/23 versus 12/24, $\chi^2=3.98$, $p=0.05$).

For many women, wanting more timeout was linked to the impossibly constant demands they felt that their work as mothers entailed.

> *Dawn Harrison* I'd like a 38 hour week (laughs), with long service. Actually I decided, seeing Nikki's nine, I've only got a year for long service anyway, as long as it's paid, and I get my three months. [Dawn was in the case group and had five children under ten.]

Dawn was making a particular point of ensuring that she had some time to herself each week, when she went swimming, though the strain of organising this timeout was also taking its toll.

> I usually go swimming one night a week and I'm finding at the moment it's getting to, dash out, do that, and come back ... I'm finding I'm losing it. I'm starting to get to the stage of saying I won't bother going, as much as I know I have to go — for sanity's sake other than anything else.

When asked what advice they would give other mothers who were depressed, just under one-third of women who themselves had experienced depression (18/60) recommended having time away from the demands of mothering as helpful to recovery. This was the second most common piece of advice women offered.

Finally, although we did not explore in any detail what timeout men had from family responsibilities or employment, it was clear from talking to women that their partners were very often involved in hobby or sporting activities, and that they were less likely to have given up their leisure-time pursuits since having children than were the women, something also found by Russell[18] when comparing mothers and fathers employed full time. Only one-third of women said that they did the same things with their 'free' time as they had done before having children, and most women talked about having to give up one or more leisure activities they had previously engaged in.

> *Josephine Cucinotta* I like to knit, but I can't sit there at it anymore 'cos this one pulls the wool, the other one pulls the knitting needle, and you find it hard to sit down and relax ...

> *Megan Appleford* I see that there's light at the end of the tunnel, because they're growing up. And I've got plans to take up my cello again, which I used to play, so I've got plans of what I'm going to do with my free time in the future, but not at the moment.

Women occasionally questioned their right to any leisure time at all. This was particularly true for women employed full time who, because of the time they already spent away from their children, felt they couldn't justify having any other 'free' time. As Katrina Peterson posed the dilemma:

> I've occasionally been taking a little bit of time lately, but basically it would usually be no [timeout]. It's very difficult — particularly now I'm working full time. When you're at home you really have to be there for them [the children].

Given women's comments about the extent of their partners' leisure pursuits it would seem that few full-time employed men suffered from such a dilemma, despite the large amounts of time they spent away from their children.

IN SUMMARY

It is difficult to read the interview transcripts and consider the reality of men's and women's working lives without concluding that there is something awry with the way in which the work of caring for children, carrying out domestic labour, and supporting the family unit economically is undertaken by men and women today. Not only does it seem unjust that 'women's work is (still) never done', but it is evident that the burdens borne by women in this uneven distribution of work, especially when accompanied by a lack of acknowledgment of their work, and little emotional support from their partners, can have serious consequences for women's emotional well-being.

Rhonda Small, Judith Lumley, Stephanie Brown

TWELVE

Three Women's Accounts of Motherhood

The follow-up interviews took us all over Melbourne and throughout much of Victoria — talking to women on farms, in tiny country towns, inner-city flats and outer-suburban housing estates. When we talked to friends and colleagues about doing these interviews, they often said 'it must be so depressing!', but it was not at all. It was sometimes harrowing, we often felt angry about the circumstances of women's lives, and sometimes there were tears — theirs and ours on a couple of occasions. But there was also laughter in every interview, and lots of shared experiences between ourselves and the women who invited us into their homes. While we quote extensively from the transcripts of the interviews in other chapters, much of the complexity and richness in women's accounts of their lives is lost or fragmented when stories are broken up in this way. For this reason, we include here longer extracts from three interviews.

Each of the women selected was in our case group; they had all been assessed as depressed when their infants were eight months old and all confirmed in the interviews that this was how they remembered this period, although only one viewed her depression as 'postnatal depression'. We deliberately chose women who had been depressed as it is their voices that are so rarely heard. Our other criteria for selection were as follows: first, there is one interview with each of the three authors who between them did most of the interviews; second, between the three women a range of factors that were found to be associated with depression are discussed — two had experienced major health problems; one had a child she experienced as difficult and this was confirmed by the Toddler Temperament Scale; one was single when her child was born; one had a partner who was absent more than fifteen hours a day; one had three children, all of whom had been sick at the time of the original survey. Third, there was, amongst the three women, a representative range of responses to depression in terms of seeking help from health professionals — one of the women selected talked to both her Maternal and Child Health nurse and her general

'DOING THINGS I HAVE NEVER DONE BEFORE IN MY LIFE'

Clare Thornton was 23 years old and lived alone with her daughter Zoe. She had separated from her husband while she was pregnant. Although she had some help from friends with household tasks and looking after Zoe, she did most of this work herself.

JUDITH	ARE YOU HAPPY WITH THE AMOUNT OF HELP YOU HAVE?
Clare	Yeah, well I'm pretty independent, I like to do as much as I can myself. There are certain jobs I just can't do.
JUDITH	SO THERE AREN'T ANY THINGS THAT YOU'D LIKE MORE HELP WITH. YOU THINK YOU'VE GOT IT ORGANISED HOW YOU LIKE?
Clare	You always like more than what you've got, that's a fact of life. But no, I'm coping on my own. I mean, there's things I want done, like, I'd like new carpet, but I just can't do it on my own.
JUDITH	DO YOU HAVE ANY TIME AWAY FROM ZOE BY YOURSELF?
Clare	Yeah, just after the New Year I left her on the Monday and picked her up on the Friday, so I had a four-day break. Mum and my sister looked after her. So I do every now and then. And then she gets minded. Yesterday I went for a driving lesson and my girlfriend minded her. And when I'm at school, I have a day away from her. So I do actually.

Although living on her own with her daughter, Clare had more support from friends and family members than many of the women in the case group. Her score for total support on the Social Support Scale was 3.15, which was above the case group mean (2.83), but still below the control group mean (3.78).

JUDITH	IS LOOKING AFTER CHILDREN HOW YOU EXPECTED?
Clare	Yeah, I find it a pleasure, I have my moments, we all do, but yeah, I like it, I enjoy it. She's worth every minute of it.
JUDITH	PRETTY MUCH AS YOU EXPECTED?
Clare	Yeah, it is. To the degree where I'm always fearful, you think of the worst, whether they're going to get sick and all that kind of stuff, but it hasn't happened yet, so, I've sort of, I made it worse than what it is, if that makes sense. Before she was born I was expecting the worst, and that hasn't happened.

JUDITH	SO IT'S ACTUALLY BEEN EASIER?
Clare	Yeah, it has.
JUDITH	WERE YOU DELIBERATELY TRYING TO THINK OF THE WORST THINGS SO ...
Clare	Yeah, well in a way. Well, when I was pregnant I broke up with my husband, and of course everything was black. So, it was easier to have everything black, and when it turned out white it was good. It was just my frame of mind at the time, that's all it was. I'm over that now.
JUDITH	WHAT STAGE IN THE PREGNANCY WAS IT WHEN YOU BROKE UP?
Clare	Five months.
JUDITH	PRETTY DIFFICULT?
Clare	Yeah, it was a bit, but that's life. I just coped with it. It just sort of, I'm glad in a lot of ways that I was that far pregnant because I had no choices. I had to have her and that was it. And I'm so glad now that I didn't have any choices. So it was worth it. Because you go through all that, 'I've got to get rid of the baby', but I'm so glad I didn't have to.
JUDITH	THAT'S GOOD.
Clare	He's actually done me a lot of favours. You think about all the financial trouble you'll be in, and there's house payments and everything, I've got none of that now. He's off with his wife, and he's happy, that's just the way it turned out.

For negative life events Clare's score on the Life Experiences Questionnaire was 14, substantially higher than both the case group mean (6.77) and the control group mean (3.84).

JUDITH	HAVE YOU BEEN PHYSICALLY WELL SINCE ZOE WAS BORN?
Clare	Yeah, I do have a back problem, but that was way back.
JUDITH	THAT WAS FROM BEFORE?
Clare	Yeah, I had an accident at work, and during my pregnancy it was really bad, and it plays up all the time. But that's nothing to do with Zoe.
JUDITH	HAS THAT HAD ANY EFFECT ON YOUR EXPERIENCE OF BEING A MOTHER?
Clare	There'll be days when I just don't want to do anything and I have to get out of bed and do it. Yeah, that's hard, but I mean I must admit, Zoe's really, I don't know what other children are like, but she's really good. If I'm not feeling well, she'll just let me go, she'll let me lie in bed, and she won't do too much terrorising. If she needs something, she'll come and get it. She's good.

JUDITH   SHE'S QUITE A BIG GIRL, DID YOU EVER HAVE PROBLEMS PICKING HER UP?
Clare   Yeah, she's pretty heavy. I do actually.

Health problems was one of the areas investigated in the Life Experiences Questionnaire — women in the case group were significantly more likely to have experienced health problems that had a negative impact on their lives. For health 'events' with a negative impact Clare scored 14, way above both the case group mean of 3.77 and the control group mean of 1.91.

JUDITH   HAS ZOE BEEN WELL SINCE SHE WAS BORN?
Clare   Yes. Last year though, she had two convulsions which really freaked me out, but that was the only major scare I've ever had. Teething I think, it was the teething. At the time the doctors kept telling me that she was an epileptic and all that stuff, and it got me into a real frenzy. And all these specialists. Never had them again, nothing's ever been wrong with her since.

JUDITH   AND THEY WERE BOTH QUITE CLOSE TOGETHER?
Clare   Yeah, it was really strange. 'Cos I lost my father in February last year, everything happened at that time. Everyone in the family, someone took ill. We don't know, but we feel it was related to that. It was just that time it happened. Nothing's happened since. Oh, she's had gastro, perforated ears, things like that. But she never, when she had the perforated ears, she never screamed, or carried on or anything. You're really good aren't you? [to child]

JUDITH   WOULD YOU DESCRIBE ZOE AS HAVING BEEN A SETTLED BABY?
Clare   Yeah, very settled. She'd cry when she wanted something and that was it. I sound like I'm bragging, but I'm not! It's true. It shocked me too, I expected to be up all night. Except if she was unwell. But she was really good.

JUDITH   WHAT DO YOU LIKE THE MOST ABOUT LOOKING AFTER HER?
Clare   Well, it's company, if that makes sense. Like we're friends. Even though she's so little. I like sharing with her. I like playing with her toys with her. Feed times, we have good fun at mealtimes. Bathtime, splashing you know. Sometimes I'll jump in the bath with her and we'll have a splash game. Play peek-a-boo, and we run round the house playing hide-and-seek. Besides, she brings out my childhood for me, it's good fun. And as far as all the cleaning and all that goes, that's just part of the game. I just accept it.

JUDITH   WHAT'S THE THING YOU LIKE LEAST ABOUT LOOKING AFTER HER?

Clare	Umm, 'I want, I want', but I accept it, and the 'NO', that's started up now. We say 'no' to everything. Overall, she pretty well does what she's told, she has her moments. She does want me, she tends to want me a lot, which is fair enough, because I feel I am away from her enough that she should want me. Just the fact, the stage she's going through. She says no, and she demands things, but I just hope that's a stage.

Zoe was rated as 'easy' on the Toddler Temperament Scale.

JUDITH	YOU'VE BEEN IN PART-TIME STUDY?
Clare	Yeah, it's classed as a full-time course, but it was pretty slack.
JUDITH	AND HOW HAS RETURNING TO STUDY AFFECTED HOW YOU FEEL ABOUT BEING A MOTHER?
Clare	Good, because I only finished in [Year] 10, and I worked at the same job until I fell pregnant. So from 16 to 21, or whatever I was, that was it. And I knew that I needed something better for her, because my wages and everything, and my commitment, it was just a matter of study. I feel like, what I was doing was a women's course, planned out for mothers who had children, so therefore it was easy to work Zoe around it. It worked in perfectly, it was much better than a job as far as hours and everything, and financially it just fitted in well. This year will be a bit of a pest (laughs)!
JUDITH	AND YOU WERE SAYING SOME GOOD THINGS ABOUT THE CRECHE. SO DO YOU THINK THAT EXPERIENCE FOR YOU AND ZOE'S BEEN POSITIVE?
Clare	Oh, definitely. The first few months I started school in '89, I had her with a very close friend of mine, and once Zoe got the convulsions she didn't want her anymore, because she had other children. And it was pot luck that I got into the creche. And when I got in there, just the difference in Zoe in a month was amazing. I learnt so much.
JUDITH	THE COURSE THAT YOU'RE STARTING, HOW LONG WILL THAT TAKE?
Clare	Well, the first year is from the start of Feb. to the end of December, and it depends on my grades whether I'm able to do the computer programming. So at the moment a year, but then I'm aiming to do the two years. I've got to be good enough.
JUDITH	AND THEN TO GET A JOB AFTER THAT?
Clare	I've got this long-term plan, I don't know if it'll work. There's this new thing coming out called the Electronic Cottage, where you work from home and that's my long-term goal. You've got to work in a business for about ten years before

	they'll give you the chance to do it, but that's what I'm aiming to do. And then after, work for myself.
JUDITH	IT'S GOOD TO HAVE SOME LONG-TERM GOALS. WOULD YOU SAY THAT BEING A MOTHER HAS BEEN WHAT YOU EXPECTED?
Clare	Really, you have no idea before they're born. You're just going on other people. I feel, I often question my raising of her because I see other children always clean, and mine's always dirty, and I think, am I doing things wrong. But then, I think, well she's happy and I think that's number one, so it's working out what I want. I wanted to bring up a child and make sure she's happy. So, so far the plan's working.
JUDITH	AND WHAT'S THE BEST THING ABOUT BEING A MOTHER?
Clare	I'd say, watching them grow. Seeing the new things popping up. All my friends thought I was mental, 'Guess what, Zoe woke up with a dry nappy' (laughs)! That was so exciting, and they go, 'Oh really, how exciting'. And it was, it's just a thrill, a new thing. And having the bottle, the day we stop the dummy, I'll probably have a party (laughs)! Just watching her grow it's magic. It really is.
JUDITH	AND WHAT ARE THE WORST THINGS?
Clare	Going through the normal things like the teething, and the crying, and the wanting, and scariness of not really knowing whether I'm going up the right path. You can do as many courses as you like, it's not going to fix your personal ... The questions in my mind are always, 'Am I doing it right? Am I going to give her a good life?'
JUDITH	SO THE RESPONSIBILITY?
Clare	Yeah, the responsibility. But then, the responsibility's also a challenge. And it's a challenge I was prepared to take on on my own. I thrive on that. I thrive on buying the house, and going through all the legal stuff.

On the Experience of Motherhood Questionnaire, Clare scored 66 — a score indicating a less positive experience of motherhood than the case group mean of 43.3 and control group mean of 37.0.

JUDITH	WHEN YOU FILLED IN THE FIRST QUESTIONNAIRE THAT YOU SENT BACK, YOUR ANSWERS TO SOME OF THE QUESTIONS SHOWED THAT YOU MIGHT HAVE BEEN DEPRESSED. IS THAT THE WAY YOU REMEMBER AT THAT TIME?
Clare	Yeah, I would've been very depressed at that time.
JUDITH	CAN YOU TELL IN A BIT MORE DETAIL ABOUT THAT TIME?

Clare	Well, I was very — I want my husband back, all that kind of thing — heartbroken. And I had a lot of decisions to make, big decisions. Do I buy — like I bought him out — I had a lot of legal things on my mind. Everything was, I got to do the best for Zoe, so I've got to do it this way. I fought for my home, I fought for this, I fought for that. And there was a lot of pressure. You know, I had this new baby, I was breast-feeding. I was doing things I had never done before in my life, and I also had the pressure of having to worry about the legal side of everything and the financial side of it. Where's my next meal coming? That sort of stuff. So it was hard, but it was a challenge. It's not me I have to worry about now, it's this little thing that's helpless. So I've got to do the best I can for her, and that kept me going. And of course I had a lot of support. Everywhere I turned I had support.
JUDITH	DID YOU TRY AND GET ANY FORMAL HELP AT THAT TIME FROM ANYBODY?
Clare	While I was pregnant I had a social worker ... And she said as soon as you have the baby come and see me. And I was on such a high when I had Zoe that I felt, I don't need a social worker, so I never went back and seen her. And then I got down to the lows, but I was too stubborn, so I never went back and seen her. And I felt guilty 'cos she was so good to me. Why didn't I go back and just show her the baby, you know? You just go through the pride, and I don't need anybody, I'm on a high, and when you're down, I don't want to show anyone I'm down.
JUDITH	SO YOU DIDN'T ACTUALLY GO AND LOOK FOR ANY HELP IN THE DOWN PHASE?
Clare	Actually, my school was that kind of help. Because they're all women, and we had assertion classes every week. So I got that help last year. Plus the new friends, and women discussing things, it was good.
JUDITH	SO DID YOU TALK ABOUT HOW YOU FEEL TO THE OTHER PEOPLE YOU MIGHT HAVE COME ACROSS, LIKE YOUR DOCTOR?
Clare	Well, actually, while I was pregnant I decided I'd tell him. Everyone said tell your doctor, because they're the person you could trust. And here I am crying on his shoulder one day and he just gave me funny looks, so from then on I never said nothing at all, 'cos I felt embarrassed. I still go to him, he's Zoe's doctor, I still go to him, but I don't feel like saying anything to him.
JUDITH	AND MATERNAL AND CHILD HEALTH, INFANT WELFARE?
Clare	Yeah, well I had all the time, right up to she was 11 months

	I went there. I just really more or less just got her weight and then say, is she healthy, and that was it. I never really got involved.
JUDITH	YOU DIDN'T SEE HER AS SOMEBODY WHO MIGHT HAVE HELPED?
Clare	No, I saw her as — this is terrible — I saw her like someone who was going to try and take my baby off me. I stayed away from anyone I thought was …
JUDITH	IF YOU KNEW OF SOMEBODY ELSE IN A SIMILAR SITUATION WHAT ADVICE WOULD YOU GIVE THEM?
Clare	Umm. Think of number one. Think if you've got a child, you have to put that child first, no matter what. That's been brainwashed from me mum, but I believe that. And then you've just got to — like my life now, in no way did I see that 15 or 18 months ago. And everyone kept telling me, you're going to have a future, you're going to find someone — and I thought, no way, no-one's going to want me, I'm ugly, blah, blah, blah. And I'd give that same advice. You've just got to keep on talking, cause there is another door and it will open. You don't see it at the time, but it's there.
JUDITH	SO HOW WOULD YOU DESCRIBE HOW YOU FEEL ABOUT THINGS IN GENERAL AT THE PRESENT TIME?
Clare	I'm happy. Yeah. Well, the bottom line is do I get this course or not? I'm determined to get my licence, I'm determined … It's full steam ahead. I've got good points in me somewhere, and I'm going to use them.
JUDITH	DO YOU SEE YOURSELF AS HAVING HAD POSTNATAL DEPRESSION?
Clare	No, I didn't.
JUDITH	YOU WERE SAYING THAT YOU WERE IN A SITUATION WHERE REALLY ANYBODY IN THAT SITUATION WOULD BE DEPRESSED?
Clare	That's right. I believe. I mean, who wouldn't be? You have a baby to have a future with that person. And all of a sudden that future's gone, it's depression number one.

Clare's score on the EPDS at the time of the follow-up interview was 10, indicating that she was no longer depressed, but still emotionally vulnerable.

JUDITH	SO, WHEN YOU WERE SAYING THAT AFTER ZOE WAS BORN YOU WERE IN A REAL HIGH STATE AT THAT TIME, HOW LONG DID IT TAKE TO …
Clare	It was funny, because she was 8 days overdue. And of course from the time she was due, it was phone calls all the time. And I had my brother living here at the time, and it was just constantly people around me, and during the hospital time,

and then say till about two weeks out of hospital. Then all of a sudden the phone calls stopped, and it just went back, and it just died. All the excitement — I was no longer in the limelight! (laughs). And it just sort of uhh.

JUDITH WHEN DO YOU THINK YOU CAME OUT OF IT?
Clare When I met Phil [boyfriend]. Yeah, I'd say that.

JUDITH SO SAY, PERHAPS, THAT'S ALMOST WHEN SHE WAS ONE?
Clare Yeah, oh she was about — we met in October — so she was about nine or ten months old. But that was still a lot of fear and a lot of being alone.

JUDITH IF YOU WERE COMPARING NOW WITH WHEN YOU GOT THE QUESTIONNAIRE WHEN SHE WAS EIGHT MONTHS OLD, HOW DO YOU FEEL COMPARED WITH THEN?
Clare Oh, much better. I'm a different person.

JUDITH AND THAT'S BEEN BECAUSE YOU'VE REALLY RESOLVED ALL THESE PROBLEMS?
Clare Yeah. I've decided what I want to do with my life. I was just a dull old meat-packer who didn't know what. I was just going along a boring road, and now I've got options and I want to take them. There's a life out there and I want to get the best out of it for both of us.

JACK WAS DIFFERENT FROM AMANDA

Caitlin Adamson lived with her husband and two children, Amanda aged five and Jack aged two. They had a new home in an outer suburb of a major rural city. Caitlin's husband, Richard, travelled to Melbourne and back every day to work and was therefore away from around 7.00 a.m. until 7.30 p.m. each week day. Richard's contribution to household tasks in the week prior to the interview was close to average for the sample for partners of women who were at home full time (score = 9), but slightly higher than average for child-care tasks (score = 26). He had not been up at all during the night to attend to Jack, although Caitlin had been up at least once every night. He had, however, shared the nappy changes over the weekend, and spent some time alone with the children twice in the previous week.

Caitlin, like many other mothers we interviewed, was happy with her husband's contributions to household tasks, and child care, 'in the circumstances'.

STEPHANIE AND ARE YOU HAPPY WITH THE CONTRIBUTION YOUR PARTNER'S MAKING TO CHILD CARE?
Caitlin Yes. Yeah, I think so, for the limited time that he's got, I think he does a pretty good job.

STEPHANIE   WHAT ABOUT THE CONTRIBUTION OF OTHERS?
Caitlin   Oh look I'm really lucky, I've got family support — really happy; two sisters and a mother and a mother-in-law are great. I was surprised when I filled out that questionnaire how much they are involved in my life, it's incredible really, it was quite interesting.

STEPHANIE   THINKING ABOUT THE TIME SINCE YOU HAD JACK, HAVE YOU BEEN PHYSICALLY WELL IN THAT TIME?
Caitlin   No I haven't. I would say well for a while. No, no, I wasn't well, I had high blood pressure and heart irregularity, and my health has just been really awful. Amanda — I was really, really sick when I had her — but I came good and I stayed good, but with him I couldn't cope at all. Twelve months and no sleep didn't help, because he didn't sleep until twelve months; and then, as I said, high blood pressure and heart irregularity — that's just happened in the last twelve months.

STEPHANIE   SO IS THAT UNDER CONTROL NOW, THE HIGH BLOOD PRESSURE AND THE HEART IRREGULARITY?
Caitlin   Yes, yes, so far, much better.

STEPHANIE   AND HOW LONG DID THAT TAKE TO RESOLVE?
Caitlin   Six months. I took one tablet for the blood pressure that suited me, and the heart irregularity has only just been solved in the last few months, so no medication for that, I'd rather stay off it — the side effects are worse than the complaint.

STEPHANIE   HOW DO YOU THINK BEING PHYSICALLY UNWELL HAS AFFECTED YOUR EXPERIENCE OF BEING A MOTHER?
Caitlin   It's really miserable just trying to cope with everyday everything; it was a real chore, it shouldn't have been that hard.

Caitlin's score for health 'events' with a negative impact was 12, much higher than the case group mean of 3.77 and the control group mean of 1.91.

STEPHANIE   COMPARED TO WHAT YOU EXPECTED BEFORE JACK WAS BORN, HAS HE BEEN MORE OR LESS DIFFICULT TO LOOK AFTER?
Caitlin   More difficult.

STEPHANIE   HAS HE? IN WHAT SORTS OF WAYS?
Caitlin   Just feeding and sleeping, he was shocking, whereas with Amanda I just fed her and it was easy and she was every four hours and she was just such a breeze, where he's been much, much more difficult. He was every two hours for the first three and four months, and then just wouldn't sleep at night, so I was feeding him all the time. So he's been difficult compared to what I expected having had a good feeder

before. He's a lot more clingy, too, than Amanda was, he was always — liked people 'round, and liked his Mum all the time, where she was quite an independent little thing right from the word go. So I expected the same and didn't get it (laughs).

STEPHANIE DID HE CRY A LOT?
Caitlin Yes. In the first four months he cried a lot.

STEPHANIE AND HAS HE HAD ANY FEEDING PROBLEMS AS WELL?
Caitlin No, just that he wanted to be fed all the time; he was a really hungry baby, really hungry, so he went onto solids at — right on three months — and pretty well accepts everything that you give him. He's pretty good like that, up until now (laughs); and now he doesn't want to eat anything, so he's gone from one extreme to the other. No, he's been good, really, as far as the feeding goes, I suppose.

STEPHANIE AND HE'S HAD SLEEPING PROBLEMS?
Caitlin Yes. He's a very light sleeper, I think, more than anything else, and if he wakes up he likes to be with somebody, he doesn't like being by himself; soft cuddly toys and sheepskin thingos — you name it, I tried everything. If he's awake, he wanted company, straight off, otherwise he'd just lay there and scream.

STEPHANIE AND HOW OFTEN WERE YOU GETTING UP AT NIGHT?
Caitlin Oh I was getting up three and four times at night, and turning him over and tucking him back in — you know, if it wasn't a feed time or whatever; and more often than not I had to resort to giving a comforter, and he was happy.

While Jack had been a healthy baby, Caitlin had found him a very difficult baby to care for. His score on the Toddler Temperament Scale indicated that he was 'difficult'.

STEPHANIE HOW WOULD YOU DESCRIBE YOUR RELATIONSHIP WITH HIM NOW THAT HE'S A TODDLER?
Caitlin Oh very loving, he's an extremely loving little boy, he's really good. He's good company but he's very tiring (laughs), mainly with his talking than his activity — I don't mind him being active, but when they talk constantly from when their eyes open until they shut (laughs), it's a bit wearing.

Since Jack was born Caitlin had been at home full time. She had no plans to return to paid work or study. Asked about this, she commented that her husband 'studies enough for both of us'. During the year after Jack was born he was finishing a graduate diploma, which meant he was often not home until after 10.30 at night.

STEPHANIE	HOW WOULD YOU DESCRIBE YOUR OVERALL EXPERIENCE THEN, OF BEING A MOTHER THIS TIME ROUND WITH JACK?
Caitlin	Difficult, that's the word that — difficult. Last time round it was much easier.
STEPHANIE	SO, IF YOU HAD TO CHARACTERISE IT IN POSITIVE/NEGATIVE TERMS, WOULD IT BE ON THE NEGATIVE SIDE?
Caitlin	It would be more on the negative than the positive. The first twelve months are we talking about or … ?
STEPHANIE	OVERALL.
Caitlin	Overall? Well he's really cute (laughs). You know, you love 'em very much but, for me — oh, I'd say half and half, really.

Caitlin's score on the Experience of Motherhood Questionnaire was 50, higher than the case mean of 43.3 and the control mean of 37 — her reflections on the changes in her life since Jack had been born confirmed the indication of the score that her life had been much changed in negative ways.

STEPHANIE	WHEN YOU FILLED IN THE QUESTIONNAIRE I SENT IN THE MAIL — NOT THIS ONE, THE ONE I SENT WHEN JACK WAS EIGHT MONTHS OLD — SOME OF THE ANSWERS TO THE QUESTIONS, THEN, INDICATED THAT YOU WERE PROBABLY FEELING A BIT DEPRESSED. IS THAT HOW YOU REMEMBER THAT PERIOD?
Caitlin	Yeah, I was, definitely. Eight months — actually I think — yes I was, and I rang and spoke to Sister —— [Maternal and Child Health Nurse], and then she put me onto —— , he's my GP and he felt that I just needed more sleep, more than anything else, 'if you can get more sleep, you'll be much happier'. That's what it kind of ended up boiling down to. But yes — it was really difficult when they cry a lot. You spend a lot of time crying, the first twelve months. But I really do think that there was postnatal depression there, but not enough to be treated drug-wise or whatever, just to talk was enough.
STEPHANIE	WOULD YOU LIKE TO DESCRIBE IN A BIT MORE DETAIL HOW YOU WERE FEELING DURING THAT TIME?
Caitlin	I didn't think I was coping terribly well, I wasn't coping with the house, definitely, that was kinda going to pack, and that really upsets me. I felt — I definitely wasn't really good with Richard [husband]. I was really super-snappy, and didn't have any time for him or whatnot. I felt like it was only me in the world that was going through it and nobody else. I didn't like going out very much 'cos I couldn't get it together; it seemed to take me ages to get there, and I'd get out there and I didn't know what I wanted. I seemed to have a high one day

and for the next four days I'd be right down in the dumps; and he [husband] kept saying to go and get help, but I really didn't want the help of any anti-depressants or anything like that, so I figured the only way you could do it was to struggle through, which we did in the end.

STEPHANIE SO WOULD YOU HAVE ANY THOUGHTS OR ADVICE FOR OTHER WOMEN WHO MIGHT BE FEELING DEPRESSED AFTER HAVING A CHILD NOW, ON THE BEST THINGS TO DO?

Caitlin Just talk to somebody, really, because once I'd spoken and admitted that I wasn't coping really well, I felt so much better. I think sitting there and thinking that you're not doing so well is the wrong thing to do. I think you should get out and talk to somebody, and you'll be feeling much, much better.

STEPHANIE CAN YOU REMEMBER, WITH JACK, WHEN YOU BEGAN FEELING DEPRESSED? YOU MENTIONED YOU HAD THE THREE-DAY BLUES — DID IT GO ON FROM THEN, OR … ?

Caitlin Well, it was really bad in hospital and I was crying and whatnot and the sweats and everything else, and then we got home and I was really buoyed up and pleased to be at home, and then about two months I got mastitis, and from then on it's been slowly downhill. I think you're on a high when you get home.

STEPHANIE MASTITIS IS AWFUL.

Caitlin It is, isn't it? I didn't have it with Amanda — I know I keep saying I never had any trouble first time round, but I honestly didn't — but that was terrible, mastitis, just shocking.

STEPHANIE I THINK IT'S MORE COMMON WHEN BABIES FEED FREQUENTLY.

Caitlin You'd think it'd be the other way round wouldn't it? Are you still feeding?

STEPHANIE MMM.

Caitlin And how old's your youngest?

STEPHANIE HE'S TEN MONTHS.

Caitlin And still feeding frequently too?

STEPHANIE NO, NOT SO MUCH NOW, BUT HE USED TO. I THINK I'VE HAD MASTITIS ABOUT SIX TIMES SINCE HE WAS BORN.

Caitlin Oh six times, that'd be agony. You poor thing. And have you got any more?

STEPHANIE YES, I'VE GOT AN ELEVEN-YEAR-OLD AS WELL … HOW LONG DID YOU GO ON FEELING DEPRESSED? OR WOULD YOU SEE YOURSELF AS STILL A BIT DEPRESSED NOW?

Caitlin No, not really now, just off days. I think I started coming good about February I'd say. I think February this year. [The interview took place in June]

STEPHANIE: THAT'S A LONG TIME.

Caitlin It is a long time, and I really don't think — I would have been better earlier, but I think I had a lot of trouble with the blood pressure tablets, they were — I didn't realise they made you depressed, some of them, and I'm not very good with medication anyway. I don't know, I don't know whether that was a side-effect of that, or whether it just took that long to get over it.

STEPHANIE: WHAT DO YOU THINK CONTRIBUTED TO YOUR FEELING DEPRESSED?

Caitlin Jack not being the same as Amanda I think, I was thinking 'Why can't I get it all together?' I was thinking back on her and how I managed her and what I did when I had her, and I was thinking 'this is wrong, I should be able to be doing a lot better than I am'. I think that doesn't help, those negative thoughts ...

Caitlin also thought that tiredness, not having any space or time to herself, and changes in the family's financial circumstances had contributed to how she had felt. On the Life Experiences Questionnaire her score for negative events was 8, slightly above the case mean of 6.77 and well above the control mean of 3.84.

Caitlin I think if I had had a little bit more time and space to myself I probably might have been a bit better, yeah. Yeah, I think so, even though I had a lot of support; I mean because I was feeding all the time, you still took what you thought was the problem with you everywhere you went. So yes, if I had have been able to leave him for a day maybe, and get off and do something, I would have been better off, yeah.

I went back to work when I had Amanda because I needed to — we just moved into the house — and I s'pose I missed the extra money and having to wangle finances and stuff. I don't think that helps at all. I think that's a contributing factor — not a major one — but I think it's an underlying one.

STEPHANIE: YOU MENTIONED THAT YOUR PARTNER HAD BEEN QUITE SUPPORTIVE. WOULD YOU BE ABLE TO DESCRIBE IN A BIT MORE DETAIL HIS RESPONSE TO HOW YOU WERE FEELING?

Caitlin He tried to be there all the time, like weekends that he would go off to the footy or whatnot, he was — tried to be at home, and he'd do the vacuuming, and he helped in that sense, and he looked after Amanda a lot for me, which was great; but that's an added pressure — you've got one wanting something while you're trying to do something. So he really looked after Amanda a lot for me in that time, and I felt guilty about that because, you know, I should have been giving her an equal amount of time, but you just couldn't spread yourself around — or I couldn't at that time anyhow. So practical support, and emotional — he'd sit down and try to talk to me about why I was feeling that I wasn't coping and things like that, he really is — he sits and listens a lot, and tries to give me any ideas of his own that might help me out of it — he's good like that. That's about all I can describe. He's just always there. Actually he quite starred in this written questionnaire (laughs). [Social support questionnaire filled in before the interview]

On the Social Support Questionnaire, Caitlin's responses gave a rating for partner support of 0.93, which was above both the case mean of 0.63 and the control mean 0.79 and confirmed Caitlin's comment in the interview that she felt well supported by her partner. This was even though her partner was never home on weeknights before 7.30 p.m., and during the first year of Jack's life often not home until 10.30 or 11.00 p.m. For support offered by all family members and friends Caitlin's score was also above the case and control means of 2.83 and 3.78. Her score was 5.41.

STEPHANIE	SO LOOKING BACK TO WHEN YOU FILLED IN OUR FIRST QUESTIONNAIRE — THE ONE I SENT YOU WHEN JACK WAS EIGHT MONTHS OLD — ARE YOU FEELING LESS DEPRESSED NOW THAN YOU WERE THEN?
Caitlin	Oh yeah, yeah.
STEPHANIE	AND WHAT DO YOU THINK ARE THE MAIN THINGS THAT HAVE CHANGED?
Caitlin	He's older, I think, less demanding. My health's better. It just seems like I've finally reached the light at the end of the tunnel. Amanda's off to school — I think that's helped a lot — just having all day with him has been good, not having — it was also the kinder year — she had three-year-old kinder — and I was trying to keep that up as well, and then last year it was four-year-old kinder, and they're horrible years, I wouldn't go through them again for anybody — the way I was feeling, anyhow.

In the interview, Caitlin described herself as feeling a lot better than she had during the first year after Jack's birth. Stephanie's personal assessment after the interview was that she was currently depressed. This was confirmed by her score on the EPDS (filled in prior to the interview); her score on this occasion was sixteen, well above the cut-off point for depression. After the tape was turned off Stephanie discussed with Caitlin the finding of the original survey that 15.4 per cent of women were depressed when their babies were eight to nine months old. They talked for some time about why so many women get depressed after having a baby, and exchanged stories about what it is like to be at home alone with a baby who cries incessantly unless being held, soothed, or having a feed.

'YOU TEETER ON THE EDGE AND COME BACK A BIT'

Camilla Jackson lived with her husband and three children — Michael aged seven, Victoria five, and Hannah two — in a major country town. At the time of the interview she was working part time and her husband, Tony, was working full time. For some time before their youngest child was born they had swapped roles — Camilla had worked full time while Tony took primary responsibility for the children. Tony's contributions to household tasks (score = 16) and child care (score = 29) in the week prior to the interview were higher than average for partners of women who were working part time. He also regularly changed nappies and got up to the children at night, although Camilla did a greater share of this work.

RHONDA	THINKING ABOUT PARENTING GENERALLY, HOW INVOLVED WOULD YOU SAY YOUR HUSBAND IS? HOW WOULD YOU DESCRIBE HIS INVOLVEMENT?
Camilla	[He does] As much as possible.
RHONDA	AND HOW DO YOU FEEL ABOUT HIS LEVEL OF INVOLVEMENT?
Camilla	Yes, I feel pretty good about it. I think he does the best he can.
RHONDA	AND HOW DO YOU FEEL THAT YOUR HUSBAND'S COPED WITH THE CHANGES BROUGHT ABOUT BY HAVING CHILDREN?
Camilla	Better than I have (laughs).
RHONDA	DO YOU WANT TO SAY A BIT MORE ABOUT THAT?
Camilla	Well he was a house-husband for two years, to let me go back full time, and he managed those two years better than I ever had, beforehand. Now I think I'm better with the third child. I think I cope a lot better than what I did with one. But he had the two home when he did it, and she was just a toddler at the time, so he had it quite hard; but I guess he didn't have people drop in — that's what he says all the time. If he's ever home he says, 'this is a constant thoroughfare'. He says, 'no wonder you don't get anything done', you know. He

considers I do, I get a lot done, I never stop — but at the same time he sees that there's not much I can do about visitors, so ... He said, 'well I never had to cope with that'; so he understands the situation a lot better because he's done it; and he budgeted a lot better. He took the kids to playgroup, even though he was the only male there.

RHONDA DO YOU EVER HAVE A BREAK FROM BEING WITH THE CHILDREN, APART FROM IF YOU'RE WORKING?

Camilla No — oh, I play basketball once a week, so that helps; and summertime is my — like we have a swap-over — like Tony plays football, so that takes a lot out of the week. So summertime he doesn't play sport and I play tennis, so therefore I get a training session and most of Saturday afternoon at tennis without the children. I can go without the children. This is the first year we've done it, the summer that's just past. It makes it a little bit easier. Usually we both play tennis and we split up the kids and that sort of thing; or whoever was going to a better venue got the kids. Now, it's just so I can get a break, so I do that and he just runs whenever it suits the family.

RHONDA AND DO YOU AND YOUR PARTNER EVER HAVE TIME TOGETHER, AWAY FROM THE CHILDREN?

Camilla We did once, last year. Mum took two of the children and his parents took one, and we had four days. That was after the three of them had chicken-pox, and Michael had refused to go to school, and we just asked; and that was the first break we've ever had.

RHONDA AND HAS HANNAH BEEN WELL SINCE SHE WAS BORN?

Camilla Yeah, she's really well. I'm just waiting for her to get asthma now. The other two have just been diagnosed.

RHONDA OH, WELL YOU MUST BE WONDERING IF IT'S GOING TO BE ALL OF THEM?

Camilla You do, but I know there's no reason to think that, but you think oh, it's gotta come in threes.

RHONDA AND COMPARED TO WHAT YOU EXPECTED BEFORE SHE WAS BORN, WOULD YOU SAY HANNAH'S BEEN MORE DIFFICULT TO LOOK AFTER, LESS DIFFICULT OR PRETTY MUCH AS YOU EXPECTED?

Camilla Oh less difficult I'd say.

RHONDA IN WHAT SORTS OF WAYS?

Camilla She entertains herself. She does for herself, she's very independent. They pick up on things a lot quicker, that third one, although you'd — oh I s'pose you don't worry so much. I mean she used to get up in the shed roof and all that sort of stuff. If it was the other two I would have dived out there, but you looked at her, gave her a look — she laughed at me — and said, 'you be careful' and that's about it. If she got up there she can get down.

RHONDA   AND WHAT DO YOU LIKE BEST ABOUT LOOKING AFTER HER, AND WHAT DO YOU LIKE LEAST?
Camilla   I s'pose that she's so adaptable; she doesn't live by routine or anything like that, she's gotta just fit in. Least: heck! Gee I don't know, I can't think. I can't think of what she does that really irritates me. Oh textas irritate me.

Hannah was rated as 'easy' on the Toddler Temperament Scale.

RHONDA   AND YOU'VE TAKEN UP EMPLOYMENT SINCE HANNAH WAS BORN?
Camilla   Yeah.

RHONDA   HOW OLD WAS SHE WHEN YOU WENT BACK TO WORK?
Camilla   She was fourteen months.

RHONDA   AND IT WAS ABOUT TWO DAYS A WEEK YOU SAID, ON AVERAGE?
Camilla   Yeah.

RHONDA   HAVE YOU FOUND RETURNING TO WORK HAS AFFECTED HOW YOU FEEL ABOUT BEING A MOTHER?
Camilla   Yeah. I would say absolutely definitely after Victoria was born. When I went back to work I was a much better person for it, but now I find that work puts a lot of pressure on. I can't be at say Michael's school mass if it occurs on that day, and I can't be everywhere at once any more. So it does put a lot more pressure on because I'm working. But I find that it's a way to get away from — sometimes it's the only time I get away from the children at all — and you do get a fresher look at things by working. But I didn't really actually want to go back to work after my third child, I had enough to do at home, trying to fit everything in.

RHONDA   WOULD YOU SAY THAT BEING A MOTHER OVERALL HAS BEEN WHAT YOU EXPECTED?
Camilla   No (laughs). You don't expect it to affect your personality as much, I don't think. I think that's the major change. Your time's not your own so — but I find that I don't laugh and burn the candle at both ends anymore. I still stay up really late, and get up late, compared to most women I would say — 'cos I don't get up 'til 8 o'clock in the morning, unless it's a work day. But personality-wise, I don't feel that I'm as carefree as what I used to be, and I s'pose that that's just responsibilties, and that's life. But at the same time you think that life should, you should be able to live it, with as much

enjoyment as you possibly can. Sometimes I have trouble finding that enjoyment — finding the positive side all the time — whereas it used to be very easy, I always lived for the positive side, I found everything positive in life, but not now.

RHONDA YOU FIND THAT HARDER SINCE YOU'VE HAD CHILDREN?
Camilla Mmm. Can't find that positive aspect of everything anymore.

RHONDA AND HOW WOULD YOU DESCRIBE YOUR OVERALL EXPERIENCE OF BEING A MOTHER, THIS TIME AROUND?
Camilla Oh yeah, wonderful. The best thing I ever did was have that third child. I think it gave me a lot more confidence, in myself.

RHONDA SO WHAT WOULD YOU SAY ARE THE BEST THINGS ABOUT BEING A MOTHER, AND WHAT ARE THE WORST?
Camilla The worst thing about being a mother is when they're sick. That's the worst. The best thing I s'pose is always having someone beside you, either in your arms, or clinging on to your leg, or pulling at your skirt, dirtying up your clothes, whatever.

Camilla scored 60 on the Experience of Motherhood Questionnaire, indicating that she had experienced many negative changes in her life since becoming a mother — her score was higher than both the case and control group means on the EMQ.

RHONDA WHEN YOU FILLED IN THE FIRST QUESTIONNAIRE — WHICH WAS WELL OVER A YEAR AGO NOW, WHEN HANNAH WOULD HAVE BEEN ABOUT EIGHT OR NINE MONTHS OLD — THE ANSWERS TO SOME OF THE QUESTIONS INDICATED THAT YOU MAY HAVE BEEN FEELING DEPRESSED AT THAT TIME. IS THAT THE WAY YOU REMEMBER IT?
Camilla Yeah. I remember it very clearly 'cos, as I said, the three of them had chicken-pox. Michael, my eldest, also got an ear infection on top of that, and I couldn't understand why he didn't want to go to school. And we had six weeks of absolute hell here, 'cos I couldn't get him to school. So I ended up — doctors and then the child psychiatrist, who sort of showed me what was actually happening. He actually advised me to get him out of the classroom he was in.

I knew this particular teacher very well from the year before, and knew she screamed at children, and knew my child was a sensitive perfectionist. It's a shocking combination, but that's what he is, and I can't change him. And he went into that classroom and he came home every night saying, 'I'm hopeless'. If a child can read novels, he's brilliant, he's a very bright child; but he was saying he was hopeless.

And it culminated in, that's how the doctor explained it to me, he said that once he was sick and had three weeks off with the chicken-pox and I said there's no way he's gonna go back to a situation like that. And I knew that I didn't have the strength or the courage to say, I don't want him there. 'Cos his teacher from the year before said, 'you've got to eventually cut the apron strings Camilla'. I thought, oh yeah, well oh God; yeah, they've gotta learn to cope by themselves, but not at that age, not in grade one.

So at the end of this year my Infant Welfare Sister said, 'be strong, be strong'; so I went down there and asked for him to go into this particular classroom, and that boy is SO different, he's just — his teacher thinks he's wonderful. He's going ahead in leaps and bounds, and I should have done that — I mean in hindsight, that's the sort of thing I do all the time. I know the right thing, but I'm not confident enough to follow my instincts and do it, do what I know to be right, at the time, 'cos I keep thinking, oh, maybe I'm not right.

RHONDA: SO, OBVIOUSLY THAT WAS A REALLY HARD TIME FOR YOU EMOTIONALLY TOO?

Camilla: Very difficult, oh yeah, very difficult time.

RHONDA: AND HOW DID YOUR HUSBAND COPE AT THAT TIME? DID HE COMMENT ON HOW YOU WERE FEELING?

Camilla: Yeah, we coped pretty well I think, for the situation. I still remembered it as the most terrible experience, yeah. I think he tried to walk away from the situation and let me deal with it too much at the time. When I look back on it now, I think he tried his hardest, but he didn't realise how desperate it was, and it took him a long time to realise how desperate it was. And STILL, it was up to me to do — you know, go and get help.

So I felt that was something he couldn't deal — well he did try — like he was the one who went up and saw the Principal, and the School Support Centre, but he was getting nowhere, so he felt that he always came to dead-ends, so it was left to me to find other avenues. So he'd done all that initial work, but we just didn't get any help.

Like the Principal admits, now, that she never had a school refusal case as bad, and never had to deal with it, so she didn't know. The School Support Centre had someone — the person that was dealing with our particular case went on sick leave, and the person that was supposed to fill in went on sick leave as well, so we had — that's why he kept running to me, 'cos he couldn't get any help that way.

But it was just — I happened to run into this child psychiatrist that I was recommended who had dealt with cases like that all the time. As soon as he explained the situation, then I realised it wasn't me, and so I could deal with it. When you're always thinking it might — 'what have I done wrong?' And school — like with people that we had from the school go, 'what's wrong at home?' and of course there's NOTHING wrong at home. I'm saying, 'there's nothing wrong'. So, once he explained what had happened, and how it came about, then I always felt I could deal with it a lot better, and I got very determined about it.

On the Social Support Questionnaire, Camilla's score for support from her partner was 0.63 which was the same as the case group mean and below the control group mean of 0.79. For support offered by all family members and friends Camilla's responses gave a score of 2.01, which was well below both the case and control group means.

RHONDA   DO YOU SEE YOURSELF AT ALL AS HAVING HAD POSTNATAL DEPRESSION?

Camilla   Yeah. Not like — I've got a girlfriend who's had it very severely, and I've looked after her children for her. When I think back on that, I think that emotionally I was never very stable, especially, yeah, I'd reckon I'm not really stable; sometimes I am on the edge. But when you speak to close friends about that sort of thing they say, 'oh yeah' or you know, 'I think most mums are', so I think, oh well, yeah alright, so we all are. But at the time I think, mmm, if we could think back — various times it might be your husband came home and you're sitting on the kitchen floor with two children crying, and you're crying too, so that's sick. It was really sick (laughs).

RHONDA   WAS THERE ANY TIME WHERE YOU FELT YOU NEEDED OUTSIDE SUPPORT OR HELP, OR YOU SOUGHT THAT?

Camilla   No, but probably I should have, but no.

RHONDA   SO YOU WOULDN'T SAY YOU'VE REALLY HAD POSTNATAL DEPRESSION THIS TIME ROUND?

Camilla   No, I don't think so. I mean there's times when you get down, but there's not — no. I don't know how you classify it. How many times have you thought you're gonna kill yourself? I mean people must think that. Yeah, I've felt that this time round too, yeah. But you work yourself through it and it's really up to you. If you fight it and get really determined about it, then you get through it.

RHONDA	SO WHAT ADVICE WOULD YOU HAVE FOR OTHER WOMEN ABOUT HOW TO DEAL WITH FEELING DEPRESSED AFTER HAVING A CHILD?
Camilla	I think you should talk about it. Put it out in the open and then you'll find that you're not all by yourself. You're not going crazy because you feel that way. Everyone feels that way at some stage unless, I think, you're supermum. I don't know, I haven't found many that haven't felt that way.
RHONDA	AND ON THE WHOLE, AT THE MOMENT, WOULD YOU SAY THAT YOU HAVE MORE GOOD DAYS THAN BAD?
Camilla	Yeah, oh — yeah (laughs).
RHONDA	FIFTY-FIFTY, OR YOU THINK IT GOES THE OTHER WAY?
Camilla	It goes the other way. I'm just thinking back to the asthma that we've had in the last two weeks. That has been pretty horrid; lining up to the doctor to get cortisone and stuff like that.

Camilla's score on the EPDS (score = 16) filled in just prior to the interview indicated that she was depressed.

RHONDA	AND THE PART OF YOUR EXPERIENCE WHERE YOU SAY YOU FEEL AS THOUGH YOU PERHAPS HAVE EXPERIENCED POSTNATAL DEPRESSION — WHEN DOES THAT START AND IS THAT SOMETHING YOU FEEL HAS PASSED NOW?
Camilla	No, look, I just — yeah, usually in the first few months you feel pretty down about things. It's just trying to cope with less sleep and feeling like a zombie, and not being able to speak to people properly because you're too tired to think, but then there's stages when the kids get older that you think — you get really down yourself, like I do, when the kids are sick. But I don't know how to cope with this situation, so then I get down about that, and then I start to entertain ideas: they'd be much better off without me; then I think, you're nuts; and you could be suffering from it but no one's ever picked it up …
RHONDA	SO YOU SEE IT AS SOMETHING THAT PERHAPS COMES AND GOES?
Camilla	Yeah. You teeter on the edge and come back a bit, and then go back to the edge again and think, oh, will you jump or not, yeah.

Stephanie Brown, Rhonda Small, Judith Lumley

THIRTEEN

What Women Do About Depression

Vivienne Welburn likens the experience of depression to having a huge load of sand dumped outside your door.

> After we have given birth it is as if we wake up to discover that a mountain of sand has been deposited in front of the doors of our home. Some women get to work energetically to dig routes out. They have friends who come along and help. They work around the sand; they find marvellously inventive ways to cope with the situation. Some women find one difficult route out and stick to that. Some try to dig a way through and get buried, others just look at it, feel defeated, retreat within their four walls and give up.[1]

As we talked with women all over Victoria who had been depressed in the weeks and months after giving birth, we were repeatedly reminded of this analogy. Women spoke about feeling they had entered a tunnel from which there seemed at the time no way out, of feeling 'like there was a rock or something sitting there that wouldn't move'. They described to us the ways they had tried to deal with these feelings, and the issues and circumstances in their lives that they believed contributed to how they were feeling.

It was clear that women had found varied ways of 'shifting the sand'; that overcoming depression was something that could be achieved in any number of ways. The individual pathways women took were contingent upon their ideas of what was making them depressed, the extent to which help was offered to them, their knowledge of places they might go for assistance, and the degree to which they felt that what they were experiencing was something for which they might seek help from other people. Many women coped alone or with very little assistance, and we return to this later in the chapter.

In carrying out the study we did not attempt to evaluate different treatments offered to women, as important as such research is. Our purpose was more exploratory. Very little is known about what recent mothers do about feeling depressed, about who they turn to for help, and what sort of help is offered. More importantly, we also wanted to find out what women found helpful. Were there common themes in what they found helpful, despite different conceptualisations of the problem? And what would they advise other mothers to do in the same situation?

SEEKING HELP FROM HEALTH PROFESSIONALS

Close to two-thirds of the women in the case group (29/45), and three-fifths of the women in the control group who had felt depressed (9/15) had not sought professional assistance concerning their depression. Only twenty women had turned to a health professional for assistance about feeling depressed. This finding is strikingly similar to that recently reported in a Glasgow study which looked at help-seeking behaviour in 60 first-time working-class mothers.[2] A little over one-third of the women in the Glasgow study who had felt depressed had turned to a health professional for help with their depression.

Table 13.1 Help sought from professional sources: cases (16/45) and controls depressed (4/15)*

Source	Sought help Cases	Controls	Total	Found it helpful Cases	Controls	Total
General Practitioner	11	2	13	8	1	9
Maternal and Child Health nurse	9	2	11	5	1	6
Psychiatrist	4	2	6	1	1	2
Psychologist	3	0	3	3	–	3
Obstetrician	2	0	2	1	–	1

*Women may have sought and/or received help from more than one source
Proportion of all women helped = 16/60
Proportion of all women in the case group helped = 13/45
Proportion of all women who had felt depressed in the control group helped = 3/15

Most women in our study who had sought professional assistance had contacted a general practitioner or their local Maternal and Child Health nurse (see table 13.1), with only a small number of women seeking out or being referred to a specialist mental health professional (8/60). Several women sought assistance from a number of sources, or were referred by one professional to another. Not all women actually found the assistance they were offered helpful. In all, thirteen women in the case group and three in the control group said they had been helped by a health professional in dealing with their feelings of depression.

When women described their experiences of turning to health

professionals for help, some very clear messages emerged about what they found helpful and what they did not. The following extracts from several interviews show that women appreciated health professionals who gave them time, acknowledged their feelings, and offered support.

Irma Cahill She'll [Maternal and Child Health nurse] just sit there and talk to you. She'll just let other people wait even ... she was I think maybe the first one to pick it up.

Katrina Peterson We spoke to the local doctor who we know really well. He has young children too, and is much our age. He was really good. I mean he always asks after both of us and how everyone's going. And he always makes a point when we take the children in of asking how we are doing. [Katrina's baby woke every two hours throughout the night for the first twelve months.]

Kerrie Sneddon I mean it wasn't the cure [talking to GP]. I think I just needed the time. But it was helpful. [Kerrie was in the control group, but visited her GP 'every second week' for a long period in the first year.]

Margit Gunn Well she [psychiatrist] offers just to talk through things. She'll ask questions, you know, and make me talk through a lot of things. And then at one stage she suggested that perhaps I'd have to go on anti-depressants, but it must have been a trigger, or whatever, because that seemed to do the trick. I seemed to snap out of it. Although she suggested I should go on anti-depressants, I really never did. Just talking — just having someone who's impartial — you could just talk through all sorts of things was good.

Dawn Harrison And then I saw my local female GP who was just wonderful. We had more of a discussion on the tablets I was taking and things. And they'd even been issued wrongly [by the hospital]. I'd been given the wrong things ... And I did a bit of counselling with her. And then finally realising that it was me who was going to do it anyway. Me that was going to solve my problems. So I slowly started to climb out.

Irma Cahill He [obstetrician attended for second pregnancy] actually had a few patients of his own that came in, and he picked it up straight away with them, and asked if I'd mind talking to them about how I felt. I had a few of them keep in touch for a while, and talked about how we felt over the phone ... It sort of let people know that you're not the only one that's going through it, and I think that helps.

As Kerrie Sneddon implied, a cure was not what most women expected when they sought help, but the experience of being heard, of being able to share their distress with someone else helped.

On the other hand, the extracts below indicate that when women's feelings are denied, when they feel unable or are not given the opportunity to talk, the experience of seeking help can be a very disheartening one.

> *Stephanie*   *Do you have a local doctor? Have you talked to him or her about it at all?*
> *Liza Rogers*   Yes, I have mentioned it.
> *Stephanie*   *Did that help you?*
> *Liza*   No, he just says, well it has to come from you. If you're unhappy about something I have to change it. I have to get my rest, or change what I don't like. I mean there's no counselling in the world that can help you with all that, can they really? It has to come from you. Things don't change, do they?

Other women had even more disheartening experiences, feeling that their level of distress was dismissed, or dealt with in a hurried and uncaring manner by professionals who appeared too busy to take a real interest.

> *Dawn Harrison*   Even at my six-week check-up, I went to the doctor [obstetrician] and said I don't feel terribly right about things. He then asked me if I was abusing my children. And I said no, and he said 'Don't worry', which I just could not believe. So after that of course, I just didn't mention it to many people. Then I found I was getting very depressed all the time ... [After some months] I took myself off to —— —— [hospital outpatients department] in Melbourne. And I came home very disheartened, because I'd sat and talked to someone for not even an hour, who'd given me some tablets and told me to come home and I'd be fine ... So I came away thinking, is that it? Am I solved? And I wasn't. It was a terrible feeling to go there and come out and feel worse than I went. I really felt I hadn't received anything.

> *Freda Holding*   Oh, I wouldn't go back to her [psychiatrist she attended for three months before being hospitalised with depression]. She was helpful, but she was always busy, like she didn't have the time to help you ... I wouldn't go back on it [medication]. I think what happened was, I think the psychiatrist, she was in a hurry that day. Without really checking me, she just gave me the medication ... She was in a hurry, she just said 'Take this, come back and see me'. Well I never got back to see her, the medication gave me a bad reaction [after which she was hospitalised].

Sometimes the advice that was offered simply didn't match up to the help women were seeking.

Melissa Dean At one stage I did [seek help from the Maternal and Child Health nurse] when I had Tracey, because she was terrible. When she got to the terrible two stage, I was really crying with her. I got really upset with her, 'cos I just couldn't control her, and they sent this nursing sister out to talk to me, but she was telling me I should try this and try that. But I was doing everything she said.

Melissa had also talked to her GP about feeling depressed, and again felt she could not take up any of his suggestions.

Melissa He just said 'Try to relax. Do yoga.' Relax! It's hard to relax with kids all the time.

Another woman who spent some time in a mother and baby hospital felt that she and her baby 'hadn't been able to fit into their system', and although she was able to decide the assistance offered was not what she wanted, she was left feeling very under-confident about her own judgements.

Well they would have put it that they had been unable to help us, but really we hadn't been able to fit into their system, which we felt was really just breaking children. It wasn't only what was happening to —— [our baby], but I think we were sensitive or we felt we were sensitive to the way they were treating the other children too, and I'm not implying cruelty or anything, but we felt it was more that you kind of break them, and that was their way of dealing with things. But that's just a different perception of child raising too I s'pose, but in spite of that, I still questioned completely my ability.

Although this woman talked to her Maternal and Child Health nurse about how things were going with the baby, and thought that her local nurse was 'a nice person', she did not ever feel her nurse detected how distressed and under-confident she was about how she was coping.

It was difficult — I don't know — I think she [Maternal and Child Health nurse] felt I was perhaps coping better than I was. I don't think she ever really knew until I ended up in —— [hospital], and I think that she was almost surprised. She'd make comments like, how well I kept the house or kept myself or kept —— [the baby], and I think she was basing it on that and just didn't know what an effort it was, and didn't know that wasn't done half the time anyway.

Often a negative experience with a health professional meant that women simply gave up asking for help. Other women were more persistent in seeking help, and talked to several health professionals before they felt happy with the help offered. Sometimes this proved a lengthy and painful process. Dawn Harrison first mentioned feeling depressed to her obstetrician at her six week check-up. When she was still feeling panicky and 'flying into tempers' some months later, she spoke to her Maternal and Child Health nurse who referred her to a public hospital outpatients clinic. At the hospital she was prescribed medication, but came home 'disheartened because I'd sat and talked to someone not even an hour, who'd given me some tablets and told me to go home and I'd be fine'. It was only when she went back to her Maternal and Child Health nurse and 'burst out crying, and cried and cried' that she was referred to a local doctor whom she felt finally listened to her story and understood. And with this assistance she was able slowly, with both medication and counselling, to begin to 'climb out' of her depression.

Sometimes problems arose because of practical difficulties — such things as getting an appointment at a manageable time — or because the woman was unsure about the treatment being offered.

> *Stephanie* *And who did you seek help from?*
> *Liza Rogers* We went to —— [community health centre]. She's a doctor, a psychiatrist.
>
> *Stephanie* *And what sort of assistance were they offering?*
> *Liza* They were offering drugs and counselling. But I haven't got the drugs yet and I don't really want to take them. I don't like the idea of taking them.
>
> *Stephanie* *The counselling, has that part of it been helpful?*
> *Liza* No, because you have to wait. Probably be lucky to get an appointment in a month. And then it's a work day ... and she's [psychiatrist] only there on Wednesdays ... And as I say, she keeps wanting me to take these pills, and I haven't had the money to buy them at the moment, and I don't like the idea of taking them. But she keeps assuring me I need them.

Although Liza had sought help, the fact that counselling could not be offered straight away or at a convenient time, and that she was both unsure about taking medication and felt that she could not afford it, meant she ended up feeling that she had received no assistance at all. Liza was one of two women among the control group who were depressed at follow-up.

In a few cases, it was evident that women's access to professional assistance was enhanced by knowing someone, either as friends or colleagues, who worked in relevant areas. Cassandra Lightfoot initially said no to our enquiry about whether she had sought any professional assistance, but reflected later in the interview that her supervisor at work had helped to put her experiences into perspective.

> Actually when I was going through that time, my supervisor who I talked to about my clients, I spoke to her about how I was feeling. I forgot about that. And what she did was basically say, she normalised it for me. She said you've been through a very traumatic experience.

Annette Flynn was able to draw on a friend who worked as a clinical psychologist to provide advice regarding her son's behaviour and her own ways of coping with this.

> Well when I went there I thought he [psychologist] might interview me about David. All he did was talk to me, and it sorted out my problems, because I was feeling down as well ... I mean my husband had been telling me that I'd been doing everything okay, everything'd turn out ... So when I went and saw someone else, and when they told me everything was alright, You're doing everything you can [to manage a sick baby and a toddler]. What you've had is a situation you didn't have control of, so there's no way you should feel guilty ... that made me feel better.

Annette contrasted this advice with the approach of her general practitioner:

> I mean with David's [toddler] anxiety he said that he'll just grow out of it and everything will be alright, but he didn't say to me 'Well you're okay, you're doing a great job, you're not causing this'.

The difference between saying it will pass, and 'you're doing a great job' was very important in enabling Annette to get on with the task of caring for her youngest child — who was constantly sick with ear infections — without feeling overwhelmed by all that she could not do for her older son given the demands of a crying baby.

Finally, it is worth emphasising that sometimes the offer of quite minimal support was all that women seemed to need. Sometimes just the offer of a telephone number, of support at the end of the phone if a woman felt really desperate, was enough to get through the most difficult times. This was Ruth Murray's experience and also Caitlin Adamson's. Once Caitlin spoke to her Maternal and Child Health nurse and her general practitioner and knew she could phone them any time, she 'felt much better'. Ruth Murray reflected that

[It was] not that she [Maternal and Child Health nurse] offered any miraculous cure, but I felt she really understood what I was talking about and that was helpful.

SEEKING HELP FROM FAMILY, FRIENDS AND COMMUNITY SOURCES

Half of the women who had felt depressed (23/45 cases, 7/15 controls) had sought help from one or more of the non-professional sources listed in table 13.2. Of the 57 women who were living with their partners and had felt depressed, only 20 turned to their partners for help. Of these, just over half had found their partners helpful. Given that feeling unsupported featured so often in women's descriptions of contributing factors, and that women in the case group turned to their partners less often for emotional support than women in the control group, it is not particularly surprising so few women asked their partners for help.

Table 13.2 Help sought from non-professional sources: cases (23/45) and controls depressed (7/15)*

Source	Sought help Cases	Controls	Total	Found it helpful Cases	Controls	Total
Partner	18	2	20	9	2	11
Mother	7	2	9	3	2	5
Other relative	2	0	2	2	–	2
Friends	15	6	21	14	4	18
Support group	4	0	4	1	–	1

*Women may have sought and/or received help from more than one source
Proportion of all women helped = 24/60
Proportion of all women in the case group helped = 19/45
Proportion of all women who had felt depressed in the control group helped = 5/15

Partners were judged as unsupportive by over 50 per cent of the women who had been depressed, and almost one in five women in the case group said that their partners had not even noticed that they were feeling depressed (see Chapter 9). Only 20 per cent of all the women with partners who had felt depressed had found their partners of assistance in dealing with the experience. However, for those women who did receive support from their partners when they felt depressed, this was clearly very important and helpful in their recovery.

Stephanie   *How did your husband react to your being depressed?*
Mary Chan   He was very supportive.
Stephanie   *In what sorts of ways?*
Mary   He'd make the effort to come home a little bit earlier and help out. He just told me one weekend to just go. If I want to get out, just go. Don't worry about the kids. I went on a week's holiday with some girlfriends, and he took the week off and minded the three boys. So he has been, and still is, very supportive. He does, and I really believe him, he does see this role as being harder than what he does at work. He knows first hand, he's done it. So in that way I can rely on him to get out any grievances I've got.

Just over one-third of women had turned to friends and this was nearly always reported as helpful. In almost every case, these friends were other women, mostly also mothers of young children who could readily identify with the feelings being experienced. The help offered was most frequently emotional or practical support, sometimes involving daily contact, as in Ruth Murray's case.

The best thing for me was that I had a very supportive friend, one in particular, who'd already had a child and was really willing to help. She used to ring every day, and offer really good advice. And she'd say there's light at the end of the tunnel. And I used to say 'No, there can't be'. Oh, but there is, there is (laughs).

Comparing the helpfulness of these two most common sources of assistance, partners and friends, friends were significantly more likely to be reported as helpful (18/21 versus 11/20).

Surprisingly few women had turned to a community support group of any kind. Only four women had made contact with a support group when looking for help related to feeling depressed. New mother's groups often held at Maternal and Child Health Centres, and playgroups of various kinds, were seen by some women as beneficial in that they enabled the sharing of experiences between mothers of babies. Angelina Razos, a young single mother, found a new mother's group very positive in this regard.

I think the thing that probably helped me the most was when Alice was six months old the health centre sister organised six of us — we all had kids the same age — and we talked things over, and getting it from other first-time mums 'Oh your kid does that too!' I mean I know it's the classic cliche ... but that helped a lot, 'cos then I realised I wasn't on my own.

However, these groups were sometimes not experienced as supportive, especially when discussions focused on children's achievements, and left unspoken the more difficult aspects of being a mother.

For some women, the notion of getting out to a group was more than they had been able to manage, particularly when they had more than one child, but also because taking the initiative of participating in a group when feeling depressed was very difficult. Amanda Joseph joined a new mother's group in order to meet other mothers in her area, but found it took her a long time to feel she could open up to any of the other mothers in the group.

> If someone came to the door I'd put on this smile and cup of tea and that, and I'd really be wishing 'Oh, I wish you'd just go'.
> *Judith So friends weren't — they didn't seem to be appropriate for finding this kind of help?*
> Amanda Well, I only met —— [friend] through the first mothers group, so you don't sort of blurt that out all at once.

'I DON'T THINK ANYONE EVER REALISED HOW BAD I WAS'

Twenty-eight women who took part in the study reported not seeking help from anyone regarding their depression. Ten women in the case group (10/45, 22 per cent) and six in the control group (6/15, 40 per cent) sought help from family members or friends, but not from professionals. The reasons women gave for not seeking help, or talking only to family and friends about how they were feeling, varied. Several women said there was no one whom they felt they could trust, or knew well enough to talk to about their distress. Amanda Joseph moved to Melbourne three years before the birth of her daughter. She felt this contributed to her isolation.

> We'd been in Melbourne three years, and I was working in the city and I really didn't have close friends there. It takes quite a while to sort of, to build up a really close friend, and that's why I joined a couple of new mother's groups and things so I could meet people. But not sort of moan and groan on their shoulders. So I had nobody I could cry to, so that's why I just cried to myself.

Even when people offered to help, Amanda found it difficult to accept assistance.

> I thought it was just me, and I tried to put on this brave face that yes, I could cope. If people came and offered to look after Emma, I wouldn't give her to them ... People were quite willing to drop meals and things around for me, but I don't think anyone ever realised how bad I was.

This was despite the fact that Amanda experienced chronic bleeding for six months after the birth, as well as frequent bouts of mastitis, and had a child who suffered with colic. Even though Amanda said she had read books that discussed the possibility of depression after having a baby, she felt she ought to be able to cope.

> I just thought it must be me; that I'm just not coping well. I'd say 'Everybody else copes, so why can't I?' But really I mean I think there's not enough [information on depression] around and maybe you're not aware that it's okay not to cope.

Amanda Joseph was not alone in putting on a 'brave face'. Several other women described how they put on their make-up before they went to the Maternal and Child Health centre, or went there on days when they were not feeling too miserable. Charlotte Williams discussed with a friend who was a nurse the possibility of spending some time in a mother and baby hospital in order to get some rest, but decided that,

> there's no way ... It wasn't so much admitting defeat or anything, but *I felt that only people who didn't cope, that were terrible mothers, did that.* [emphasis added]

For other women, it was more a matter of feeling people wouldn't understand.

> *Rhonda Did your partner notice or comment on how you were?*
> Kaylene Shaw He may notice I guess. He's more likely to get annoyed with me and say 'Wake up to yourself!', you know, rather than try and solve the problem. So I guess I don't talk to him a lot about why I'm feeling depressed. I just generally try to work it through myself or I'll go and talk to Mum.

Kaylene's isolation was compounded by the distance she had to travel to gain access to local services in the country area where she lived, and by the responsibility she felt to be available to assist her husband with farm work, which meant she was reluctant to leave the farm.

Some women who had been depressed, but saw this as directly linked to their baby's ill-health or constant crying, chose not to talk to anyone about their feelings, thinking that 'once they fixed the baby, I'd come good', although this did not always follow. One woman refrained from seeking help for herself, commenting that 'there was really no answer. I don't think anybody knows why some babies are good sleepers and others aren't.'

Crying babies were also experienced as an obstacle to going out and being amongst people who might help. Amanda Joseph described how she 'used to be paranoid about taking Emma anywhere because she'd cry a lot'. Another woman said that whenever the children were asleep, this time was precious and she did not want to use it by talking to someone.

> I guess every minute counted. If I had both of them asleep, I was gonna lay down myself. I just wasn't going to bother picking up the phone and talking to somebody.

Other women spoke about lack of confidence as a major obstacle to seeking help. In the following extract, a woman describes how in hindsight she felt she would have gained a great deal from joining a new mothers group, but at the time she had been unable to do this.

> Something I've always wanted to do but never been quite an open enough person to do is go to the health centre and go to these, like, mother's meetings that they have down there.

Another reason for not speaking about their distress was fear of being considered an unfit mother and of having their children removed from their care. Two women, Clare Thornton and Georgia Trembath, spoke about their fears that Maternal and Child Health nurses were there to check up on their mothering abilities, rather than to provide support and a listening ear.

Often women had very low expectations of anyone being interested in their experiences as mothers, or that anyone would think that these experiences were important. Over and over again, as we thanked women for their time and trouble in participating in the study they insisted that it was *they* who were grateful for the interest we had shown in their experiences. Some women said no one had ever bothered to ask them about the birth, or about how they felt about their lives as mothers. Others thanked us for taking up issues that were critical to them, but seemed to be of low social priority.

ADVICE TO OTHER MOTHERS

Towards the end of each interview, we asked women who had been depressed what advice they would give to other mothers having a similar experience. Table 13.3 documents the advice women gave, with their most frequent suggestions listed first. Reflecting upon their own experiences, the advice women most often gave was to find someone to talk to about feeling depressed, and to try to organise some time out from mothering. These responses were also most likely to be mentioned first. Women were three times as likely to recommend talking to someone as they were to suggest seeking medical help.

Table 13.3 Advice to other mothers about dealing with depression from women who had felt depressed themselves (n=60)

Advice	Frequency of response	First mentioned response
Find someone to talk to	30	19
Find time for self	18	12
Get out among people	12	3
Seek counselling	10	5
Seek medical help	8	4
See a support group	8	2
See a Maternal and Child Health nurse	6	1
No advice	6	6
Just get through it	4	1
Will end	2	0
Other advice	20	2
Missing	5	5

Combining all the suggestions that involve talking and interaction with others (finding someone to talk to, seeking counselling, talking to a Maternal and Child Health nurse, joining a support group, getting out among people), over 75 per cent of women (32/45 cases and 14/15 controls who had been depressed) mentioned contact with other people and/or 'talking about it' in their suggestions to other women. However, as we have already seen, many women found these things difficult to do at the time, requiring lots of encouragement and interest shown by health professionals or friends and family members before they felt they could comfortably and legitimately talk about how they were feeling.

FINDING ROUTES OUT

To some extent this chapter paints a depressing picture. Many women did not receive the kind of encouragement to talk about their feelings or the assistance from either their partners, friends or health professionals that might have enabled some clearing of the sand deposited on their front doorstep around the time that their baby was born. The problems women experienced — poor physical health, adverse life experiences, a sick child or a child with a difficult temperament — often seemed intractable. On the other hand, the kinds of assistance that in hindsight women believed might have helped them, or did indeed help them deal with these and other difficulties were often quite simple: acknowledgment that these problems were real and their feelings about them understandable; someone (anyone?) being prepared to listen to their thoughts on what was happening in their lives; to be told they were doing a good job, or that they are a good mother, or that it is okay to feel one needs a break from children; that children survive and possibly benefit when their mothers have a break from them; and *not* being told they are 'crazy' for finding motherhood difficult at times. Explicit recognition by someone else that the demands of looking after one or more children who wake frequently at night, cry when not being held or soothed, or suffer from frequent ill-health; or that other circumstances in women's lives such as partners who are absent most of the day, financial difficulties, or their own poor health, may be more than they can manage was very helpful when it was given.

The overwhelming view from women who had been depressed was that talking about it helped. In recent years, intervention studies have begun to demonstrate the value of strategies built around acknowledging women's feelings, supportive counselling and offering a 'listening ear' in reducing levels of depression among recent mothers.[3] This is not to deny the potency of the difficult circumstances that surrounded many women's experiences of motherhood. The way in which fathers contribute to child care and household work, the structural and psychological barriers to men spending more time at home with children, the social and emotional barriers to women being involved in paid employment and/or having other 'timeout' from mothering responsibilities, and the poor response of health services to the physical health problems women often suffer after childbirth also need to change.

But there is also much that health professionals, the partners, friends and relatives or women who have recently had a baby, and women themselves can learn from this study. Depression after childbirth is a very common experience; listening to what women say about their lives as mothers and acknowledging the validity of these feelings — believing women — may make an enormous difference to women currently dealing with the sorts of difficulties experienced by the women in this study.

Rhonda Small, Stephanie Brown, Judith Lumley

AN AFTERWORD

What does the phrase, 'a motherhood statement', now in such widespread use that it qualifies as a cliche, actually mean? Is it a statement that everyone agrees with but no one is going to do anything about? Does it imply wishful thinking? Is it a critique about escaping from the harsh realities of a situation or an argument? Whatever the intent may be on a particular occasion, the phrase 'a motherhood statement', particularly in its common form 'just a motherhood statement', carries a freight of meaning: trivial, unimportant, able to be dismissed or disregarded, off the point, irrelevant to the main purpose. The phrase is thus a true representation of what many women perceived and described to us as the experience of being a mother: motherhood often brought with it a sense that what one was doing or feeling or saying was being dismissed as trivial, disregarded as unimportant, or even not heard at all. This is accentuated in this study by the fact that more than half of the women interviewed had been depressed, so that the darker shades of women's experiences as mothers are given full weight, rather than being discounted.

What women wanted most was the recognition that someone was listening. The Chinese ideogram for 'listening' is composed from the four signs for ear, eyes, heart and undivided attention.

> It is as though he listened and such listening as his enfolds us in a silence in which at last we begin to hear what we are meant to be.
> (Lao-Tze Tâo Teh King)

It was this 'being heard' that women, especially women who were depressed, sought from their partners, their friends, their families and the health professionals with whom they came into contact. Some of them found it.

It is our hope that the 'motherhood statements' in this book, the powerful and moving accounts of what it is like to be a mother, will be heard and will make it easier for other mothers to find someone who 'listens' to them with eyes, ears, heart and undivided attention.

Judith Lumley

APPENDIX 1

Other Research Issues

ASSESSING SATISFACTION AND DISSATISFACTION

Interpreting measures of satisfaction needs to be approached with caution. As Ann Jacoby and Ann Cartwright have commented, satisfaction is both 'difficult to define and to measure in a meaningful way'.[1] A repeated finding in studies of satisfaction with maternity care is that general questions about how women feel about the care they received elicits high levels of expressed satisfaction. Over 60 per cent of women interviewed in one of the British studies said they were satisfied with the way their labours were managed, 33 per cent said their labour was managed as they liked in some ways and not in others. Only 6 per cent said their labours were not managed as they liked.[2] Even higher rates of satisfaction were reported in a representative sample of recent mothers surveyed in Arizona by the Department of Health: 93 per cent reported themselves as satisfied or very satisfied with antenatal care; 90 per cent rated their care during labour and delivery in the same way.[3]

Such global measures of satisfaction, it has been argued, may mask important differences in satisfaction with particular aspects of care.[4] The first postal questionnaire included several questions relating to overall satisfaction with antenatal care, the management of labour, kindness of staff and so on, together with more specific questions about particular aspects of care, such as access to information, continuity of care-givers at antenatal appointments, and time spent waiting for check-ups. Comparisons of this kind confirm the findings of other studies that women may express high levels of satisfaction in response to general questions, while simultaneously reporting high levels of dissatisfaction with particular aspects of their care.

WHY A POPULATION SAMPLE?

Why did we bother to study a sample of the complete population of women giving birth in a given period? It would have been easier to go to the nearest large hospital and arrange to send questionnaires to, or even to visit, one thousand of their recent mothers. Many studies have used hospital-based samples,[5] but in Australia it is highly unlikely that a city hospital will be truly representative of the community. The largest ones have a very mixed clientele: women at high risk of complications, women living in the inner city, above average proportions of recent immigrants, refugees and women without partners, and increasingly, a private section with a high proportion of women over 35 years of age. In many ways this is very different from the whole population.

Hospital-based samples may also have too little variation in the patterns of obstetric care to enable analysis of associations between these factors and emotional well-being,[6] and a study at a single location would not allow comparison between the experiences of women living in the city and the country. Very few studies of depression after birth have included any women living outside cities and large towns.

Our population sample did exclude women whose babies died before birth or between birth and the time of the survey. The reasons for excluding these women were two-fold: first, we thought the approach might upset and distress them, and second, the questionnaire did not deal with specific concerns they might have had about procedures or staff attitudes around the death of their child. In terms of satisfaction with care and depression after birth these women are a very important group, but their numbers in a single week of births (between 10 and 20) are too few for separate analysis. Any conclusions that could be drawn from the study cannot be generalised to include women whose babies died.

Many other studies of depression have excluded large groups of women. The commonest are women who have had a previous child; a surprising category, since such women are a majority of women giving birth. Perhaps it is to simplify the research questions by not having to take into account women's experiences after an earlier birth. This exclusion certainly reduces the generalisability of findings, and it may be a contributing factor to the not uncommon view that depression after birth is a problem of first-time mothers only, and hence readily explained by lack of knowledge about parenthood or 'unreal expectations'.

Many studies have excluded women without partners and some have excluded migrant women. It is likely that these exclusions have also been carried out to simplify the research questions. Unfortunately, the exclusion of powerful social differences (the presence of other children, the lack of a partner, being in a country far from family and friends) necessarily leads to a focus on intrapsychic and interpersonal factors in the development of depression.

COMMUNITY STUDIES AND CLINICAL STUDIES
In the course of these research projects we often came across the

view that depression after birth was mostly a problem of first-time mothers. Other people were equally convinced that women living in poverty, women with poor housing, or those with little or no access to transport would be most likely to be affected. The extent to which any of the stereotypes were borne out by the evidence in this project is discussed in Chapter 6, but it can briefly be said here that these factors were not at all powerful.

One reason why there can be a big gulf between the picture gained in a community- or population-based study and the views held even by health professionals is that only a small proportion of women with depression seek any professional help, and an even smaller proportion seek help from a mental-health professional.

The clinical sample — those seen by a health professional — are not necessarily those with the most severe or sustained symptoms. In our study there were no differences in EPDS scores between those who sought professional help and those who did not. The processes by which they had reached a general practitioner or a Maternal and Child Health nurse were quite diverse but all required the woman herself (or a close friend or relative) to identify that 'something was wrong', and that this 'something' was a health issue rather than a case of domestic incompetence, a family secret, or a moral failing. The further steps whereby some women went on to be referred to a psychologist or a psychiatrist are even more complex. It is these recognition and referral practices, including personal and social barriers, that determine who enters the clinical sample of depressed women.[7]

Babies with feeding, sleeping, or crying problems — 'unhappy' babies — are likely to have unhappy mothers. Almost 40 per cent of mothers whose babies were admitted to a mother and baby Karitane hospital in New South Wales scored as depressed on the EPDS, using the same cut-off score as we did. These mothers were predominantly first-time mothers, and only 10 per cent had experienced a caesarean birth.[8] A comparison of these two factors (parity and operative delivery) in the hospital clinical sample with the same factors in the whole population[9] (see Chapter 6), shows how misleading it would be to infer that having a first child was a major risk for depression, while having a caesarean birth was protective!

Equally it would be hazardous to extrapolate from the Karitane hospital admissions that all women who are depressed have unhappy or difficult babies. Some do, most do not. The Karitane sample did not include a high proportion of women with prior psychiatric problems: the proportion (13 per cent) was close to expected community rates and lower than the proportion in our population sample of women depressed at eight to nine months (20 per cent).

This raises the possibility that women who have previously received psychiatric treatment may be more likely to approach mental-health services if they develop depression after birth, rather than a mother and baby hospital or a paediatrician.

Brown and Harris, in their classic study of depression in women, involving both clinical and community samples, found significant differences between the two groups and they caution about this very issue:

> ... we begin to doubt the usefulness of much social and clinical research with psychiatric patients — at least with the more common conditions — without parallel investigations of those not receiving psychiatric care.[10]

The postal questionnaire and the follow-up study provide that parallel investigation into the circumstances and experiences of the majority of women with depression after birth.

CAUSES

The diseases that were once the most familiar, the infectious diseases, were also relatively straightforward and easy to understand. Although there were obviously aspects of the individual that affected whether or not she or he became ill when exposed to an infectious agent — such as malnutrition, or immunity from a previous exposure — the infectious agent was an essential factor. It was a necessary cause of the infection even if it was not in itself a sufficient cause.

With rare exceptions the major diseases and disorders of contemporary life do not have single necessary causes. For example, coronary heart disease is more common in men and women who have a strong family history of the problem, and even more common in families with specific genetic disorders, but the majority of people who develop this problem do not have a family history of it. Cigarette smoking is a definite risk factor for coronary heart disease, to an extent which depends on the number of cigarettes smoked per day and the number of years of smoking. The association of smoking with heart disease is consistent when studied in different places with different methods. Ex-smokers begin to lose their extra risks the longer it is since they quit. There is a large body of research as to what the mechanisms might be. Yet we probably all know many non-smokers with heart disease. Smoking is not a sufficient cause of heart disease. It is not even a necessary cause. Nor is fat consumption, nor being overweight, nor being a couch potato a necessary cause, though all are risk factors. They are factors that increase the chance that a person will develop heart disease.

In discussing depression after birth we look at the factors that make depression more likely to occur. None of them is a necessary factor, and only occasionally will any single factor be sufficient to lead to depression. That is why we use words like 'associated with' and 'factor', rather than 'cause', throughout the book.

RISKS: ABSOLUTE, RELATIVE AND ATTRIBUTABLE

The *absolute* risk of giving birth by caesarean section is about 17 in 100 births for women in Australia. This absolute risk differs a little across the States and Territories, being higher in South Australia (21.4 per cent) than in Tasmania (14.7 per cent).[11] The *relative* risk of having a caesarean birth in South Australia, compared with Tasmania, is the ratio of these two (21.4/14.7, i.e. 1.46) and many relative risks are presented throughout the book. Often the relative risk is expressed in terms of 'odds' as in betting. These terms are described at more length in Appendix 2.

The proportion of cases in the community explained by a specific factor is the risk attributable to that factor, or the *attributable* risk. A factor with a large relative risk may or may not be important in explaining a high proportion of cases. The other key component will be how common the factor itself is in the population. Chapter 6 summarises the evidence that mothers over 34 years of age having their first child do have a high odds of depression (more than nine-fold). Yet these women make up only 2.4 per cent of women giving birth, so this factor in itself accounts for relatively few cases. The *attributable* risk of older first-mothers for depression in the community is negligible. By contrast, the *attributable* risk of operative delivery for depression is much greater, since although the odds of depression are not as high in this latter group, the proportion of women experiencing a caesarean, forceps or vacuum extraction birth is almost one in three.

CODING

A structured coding schedule was developed for the home interviews before we began. After completing the first ten interviews we modified the coding, taking into account women's ways of responding to our questions. For example, a common reply to the question of how much the women had known about children before having their own was 'nothing at all' — which we had not predicted.

A further revision was made at the end of the interviews. This revised schedule was trialled by three of the authors via a process of triple coding the same six interviews followed by extensive discussion about any differences in coding and interpretation. Alterations were made to the coding schedule as a result to ensure the accuracy and comparability of coding between the authors. Following this, each author coded her own interviews using the interview transcripts and the notes she had made at the time of interview.

Coding the open-ended questions was more challenging. The process developed for looking at the question 'How would you describe a "good" mother?' gives a sense of the process. We tackled the task of analysing women's comments in a series of steps that employed both qualitative and quantitative approaches. The first step was to develop a coding schedule for this section of the interviews.

A preliminary coding schedule was developed by two of the research team after reading through twenty of the transcripts. One member of the team then began coding the transcripts using this schedule. Prior to coding, the transcripts were shuffled so that the order for coding did not reflect the order in which interviews had been undertaken, and to ensure that women in the case and control groups were not grouped together. The only identifying information on the transcripts was a number which did not indicate the woman's group status. In this first round of coding the categories we applied were fairly broad, and it was apparent that many women's responses did not fit within the framework we were using. As a result, we re-worked the coding categories and coded the transcripts again, this time with double the number of categories we had used in the preliminary schedule. After a further attempt, we decided to code women's responses in three domains. These were: qualities and attributes; a somewhat shorter list of tasks; and a third section in which we recorded comments from a few women who talked about how 'good' mothers balance their own needs with those of their children. This formed the basis of the final coding schedule.

The coding categories were revised (and the interview transcripts re-coded) four times before we were confident that they adequately covered what women had said. Anne Potter, a staff member at the Centre, but not a member of the research team, then spent a day reading and independently coding the transcripts. Any differences in coding were discussed with a member of the research team and agreement reached about the most appropriate coding in each case. There were five cases where agreement could not be reached, and these were referred back to the full research team. Having the interviews independently coded in this way enabled us to feel confident that our own knowledge of individual women was not leading to biased judgements about their comments. Even though the group status of individual women had been removed from the transcripts, just reading a small segment of a transcript was often enough for the interviewer to recall the woman's circumstances and status as either a case or control. As we were interested in looking for possible differences among women in the original case and control groups, and between women depressed and not depressed at follow-up, independent coding was an important step in the analysis.

APPENDIX 2

Glossary of Statistical Terms

Chi-Square (χ^2) test   Any statistical test based on comparison of a test statistic to a chi-square distribution. The oldest and most common chi-square tests are for detecting whether two or more population distributions differ from one another; these tests usually involve counts of data, and may involve comparison of samples from the distributions under study, or the comparison of a sample to a theoretically expected distribution.

Confidence interval   A range of values for a variable of interest constructed so that this range has the specified probability of including the true value of the variable. The specified variability is called the confidence level and the end points of the confidence interval are called the confidence limits.

Confounding   1. A situation in which the effects of two processes are not separated. The distortion of the apparent effect of an exposure on risk brought about by the association with other factors that can influence the outcome. 2. A relationship between the effects of two or more causal factors as observed in a set of data, such that it is not logically possible to separate the contribution that any single causal factor has made to the effect. 3. A situation in which a measure of the effect of an exposure on risk is distorted because of the association of exposure with other factors that influence the outcome under study.

Correlation   The degree to which variables change together.

Correlation coefficient.   A measure of association that indicates the degree to which two variables have a linear relationship. This coefficient, represented by the letter r, can vary between +1 and −1.

Interaction   1. The interdependent operation of two or more causes to produce or prevent an effect. 2. Differences in the effects of one or more factors according to the level of the remaining factor(s).

Mean (average)   The sum of the individual values of a variable divided by the number of individual values.

Median   The simplest division of a set of measurements is into two parts — the lower and the upper half. The median is the point on the scale that divides the group in this way.

Odds   The ratio of the probability of the occurrence of an event to that of non-occurrence or the ratio of the probability that something is so, to the probability that it is not so. *Odds ratio (relative odds)*   The ratio of two odds.

p (probability) value   The probability that a test statistic would be as extreme, or more extreme, than observed if the null hypothesis were true. *P ns* is a statement of the probability that the difference observed could have occurred by chance. A study result whose probability is less than 5 per cent (p<0.05) or 1 per cent (p<0.01) is considered sufficiently unlikely to have occurred by chance to justify the designation 'statistically significant'.

Regression analysis   Given data on a dependent variable and one or more independent variables regression analysis involves finding the 'best' mathematical model (within some restricted class of models) to describe the dependent variable as a function of the independent variables or to predict the dependent variable from the independent variables. The most common form is a linear model; in epidemiology *logistic* models are also common.

Relative risk (risk ratio)   The ratio of the risk of disease or death among the exposed to the risk among the unexposed.

Risk factor   An aspect of personal behaviour or lifestyle, an environmental exposure, or an inborn or inherited characteristic, which on the basis of epidemiologic evidence is known to be associated with health-related condition(s) considered to be important to prevent.

Sample   A selected subset of a population. A sample may be random or non-random and may be representative or non-representative.

Standard deviation   A measure of dispersion or variation. It is the most widely used measure of dispersion of a frequency distribution. It is equal to the positive square root of the variance. The mean tells where the values for a group are centred. The standard deviation is a summary of how widely dispersed the values are around this centre.

Statistical significance   Statistical methods allow an estimate to be made of the probability of the observed or greater degree of association between independent and dependent variables under the null hypothesis. From this estimate, in a sample of given size, the 'statistical significance' of a result can be stated. Usually, the level of statistical significance is stated by the *p value*.

Stratification The process or result of separating a sample into several sub-samples according to specified criteria such as age groups, socioeconomic status, etc. The effect of confounding variables may be controlled by stratifying the analysis of results.

t-test The *t*-test uses a statistic that, under the null hypothesis, has the *t*-distribution, to test whether two means differ significantly, or to test linear regression or correlation coefficients.

These definitions are taken from *A Dictionary of Epidemiology*, 2nd edition, edited by John Last, sponsored by the International Epidemiology Association, Oxford University Press, New York, 1988.

APPENDIX 3

Standardised Questionnaires and Obstetric Procedure Score

A brief descripion of the five standardised questionnaires used in the follow-up study is given below, including some examples of questions as well as the mean scores obtained on each questionnaire by women in the case and control groups at the time of follow-up.

Edinburgh Postnatal Depression Scale (EPDS)
[J.L. Cox, J.M. Holden, R. Sagovsjy, 'Detection of Postnatal Depression: Development of the 10-item Edinburgh Postnatal Depression Scale', *British Journal of Psychiatry* 150, 1987, 782–6]

The EPDS is a 10-item questionnaire in which women were asked to underline the answers that came closest to how they were feeling in the previous seven days. The cut-off score for depression was a score of thirteen or more.

Examples:
I have looked forward with enjoyment to things
    As much as I ever did
    Rather less than I used to
    Definitely less than I used to
    Hardly at all

Things have been getting on top of me
    Yes, most of the time I haven't been able to cope at all
    Yes, sometimes I haven't been coping as well as usual
    No, most of the time I have coped quite well
    No, I have been coping as well as ever

Mean score for the case group at follow-up: 11.3
Mean score for the control group at follow-up: 5.4

Experience of Motherhood Questionnaire (EMQ)
[J. Astbury, 'Making Motherhood Visible: The Experience of Motherhood Questionnaire', *Journal of Reproductive and Infant Psychology* (in press)]

The EMQ is a 20-item questionnaire that asks women to circle a number corresponding to their level of agreement with a range of statements about the changes brought about in their lives by having children. The numbers indicated agreement as follows: 1 = Not at all; 2 = Somewhat; 3 = Moderately so; 4 = Very much so. Higher scores obtained on the questionnaire indicate less positive experiences of motherhood.

Examples:
I find the trouble of organising a babysitter takes the pleasure out of going out

I have greater confidence since becoming a mother

I have little to talk about besides the child(ren)

Mean score for the case group: 43.3
Mean score for the control group: 37.0

Social Support Questionnaire (SSQ)
[I.G. Sarason, H.M. Levine, R.G. Basham, B.R. Sarason, 'Assessing Social Support: The Social Support Questionnaire', *Journal of Personal and Social Psychology* 44, 1983, 127–39]

The SSQ is a 27 item questionnaire that asks about people who provide help or support. Each question has two parts: one which requires the listing of all people (up to a maximum of nine) relied on for support in the manner described in the question and the second part is a rating of satisfaction with that support on a scale from very satisfied to very dissatisfied. Higher support scores indicate better levels of support.

Examples:
Whom can you really count on to listen to you when you need to talk?

Whom can you really count on to distract you from your worries when you feel under stress?

Mean social support score for the case group: 2.8
Mean social support score for the control group: 3.8

Mean partner support score for the case group: 0.6
Mean partner support score for the control group: 0.8

Mean satisfaction with support score for the case group: 5.0
Mean satisfaction with support score for the control group: 5.5

Life Experiences Questionnaire (LEQ)
[I.G. Sarason, J.H. Johnson, J.M. Siegel, 'Assessing The Impact of Life Changes: Development of the Life Experiences Survey', *Journal of Consulting and Clinical Psychology* 46, 1978, 932–46; J.S. Norbeck, 'Modification of Life Event Questionnaires

For Use with Female Respondents', *Research in Nursing and Health* 7, 1984, 61–71]

The LEQ is a 77-item questionnaire covering possible life events grouped in the following areas: health, work, study, love and marriage, family and close friends, parenting, personal and social, financial, crime and legal matters. It also includes provision to list further events not covered by the questionnaire. Women were asked to tick any events that had occurred since the child's birth and rate each one from –3 to +3 to indicate the degree of negative or positive impact on life at the time the event occurred (with nought indicating no impact).

Examples:
Major personal illness or injury (health)
Beginning/resuming work outside the home (work)
A change in closeness with your spouse or partner (love and marriage)

Mean number of positive life events for the case group: 5.3
Mean number of positive life events for the control group: 4.0

Mean number of negative life events for the case group: 6.8
Mean number of negative life events for the control group: 3.8

Mean positive impact score for the case group: 11.8
Mean positive impact score for the control group: 10.2

Mean negative impact score for the case group: 13.9
Mean negative impact score for the control group: 6.14

Toddler Temperament Scale (TTS)
[J. Sewell, F. Oberklaid, M. Prior, A. Sanson, M. Kyrios, 'Temperament in Australian Toddlers', *Australian Paediatric Journal* 24, 1988, 343–5]

The TTS is a 97-item scale intended to measure a child's behavioural style in interacting with his or her environment. For each question mothers were asked to circle the number that best corresponded to their child's recent and current behaviour. Statements felt not to apply to the child at all could be deleted. The numbers for rating the child's behaviour were as follows: 1 = Almost never; 2 = Rarely; 3 = Variable, usually not; 4 = Variable, usually does; 5 = Frequently; 6 = Almost always. The TTS enables a categorisation of the child as 'easy', 'difficult', 'slow to warm up' or 'intermediate'. It is also possible to calculate a score for a continuous variable of 'difficultness' with higher scores indicating greater 'difficultness'.

Examples:
The child accepts delays for several minutes for desired objects (snacks, rewards, gifts)

The child stops eating and looks up when a person walks by

The child plays actively (bangs, throw, runs) with toys indoors

Mean 'difficultness' score for the case group children: 16.6
Mean 'difficultness' score for the control group children: 15.9

Obstetric Procedure Score
[Adapted from S. Elliot, M. Anderson, D. Brough, J. Watson and A. Rugg, 'Relationship Between Obstetric Outcome and Psychological Measures in Pregnancy and the Postnatal Year', *Journal of Reproductive and Infant Psychology* 2, 1984, 19–22]

Details of the scoring system applied to obstetric procedures are as follows:

Procedure	*Score*
Pethidine	1
Episiotomy or tear requiring stitches	1
Induction	2
Augmentation	2
Epidural	4
Forceps	5
General Anaesthetic	6
Caesarean Section	10

NOTES

ACKNOWLEDGEMENTS

1 S. Brown and J. Lumley, 'Antenatal Care: A Case of the Inverse Care Law?', *Australian Journal of Public Health* 17, 1993, 95–102; J. Astbury, S. Brown, J. Lumley and R. Small, 'Birth Events, Birth Experiences and Social Difference in Depression After Birth', *Australian Journal of Public Health* 18, 1994, 176–84.
2 J. Lumley and S. Brown, 'Attenders and Non-Attenders at Childbirth Education Classes in Australia: How Do They and Their Births Differ?', *Birth*, 1993, 123–9; S. Brown and J. Lumley, 'Satisfaction with Care in Labor and Birth: A Survey of 790 Australian Women', *Birth* 21, 1994, 4–13.
3 J. Astbury, 'Making Motherhood Visible: The Experience of Motherhood Questionnaire', *Journal of Reproductive and Infant Psychology* (in press); R. Small, S. Brown, J. Lumley and J. Astbury, 'Missing Voices: What Women Say and Do About Depression After Childbirth', *Journal of Reproductive and Infant Psychology* (in press).
4 R. Small, J. Astbury, S. Brown and J. Lumley, 'Depression After Childbirth: Does Social Context Matter?', *Medical Journal of Australia* 161, 1994 (in press).
5 R. Small, J. Lumley and S. Brown, 'To Stay Or Not To Stay: Are Fears About Shorter Postnatal Hospital Stays Justified?', *Midwifery* 8, 1992, 170–7.
6 J. Lumley, 'Gatekeeping by Ethics Committees', in V. A. Brown and G. Preston (eds), *Choice and Change: Ethics, Politics and Economics of Public Health*, Public Health Association of Australia, Canberra, 1993, 72–6; S. Brown, J. Lumley, R. Small and J. Astbury, 'The Social Costs of Intervention in Childbirth', in Brown and Preston (eds), *Choice and Change*, 133–40.
7 J. Last (ed.), *A Dictionary of Epidemiology*, 2nd edn, Oxford University Press, New York, 1988.

PREFACE ON BELIEVING WOMEN

1 J.S. Mill, 'The Subjection of Women', in *On Liberty, Representative Government, the Subjection of Women*, Oxford University Press, London, 1974, 454.
2 A. Oakley, *Women Confined: Towards a Sociology of Childbirth*, Martin Robertson, Oxford, 1980.
3 J. Astbury and B. Bajuk, 'Psychological Aspects of Preterm Birth', in V. Y. H. Yu and E. C. Wood (eds), *Prematurity*, Churchill Livingstone, Melbourne, 1987.
4 S. Harding (ed.), *Feminism and Methodology*, Indiana University Press, Bloomington, and Open University Press, Milton Keynes, 1987.
5 J.L. Cox, A. Rooney, P.F. Thomas and R.W. Wrate, 'How Accurately Do Mothers Recall Postnatal Depression: Further Data From a 3 Year Follow-Up Study', *Journal of Psychosomatic Obstetrics and Gynaecology* 3, 1984, 185–9.

6 B.K. Armstrong, E. White and R. Saracci, 'Methods of Exposure Measurement', in *Principles of Exposure Measurement in Epidemiology*, Oxford University Press, Oxford, 1992, 22–48.
7 C.J. Martin, 'Monitoring Maternity Services by Postal Questionnaire: Congruity between Mothers' Reports and Their Obstetric Records', *Statistics in Medicine* 6, 1987, 613–27; A. Cartwright and C. Smith, 'Some Comparisons of Data from Medical Records and From Women Who Recently Had a Live Birth or Stillbirth', *Journal of Biosocial Science* 11, 1979, 49–64; M. Joffe and J.A. Grisso, 'Comparison of Antenatal Hospital Records with Retrospective Interviewing', *Journal of Biosocial Science* 17, 1985, 113–19; D. Hewson and A. Bennett, 'Childbirth Research Data: Medical Records or Womens' Reports?', *American Journal of Epidemiology* 125, 1987, 484–91; L.J. Lauren, M.R. Forman, G.L. Hundt et al., 'Maternal Recall of Infant Feeding Events is Accurate', *Journal of Epidemiology and Community Health* 46, 1992, 203–6; S.D. Harlow and M.S. Linet, 'Agreement Between Questionnaire Data and Medical Records: The Evidence for Accuracy of Recall', *American Journal of Epidemiology* 129, 1989, 233–48.
8 Harding, *Feminism and Methodology*.
9 J.W. Ratcliffe, 'Analyst Biases in KAP Surveys: A Cross Cultural Comparison', *Studies in Family Planning* 7, 1976, 322–30.
10 E. Lord, L. Ross and M.R. Lepper, 'Biased Assimilation and Attitude Polarization: The Effects of Prior Theories on Subsequently Considered Evidence', *Journal of Personality and Social Psychology* 37, 1979, 2098–109.
11 M.J. Gitlin and R.O. Pasnau, 'Psychiatric Syndromes Linked to Reproductive Function in Women: A Review of Current Knowledge', *American Journal of Psychiatry* 146, 1989, 1413–22.
12 Gitlin and Pasnau, 'Psychiatric Syndromes'.
13 Gregg et al., Cited in J.W. Ratcliffe and A. Gonzalez-del-Valle, 'Rigor in Health Related Research: Toward an Expanded Conceptualization', *International Journal of Health Services* 18, 1988, 361–92.
14 A. Wieck, 'Endocrine Aspects of Postnatal Mental Disorders', *Bailliéres Clinics in Obstetrics and Gynaecology* 3, 1989, 857–77.

1 RESEARCHING PREGNANCY, BIRTH, MOTHERHOOD AND DEPRESSION

1 J. Lumley, R. Small and J. Yelland, *Having a Baby in Victoria: Final Report of the Ministerial Review of Birthing Services in Victoria*, Health Department of Victoria, Melbourne, 1990; R.P. Shearman, *Maternity Services in New South Wales: Final Report of the Ministerial Task Force on Obstetric Services in New South Wales*, 3 vols, New South Wales Department of Health, Sydney, 1989; C. Michael, *Report of the Ministerial Task Force to Review Obstetric, Neonatal and Gynaecological Services in Western Australia*, 3 vols, Health Department of Western Australia, Perth, 1990.
2 A. Bennett, 'The Birth of a First Child: Do Women's Reports Change Over Time?', *Birth* 12, 1985, 153–8; L. Erb, G. Hill and D. Houston, 'A Survey of Parents' Attitudes Towards Their Caesarean Births in Manitoba Hospitals', *Birth* 10, 1983, 85–92.
3 Erb et al., 'A Survey of Parents' Attitudes Towards Their Caesarean Births'.
4 A. Cartwright, 'Some Experiments With Factors That Might Affect the Response of Mothers to a Postal Questionnaire', *Statistics in Medicine* 5, 1986, 607–17.

5 A. Cartwright, 'Interviews or Postal Questionnaires? Comparison of Data About Women's Experiences with Maternity Services', *Milbank Memorial Fund Quarterly* 66, 1988, 172–89.
6 Cartwright, 'Some Experiments with Factors that Might Affect the Response of Mothers to a Postal Questionnaire'; Cartwright, 'Interviews or Postal Questionnaires'.
7 Michael, *Report of the Ministerial Task Force to Review Obstetric, Neonatal and Gynaecological Services in Western Australia*.
8 Lumley et al., *Having a Baby in Victoria*.
9 J. Lumley, S. Baskin and S. Rigoni, *Rights and Wrongs: A Validation Study of the Perinatal Morbidity Statistics Form*, Health Department of Victoria, Melbourne, 1984.
10 Consultative Council on Obstetric and Paediatric Mortality and Morbidity, *Annual Report on Maternal and Perinatal Deaths in Victoria, 1989 and 1990*, Health Department of Victoria, 1991 and 1992.
11 D. Sullivan, R. Beeman, 'Satisfaction with Maternity Care: A Matter of Communication and Choice', *Medical Care* 20, 1982, 321–30; A. Cartwright, 'Who Responds to Postal Questionnaires?', *Journal of Epidemiology and Community Health* 40, 1986, 267–73; A. Taylor, 'Maternity Services: The Consumers' View', *Journal of the Royal College of General Practitioners* 36, 1986, 157–60; 'Measuring Maternity Services: Quality and Outcome', *Report of a Maternity Services Outcome Indicators Project*, Illawarra Area Health Service, 1993.
12 H. Bartlett and D. Pennebaker, 'Consumer Views of Maternity Services in Western Australia', in *Report of the Ministerial Task Force to Review Obstetric, Neonatal and Gynaecological Services in Western Australia*, vol. III, *Survey Reports*, Health Department of Western Australia, Perth, 1990.
13 Cartwright, 'Who Responds to Postal Questionnaires?'; Bartlett and Pennebaker, 'Consumer Views of Maternity Services in Western Australia'.
14 R. Bell, J. Lumley, 'Alcohol Consumption, Cigarette Smoking and Fetal Outcome in Victoria', 1985, *Community Health Studies* 13, 1989, 484–91.
15 B. K. Armstrong, E. White and R. Saracci, 'Response Rates and Their Maximisation', in *Principles of Exposure Measurement in Epidemiology*, Oxford University Press, Oxford, 1992, ch. 11, 294–321.
16 B. K. Armstrong, E. White and R. Saracci, 'Methods of Exposure Measurement', in *Principles of Exposure Measurement in Epidemiology*, ch. 2, 22–48.
17 P. Simkin, 'Just Another Day in a Woman's Life? Part II: Nature and Consistency of Women's Long Term Memories of their First Birth Experience', *Birth* 19, 1992, 64–81.
18 J. L. Cox, J. M. Holden and R. Sagovsky, 'Detection of Postnatal Depression: Development of the 10-item Edinburgh Postnatal Depression Scale', *British Journal of Psychiatry* 150, 1987, 782–6.
19 I. G. Sarason, H. M. Levine, R. B. Basham and B. R. Sarason, 'Assessing Social Support: The Social Support Questionnaire', *Journal of Personal and Social Psychology* 44, 1983, 127–39.
20 J. Sewell, F. Oberklaid, M. Prior, A. Sanson and M. Kyrios, 'Temperament in Australian Toddlers', *Australian Paediatric Journal* 24, 1988, 343–5.
21 I. G. Sarason, J. H. Johnson and J. M. Siegel, 'Assessing the Impact of Life Changes: Development of the Life Experiences Survey', *Journal of Consulting and Clinical Psychology* 46, 1978, 932–46; J. S. Norbeck, 'Modification of

Life Event Questionnaires For Use with Female Respondents', *Research in Nursing and Health* 7, 1984, 61–71.
22 J. Astbury, 'Making Motherhood Visible: The Experience of Motherhood Questionnaire', *Journal of Reproductive and Infant Psychology* (in press).
23 A. Oakley, 'Interviewing Women: A Contradiction in Terms?', in H. Roberts (ed.), *Doing Feminist Research*, Routledge & Kegan Paul, London, 1981.
24 Cox et al., 'Detection of Postnatal Depression', 782–6; B. Harris, P. Huckle, R. Thomas, S. John and H. Fung, 'The Use of Rating Scales to Identify Postnatal Depression', *British Journal of Psychiatry* 154, 1989, 813–17; L. Murray and A. D. Carothers, 'The Validation of the Edinburgh Post-natal Depression Scale on a Community Sample', *British Journal of Psychiatry* 157, 1990, 288–90.
25 P. Boyce, R. Stubbs and A. Todd, 'The Edinburgh Postnatal Depression Scale: Validation in an Australian Sample', *Australian and New Zealand Journal of Psychiatry* 27, 1993, 472–6.
26 Sewell et al., 'Temperament in Australian Toddlers'.
27 Astbury, 'Making Motherhood Visible'.
28 Sarason et al., 'Assessing the Impact of Life Changes'; Norbeck, 'Modification of Life Events Questionnaire For Use with Female Respondents'.

2 CARE IN PREGNANCY

1 A. Oakley, *Becoming a Mother*, Martin Robertson, Oxford, 1979.
2 J. Lumley, R. Small and J. Yelland, 'Birth in Victoria: A Statistical Overview', in *Having a Baby in Victoria: Final Report of the Ministerial Review of Birthing Services in Victoria*, Health Department of Victoria, Melbourne, 1990.
3 Lumley et al., 'Birth in Victoria'.
4 A. Oakley, 'The Origins and Development of Antenatal Care', in M. Enkin and I. Chalmers (eds), *Effectiveness and Satisfaction in Antenatal Care*, Heinemann, London, 1982, 1–21.
5 Oakley, *Becoming a Mother*; C. Martin, 'How Do You Count Maternal Satisfaction? A User-commissioned Survey of Maternity Services', in M. Roberts (ed.), *Women's Health Counts*, Routledge, London, 1990, 147–66; A. Taylor, 'Maternity Services: The Consumer's View', *Journal of the Royal College of General Practitioners* 36, 1986, 157–60.
6 J. Garcia, 'Women's Views of Their Antenatal Care', in Enkin and Chalmers (eds), *Effectiveness and Satisfaction in Antenatal Care*, 81–91.
7 A. Jacoby and A. Cartwright, 'Finding Out About the Views and Experiences of Maternity Service Users', in J. Garcia, R. Kilpatrick and M. Richards (eds), *The Politics of Maternity Care Services for Childbearing Women in Twentieth Century Britain*, Oxford University Press, Oxford, 1990, 238–55; D. Locker and D. Dunt, 'Theoretical and Methodological Issues in Sociological Studies of Consumer Satisfaction with Medical Care', *Social Science and Medicine* 12, 1979, 283–92.
8 Oakley, *Becoming a Mother*; A. Oakley, *Women Confined: Towards a Sociology of Childbirth*, Martin Robertson, Oxford, 1980; H. Graham and L. McKee, 'The First Months of Motherhood: Summary Report of a Survey of Women's Experiences of Pregnancy', quoted in J. Garcia, 'Women's Views of their Antenatal Care'; M. E. Reid and G. M. McIlwaine, 'Consumer Opinion of a Hospital Antenatal Clinic', *Social Science and Medicine* 14a, 1980, 363–8.
9 Garcia, 'Women's Views of their Antenatal Care'.

10 Garcia, 'Women's Views of their Antenatal Care'.
11 M. Richards, 'The Trouble with "Choice" in Childbirth', *Birth* 9, 1982, 253–60; A. Bennett, W. Etherington and D. Hewson (eds), *Childbirth Choices*, Penguin, Ringwood, 1993.
12 Richards, 'The Trouble with "Choice" in Childbirth'.
13 A. Jacoby, 'Women's Preferences For and Satisfaction With Current Procedures in Childbirth: Findings from a National Study', *Midwifery* 3, 1987, 117–24.
14 H. Bartlett and D. Pennebaker, 'Consumer Views of Maternity Services in Western Australia', in *Report of the Ministerial Task Force to Review Obstetric, Neonatal and Gynaecological Services in Western Australia*, vol. III, *Survey Reports*, Health Department of Western Australia, Perth, 1990.
15 Martin, 'How Do You Count Maternal Satisfaction?'.
16 W. Giles, J. Collins, F. Ong and R. MacDonald, 'Antenatal Care of Low Risk Obstetric Patients by Midwives: A Randomised Trial', *Medical Journal of Australia* 157, 1992, 158–61; U. Waldenström and C. A. Nilsson, 'Women's Satisfaction with Birth Center Care: A Randomized, Controlled Study', *Birth* 20, 1993, 3–13.

3 THOUGHTS ABOUT THE BIRTH EIGHT MONTHS LATER

1 J. Lumley, R. Small and J. Yelland, 'Birth in Victoria: A Statistical Overview', in *Having a Baby in Victoria: Final Report of the Ministerial Review of Birthing Services in Victoria*, Health Department of Victoria, Melbourne, 1990.
2 Consultative Council on Obstetric and Paediatric Mortality and Morbidity, *Annual Report for the Year 1991*, Department of Health and Community Services, Melbourne, 1992.
3 C. MacArthur, M. Lewis and E. Knox, *Health After Childbirth*, HMSO, London, 1991.
4 Lumley et al., *Having a Baby in Victoria*.
5 H. Bastian and P. Lancaster, *Homebirths in Australia 1985–1987*, National Perinatal Statistics Unit, Sydney, 1990.
6 M. Pym, R. Nguyen, L. Taylor and L. Houlahan, *New South Wales Midwives Data Collection 1992*, Epidemiology and Health Services Evaluation Branch, Public Health Division, New South Wales Health Department, Sydney, 1993.
7 L. Kozak, 'Surgical and Non-surgical Procedures Associated with Hospital Delivery in the United States: 1980–1987', *Birth* 16, 1989, 209–13.
8 J. Lumley, R. Small and J. Yelland, 'Intervention', in *Having a Baby in Victoria: Final Report of the Ministerial Review of Birthing Services in Victoria*, Health Department of Victoria, Melbourne, 1990.
9 World Health Organisation, 'Appropriate Technology for Birth', *Lancet* 2, 1985, 436–7.
10 Lumley et al., 'Intervention'.
11 I. Chalmers, M. Enkin and M. Keirse (eds), *Effective Care in Pregnancy and Childbirth*, Oxford University Press, Oxford, 1989.
12 Lumley et al., 'Intervention'.
13 P. Lancaster and E. Pedisich, *Caesarean Births in Australia, 1985–1990*, Australian Institute of Health and Welfare National Perinatal Statistics Unit, Sydney, 1993.
14 Lumley et al., 'Intervention'.

15 J. Lumley, 'Assessing Satisfaction with Childbirth', *Birth* 12, 1985, 141–5; M. Shearer, 'The Difficulty of Defining and Measuring Satisfaction with Perinatal Care', *Birth* 10, 1983, 77; M. Porter and S. Macintyre, 'What Is Must Be Best: A Research Note on Conservative or Deferential Responses to Antenatal Care Provision', *Social Science and Medicine* 19, 1984, 1197–200; A. Oakley, 'Social Consequences of Obstetric Technology: The Importance of Measuring "Soft" Outcomes', *Birth* 10, 1983, 99–108; D. Locker and D. Dunt, 'Theoretical and Methodological Issues in Sociological Studies of Consumer Satisfaction with Medical Care', *Social Science and Medicine* 12, 1978, 283–92; I. Bramadat and M. Dreidger, 'Satisfaction with Childbirth: Theories and Methods of Measurement', *Birth* 20, 1993, 22–9.

16 Locker and Dunt, 'Theoretical and Methodological Issues in Sociological Studies of Consumer Satisfaction with Medical Care'; Bramadat and Dreidger, 'Satisfaction with Childbirth'; S. Strasser and R. Davis, *Measuring Patient Satisfaction for Improved Patient Services,* Health Administration Press, United States, 1991; M. Shearer, 'Commentary: How Well Does the LADSI Measure Satisfaction with Labor and Delivery?', *Birth* 14, 1987, 125–9.

17 Shearer, 'The Difficulty of Defining and Measuring Satisfaction with Perinatal Care'.

18 P. Simkin, 'Just Another Day in a Woman's Life? Part II: Nature and Consistency of Women's Long Term Memories of their First Birth Experiences', *Birth* 19, 1992, 64–81.

19 C. Naaktgeboren, 'The Biology of Childbirth', in Chalmers et al. (eds), *Effective Care in Pregnancy and Childbirth*, 795–803.

20 J. Lumley, 'Trends in Birthstyle in Australia', in D. Tudehope and J. Chenoweth (eds), *Perinatal Medicine, Journal of the Australian Perinatal Society*, Proceedings of the Fourth Congress, Brisbane, 1986, 61–5.

21 M. J. N. C. Keirse, M. Enkin and J. Lumley, 'Social and Professional Support During Childbirth', in Chalmers et al. (eds), *Effective Care in Pregnancy and Childbirth*, 805–14.

22 S. Elliot, M. Anderson, D. Brough, J. Watson and A. Rugg, 'Relationship Between Obstetric Outcome and Psychological Measures in Pregnancy and the Postnatal Year', *Journal of Reproductive and Infant Psychology* 2, 1984, 18–22.

23 A. Jacoby, 'Women's Preferences For and Satisfaction With Current Procedures in Childbirth: Findings from a National Study', *Midwifery* 3, 1987, 117–24; C. Martin, 'How Do You Count Maternal Satisfaction?: A User-Commissioned Survey of Maternity Services', in M. Roberts (ed.), *Women's Health Counts*, Routledge, London, 1990, 147–66.

24 A. Cartwright, *The Dignity of Labor? A Study of Childbearing and Induction*, Tavistock Press, London, 1979; D. Sullivan and R. Beeman, 'Satisfaction with Maternity Care: A Matter of Communication and Choice', *Medical Care* 10, 1982, 321–30; J. Green, V. Coupland and J. Kitzinger, 'Expectations, Experiences and Psychological Outcomes of Childbirth: A Prospective Study of 825 Women', *Birth* 17, 1990, 15–24; B. Morgan, C. Bulpitt, P. Clifton and P. Lewis, 'Analgesia and Satisfaction in Childbirth (The Queen Charlotte's 1000 Mother Survey)', *Lancet* ii, 1982, 808–11; D. Hewson, A. Bennett, S. Holliday and E. Booker, 'Childbirth in Sydney Teaching Hospitals: A Study of Low-risk Primiparous Women', *Community Health Studies* 10(3), 1985, 195–201.

25 Green et al., 'Expectations, Experiences and Psychological Outcomes of Childbirth'.
26 Green et al., 'Expectations, Experiences and Psychological Outcomes of Childbirth'.
27 Chalmers et al. (eds), *Effective Care in Pregnancy and Childbirth*.
28 J. Green, J. Kitzinger and V. Coupland, 'Stereotypes of Childbearing Women: A Look at Some Evidence', *Midwifery* 6, 1990, 125–32; I. Bowler, 'Stereotypes of Women of Asian Descent in Midwifery: Some Evidence', *Midwifery* 9, 1993, 7–16.
29 P. Steer, 'The House of Commons Health Committee Report on the Maternity Services: A Personal View', *British Journal of Obstetrics and Gynaecology* 99, 1992, 445–51; J. Lumley and S. Brown, 'The House of Commons Health Committee Report on the Maternity Services: A Personal View' (letter), *British Journal of Obstetrics and Gynaecology* 100, 1993, 193.
30 Porter and Macintyre, 'What Is Must Be Best'.

4 CHILDBIRTH CLASSES: MAKING A DIFFERENCE?

1 J. Lumley and J. Astbury, 'Childbirth Education', in *Birth Rites, Birth Rights*, Thomas Nelson, Melbourne, 1980, 27–38.
2 J. Lumley, R. Small, J. Yelland, *Having a Baby in Victoria: Final Report of the Ministerial Review of Birthing Services in Victoria*, Health Department of Victoria, Melbourne, 1990, 60–71.
3 R. P. Shearman, *Maternity Services in New South Wales: Final Report of the Ministerial Task Force on Obstetric Services in New South Wales*, 3 vols, New South Wales Department of Health, Sydney, 1989, 115 (Appendices).
4 P. Simkin, M. Enkin, 'Antenatal Classes', in I. Chalmers, M. Enkin and M. J. N. C. Keirse (eds), *A Guide to Effective Care in Pregnancy and Childbirth*, Oxford University Press, Oxford, 1989, 24–7.
5 C. Michael, *Report of the Ministerial Task Force to Review Obstetric, Neonatal and Gynaecological Services in Western Australia*, 3 vols, Health Department of Western Australia, Perth, 1990.
6 S. Redman, S. Oak, P. Booth, J. Jensen and A. Saxton, 'Evaluation of an Antenatal Education Programme: Characteristics of Attenders, Changes in Knowledge and Satisfaction of Participants', *Australian and New Zealand Journal of Obstetrics and Gynaecology* 31, 1991, 310–16.
7 Simkin and Enkin, 'Antenatal Classes'.
8 Simkin and Enkin, 'Antenatal Classes'.
9 Redman et al., 'Evaluation of an Antenatal Programme'.
10 R. K. McGraw and J. M. Abplanalp, 'Motivation to Take Childbirth Education: Implications for Studies of Effectiveness', *Birth* 9, 1982, 179–82.
11 M. H. Shearer, 'Effects of Prenatal Education Depend on the Attitudes and Practices of Obstetric Caregivers', *Birth* 17, 1990, 73–4.
12 J. Lumley, J. Astbury, 'The Medical Model for Birth', in *Birth Rites, Birth Rights*, 91.
13 Redman et al., 'Evaluation of an Antenatal Education Programme'.
14 Redman et al., 'Evaluation of an Antenatal Education Programme'.
15 Simkin and Enkin, 'Antenatal Classes'.
16 Redman et al., 'Evaluation of an Antenatal Education Programme'.
17 P. A. St Clair and N. A. Anderson, 'Social Network Advice During Pregnancy: Myths, Misinformation and Sound Counsel', *Birth* 16, 1989, 103–7.

18 A. Oakley, 'Sickness in Salonica and Other Stories', in *Social Support and Motherhood*, Blackwells, Oxford, 1992, ch. 3, 76–92; W. A. Silverman, *Human Experimentation: A Guided Step into the Unknown*, Oxford University Press, Oxford, 1985.
19 Simkin and Enkin, 'Antenatal Classes'.
20 M. Porter, S. Macintyre, 'What Is Must Be Best: A Research Note on Conservative or Deferential Responses to Antenatal Care Provision', *Social Science and Medicine* 19, 1984, 1197–200.

5 THROWN INTO A NEW JOB

1 A. Woollett and N. Dosanjh-Matwala, 'Postnatal Care: The Attitudes and Experiences of Asian Women in East London', *Midwifery* 6, 1990, 178–84; P. Moss, G. Bolland, R. Foxman et al., 'The Hospital Inpatient Stay: The Experience of First Time Parents', *Child: Care, Health and Development* 13, 1983, 153–67.
2 Obstetric Physiotherapy Society, Hospital Questionnaire, February 1977 [unpublished survey].
3 J. Lumley and B. A. Davey, 'Do Hospitals with Family-Centred Maternity Care Have Lower Intervention Rates?', *Birth* 14, 1987, 132–4; [and additional unpublished data from B. A. Davey, Family-centred Birth in Melbourne, Survey, March 1984].
4 Obstetric Physiotherapy Society, Hospital Questionnaire.
5 C. Drapac and A. Rubinstein, 'Choices of Childbirth: A Survey of Practice in Melbourne Maternity Hospitals', *Australian Journal of Physiotherapy* 30, 1984, 52–9.
6 Woollett and Dosanjh-Matwala, 'Postnatal Care'; A. Taylor, 'Maternity Services: The Consumer's View', *Journal of the Royal College of General Practitioners* 36, 1986, 157–60.
7 P. L. Rice, 'My Forty Days: A Cross-cultural Resource Book for Health Care Professionals in Birthing Services', Vietnamese Antenatal/Postnatal Support Project, Melbourne, 1993, 67–9.
8 Rice, 'My Forty Days'.
9 Woollett and Dosanjh-Matwala, 'Postnatal Care'.
10 L. Wadd, 'Vietnamese Postpartum Practices: Implications for Nursing in the Hospital Setting', *Journal of Obstetric and Gynecological Nursing*, Jul/Aug, 1983, 252–8.
11 *Annual Reports of Maternal and Infant Health 1971–1980*, Health Commission of Victoria, Melbourne, 1972–82 [and unpublished data from the Maternal and Child Health Program, Department of Health and Community Services].
12 Obstetric Physiotherapy Society, Hospital Questionnaire.
13 Lumley and Davey, 'Do Hospitals with Family-Centred Maternity Care Have Lower Intervention Rates?'.
14 Obstetric Physiotherapy Society, Hospital Questionnaire.
15 Lumley and Davey, 'Do Hospitals with Family-Centred Maternity Care Have Lower Intervention Rates?'.
16 D. A. Sullivan, 'Satisfaction with Postpartum Care: Opportunities for Bonding, Reconstructing the Birth and Instruction', *Birth and the Family Journal* 8, 1981, 153–9.

17 J. Lumley, R. Small and J. Yelland, *Having a Baby in Victoria: Final Report of the Ministerial Review of Birthing Services in Victoria*, Health Department of Victoria, Melbourne, 1990, 123.
18 Lumley et al., *Having a Baby in Victoria*, 124.
19 K. F. Norr and K. Nacion, 'Outcomes of Postpartum Early Discharge, 1960–1986: A Comparative Review', *Birth* 14, 1987, 135–41; U. Waldenström, C. Sundelin and G. Lindmark, 'Early and Late Discharge After Hospital Birth: Health of Mother and Infant in the Postpartum Period', *Uppsala Journal of Medical Science* 92, 1987, 301–14; C. T. Beck, 'Early Postpartum Discharge Programs in the United States: A Literature Review and Critique', *Women and Health* 17, 1991, 125–38.
20 Moss et al., 'The Hospital Inpatient Stay'.
21 U. Waldenström, C. Sundelin and G. Lindmark, 'Early and Late Discharge After Hospital Birth: Breastfeeding', *Acta Paediatrica Scandinavica* 76, 1987, 727–32; E. M. Carty and C. F. Bradley, 'A Randomized, Controlled Evaluation of Early Postpartum Hospital Discharge', *Birth* 17, 1990, 199–204.
22 Carty and Bradley, 'A Randomized, Controlled Evaluation of Early Postpartum Hospital Discharge'; I. Burnell, M. McCarthy, G. V. P. Chamberlain, D. F. Hawkins and D. Elbourne, 'Patient Preference and Postnatal Hospital Stay', *Journal of Obstetrics and Gynaecology* 3, 1982, 43–7; M. L. James, C. N. Hudson, V. J. Gebski, L. H. Browne, G. R. Andrews, S. E. Crisp, D. Palmer and J. L. Beresford, 'An Evaluation of Planned Early Postnatal Transfer Home with Nursing Support', *Medical Journal of Australia* 147, 1987, 434–8.
23 Carty and Bradley, 'A Randomized, Controlled Evaluation of Early Postpartum Hospital Discharge'.
24 K. F. Norr, K. Nacion and R. Abramson, 'Early Discharge with Home Follow-up: Impacts on Low-Income Mothers and Infants', *Journal of Obstetrical Gynecological and Neonatal Nursing*, Mar/Apr, 1989, 133–41.
25 Waldenström et al., 'Early and Late Discharge After Hospital Birth: Breastfeeding'; Carty and Bradley, 'A Randomized, Controlled Evaluation of Early Postpartum Hospital Discharge'.
26 M. Porter and S. Mcintyre, 'What Is Must Be Best: A Research Note on Conservative or Deferential Responses to Antenatal Care Provision', *Social Science and Medicine* 19, 1984, 1197–200.

6 ONE IN SEVEN: DEPRESSION AFTER BIRTH

1 G. Stein, 'The Maternity Blues', in I. F. Brockington and R. Kumar (eds), *Motherhood and Mental Illness*, Academic Press, London, 1982, ch. 5, 119–54.
2 I. F. Brockington, G. Winokur and C. Dean, 'Puerperal Psychosis', in Brockington and Kumar, *Motherhood and Mental Illness*, 37–69.
3 S. Day, 'Is Obstetric Technology Depressing?', *Radical Science Journal* 12, 1982, 17–45.
4 P. Romito, 'Unhappiness After Childbirth', in I. Chalmers, M. Enkin and M. J. N. C. Keirse (eds), *Effective Care in Pregnancy and Childbirth*, Oxford University Press, Oxford, 1989, 1433–46.
5 Romito, 'Unhappiness After Childbirth'.
6 J. L. Cox, M. J. Holden and R. Sagovsky, 'Detection of Postnatal Depression: Development of the 10-item Edinburgh Postnatal Depression Scale', *British Journal of Psychiatry* 150, 1987, 782–6.

7 P. Snaith, 'What Do Depression Rating Scales Measure?', *British Journal of Psychiatry* 163, 1993, 293–8.
8 P.N. Nott and S. Cutts, 'Validation of the 30-item General Health Questionnaire in Postpartum Women', *Psychological Medicine* 12, 1982, 409–13.
9 Cox et al., 'Detection of Postnatal Depression'; B. Harris, P. Huckle, R. Thomas, S. John and H. Fung, 'The Use of Rating Scales to Identify Postnatal Depression', *British Journal of Psychiatry* 154, 1989, 813–17; L. Murray and A. D. Carothers, 'The Validation of the Edinburgh Post-natal Depression Scale on a Community Sample', *British Journal of Psychiatry* 157, 1990, 288–90.
10 P. Boyce, R. Stubbs and A. Todd, 'The Edinburgh Postnatal Depression Scale: Validation in an Australian Sample', *Australian and New Zealand Journal of Psychiatry* 27, 1993, 472–6.
11 A. Roy, P. Garg, K. Cole et al., 'Use of the Edinburgh Postnatal Depression Scale in a North American Population', *Progress in Neuropsychopharmacology and Biological Psychiatry* 17, 1993, 501–4.
12 M. Thome, 'Screening of Postnatal Depression by Community Nurses in Iceland', Fifth International Conference of the Marcé Society: Childbearing and Mental Health, York, 1990.
13 V.J. Pop, I. H. Komproe and M. J. van Son, 'Characteristics of the Edinburgh Post Natal Depression Scale in the Netherlands', *Journal of Affective Disorders* 26, 1992, 105–10.
14 T. Dragonas, K. Thorpe and J. Golding, 'Transition to Fatherhood: A Cross-cultural Comparison', *Journal of Psychosomatic Obstetrics and Gynaecology* 13, 1992, 1–19.
15 J.L. Cox, D. Murray and G. Chapman, 'A Controlled Study of the Onset, Duration and Prevalence of Postnatal Depression', *British Journal of Psychiatry* 163, 1993, 27–31; K. Thorpe, 'A Study of the Use of the Edinburgh Postnatal Depression Scale with Parent Groups Outside the Postpartum Period', *Journal of Reproductive and Infant Psychology* 11, 1993, 119–25.
16 Thorpe, 'A Study of the Use of the Edinburgh Postnatal Depression Scale with Parent Groups Outside the Postpartum Period'.
17 Thorpe, 'A Study of the Use of the Edinburgh Postnatal Depression Scale with Parent Groups Outside the Pospartum Period'.
18 Cox et al., 'A Controlled Study of the Onset, Duration and Prevalence of Postnatal Depression'.
19 Murray and Carothers, 'The Validation of the Edinburgh Post-natal Depression Scale on a Community Sample'.
20 Cox et al., 'Detection of Postnatal Depression'; Murray and Carothers, 'The Validation of the Edinburgh Post-natal Depression Scale on a Community Sample'.
21 R. M. Kumar and K. Robson, 'A Prospective Study of Emotional Disorders in Childbearing Women', *British Journal of Psychiatry* 144, 1984, 34–47.
22 M.W. O'Hara, E.M. Zekoski, L.H. Philipps and E.J. Wright, 'Controlled Prospective Study of Postpartum Mood Disorders: Comparison of Childbearing and Non-childbearing Women', *Journal of Abnormal Psychology* 99, 1990, 3–15.
23 Kumar and Robson, 'A Prospective Study of Emotional Disorders in Childbearing Women'; G.W. Brown and T. Harris, *Social Origins of Depression: A Study of Psychiatric Disorders in Women*, Tavistock Press, London, 1978; J.P. Watson, S.A. Elliott, A.J. Rugg et al., 'Psychiatric Disorder in Pregnancy and the First Postnatal Year', *British Journal of Psychiatry* 144,

1984, 453–62; P. Bebbington, J. Hurry, C. Tennant et al., 'Epidemiology of Mental Disorders in Camberwell', *Psychological Medicine*, 1981, 561–97; P. J. Cooper, E. A. Campbell, A. Day et al., 'Non-psychotic Psychiatric Disorder After Childbirth', *British Journal of Psychiatry* 152, 1988, 799–806; P. G. Surtees, C. Dean, J. G. Ingham et al., 'Psychiatric Disorder in Women from an Edinburgh Community: Associations with Demographic Factors', *British Journal of Psychiatry* 142, 1983, 238–46.

24 Cox et al., 'A Controlled Study of the Onset, Duration and Prevalence of Postnatal Depression'.

25 Cox et al., 'A Controlled Study of the Onset, Duration and Prevalence of Postnatal Depression'.

26 Romito, 'Unhappiness After Childbirth'; M. W. O'Hara and E. Zekoski, 'Postpartum Depression: A Comprehensive Review', in *Motherhood and Mental Illness 2*, ch. 2, 17–63.

27 Romito, 'Unhappiness After Childbirth'.

28 S. Elliot, M. Anderson, D. Brough, G. Watson and A. Rugg, 'Relationship Between Obstetric Outcome and Psychological Measures in Pregnancy and the Postnatal Period', *Journal of Reproductive and Infant Psychology* 2, 1984, 18–32.

29 S. E. Romans-Clarkson, V. A. Walton, G. P. Herbison and P. E. Mullen, 'Psychiatric Morbidity Among Women in Urban and Rural New Zealand: Psychosocial Correlates', *British Journal of Psychiatry* 156, 1990, 84–91.

30 D. Blazer, L. K. George, R. Landerman, M. Pennybacker, M. Melville, M. Woodbury et al., 'Psychiatric Disorders: A Rural/Urban Comparison', *Archives of General Psychiatry* 42, 1985, 651–6; B. A. Crowell, L. K. George, D. Blazer and R. Landerman, 'Psychosocial Risk Factors and Urban/Rural Differences in the Prevalence of Major Depression', *British Journal of Psychiatry* 149, 1986, 307–14.

31 Romito, 'Unhappiness After Childbirth'; O'Hara and Zekoski, 'Postpartum Depression'.

32 H. Williams and A. Carmichael, 'Depression in Mothers in a Multi-Ethnic Urban Industrial Municipality of Melbourne: Aetiological Factors and Effects on Preschool Children', *Journal of Child Psychology and Psychiatry* 26, 1989, 277–88.

33 Romito, 'Unhappiness After Childbirth'.

34 A. Oakley and L. Rajan, 'Social Class and Social Support: The Same or Different?', *Sociology* 25, 1991, 31–59.

35 A. Stein, P. J. Cooper, E. A. Campbell, A. Day and P. M. E. Altham, 'Social Adversity and Perinatal Complications: Their Relation to Postnatal Depression', *British Medical Journal* 298, 1989, 1073–4.

36 J. Green, V. Coupland and J. Kitzinger, 'Expectations, Experiences, and Psychological Outcomes of Childbirth: A Prospective Study of 825 Women', *Birth* 17, 1990, 15–23.

37 P. Hannah, D. Adams, A. Lee, V. Glover and M. Sandler, 'Links Between Early Postpartum Mood and Post-Natal Depression', *British Journal of Psychiatry* 160, 1992, 777–80; T. O'Neill, P. Murphy and V. T. Greene, 'Postnatal Depression: Aetiological Factors', *Irish Medical Journal* 83, 1990, 17–18.

38 P. M. Boyce and A. L. Todd, 'Increased Risk of Postnatal Depression After Emergency Caesarean Section', *Medical Journal of Australia* 157, 1992,

172–4; J. Fisher, 'Obstetric Intervention: Psychological Predictors and Psychological Consequences', PhD thesis, University of Melbourne (submitted 1994).
39 B. Harris, S. John, H. Fung, R. Thomas, R. Walker, G. Read et al., 'The Hormonal Environment of Postnatal Depression', *British Journal of Psychiatry* 154, 1989, 660–7.
40 C. MacArthur, M. Lewis and E. G. Knox, *Health After Childbirth*, HMSO, London, 1991.
41 B. Pitt, 'Atypical Depression Following Childbirth', *British Journal of Psychiatry* 114, 1968, 1325–35.
42 K. Dalton, 'Prospective Study into Puerperal Depression', *British Journal of Psychiatry* 118, 1971, 689–92.
43 Hannah et al., 'Links Between Early Postpartum Mood and Postnatal Depression'.
44 Harris et al., 'The Hormonal Environment of Postnatal Depression'.
45 E. M. Alder and J. L. Cox, 'Breastfeeding and Post-natal Depression', *Journal of Psychosomatic Research* 27, 1983, 139–44.
46 E. M. Alder and J. Bancroft, 'The Relationship Between Breast Feeding Persistence, Sexuality and Mood in Postpartum Women', *Psychological Medicine* 18, 1988, 386–96.
47 Alder and Bancroft, 'The Relationship Between Breast Feeding Persistence, Sexuality and Mood in Postpartum Women'.
48 E. M. Alder, A. Cook, D. Davidson, C. West and J. Bancroft, 'Hormones, Mood and Sexuality in Lactating Women', *British Journal of Psychiatry* 148, 1986, 74–9.
49 T. Tamminen, 'The Impact of Mother's Depression on Her Breastfeeding Attitudes and Experience', *Journal of Psychosomatic Obstetrics and Gynaecology* Suppl. 10, 1989, 69–78.
50 G. E. Stamp and C. Crowther, 'Postnatal Depression: A South Australian Prospective Survey', *Australian and New Zealand Journal of Obstetrics and Gynaecology* 34, 1994, 164–7.
51 P. J. Cooper, L. Murray and A. Stein, 'Psychological Determinants of Early Termination of Breast Feeding', *Journal of Psychosomatic Research* 37, 1993, 171–6.
52 Dalton, 'Prospective Study into Puerperal Depression'.
53 Alder and Cox, 'Breastfeeding and Post-Natal Depression'.
54 Alder and Cox, 'Breastfeeding and Post-Natal Depression'.
55 Harris et al., 'The Hormonal Environment of Post-Natal Depression'.
56 L. Dennerstein, P. Lehart and F. Riphagen, 'Postpartum Depression: Risk Factors', *Journal of Psychosomatic Obstetrics and Gynaecology* Suppl. 10, 1989, 53–65.
57 Harris et al., 'The Hormonal Environment of Post-Natal Depression'.
58 A. George and M. Sandler, 'Endocrine and Biochemical Studies in Puerperal Mental Disorders', in Kumar and Brockington (eds), *Motherhood and Mental Illness 2*, 78–112.
59 George and Sandler, 'Endocrine and Biochemical Studies in Puerperal Mental Disorders'.
60 M. Shearer, 'Commentary: Pondering the Study of Women's Psychological Outcomes', *Birth* 17, 1990, 24.
61 Shearer, 'Commentary'.

THE FOLLOW-UP STUDY   INTRODUCTION

1. Australian Bureau of Statistics, 'Labour Force Australia', Catalogue No. 6204. 0.
2. Australian Bureau of Statistics, 'Weekly Earnings of Employees (Distribution Australia)', Catalogue No. 6310. 0.
3. J. Martin, 'Non-English Speaking Migrant Women in Australia', in N. Grieve and A. Burns, *Australian Women: New Feminist Perspectives*, Oxford University Press, Melbourne, 1986.
4. The Consultative Council on Obstetric and Paediatric Mortality and Morbidity, *Annual Report for the Year 1989*, Health Department of Victoria, Melbourne, 1990.
5. P. Raskall, 'Widening Income Disparities in Australia', in S. Rees, G. Rodley and S. Stilwell (eds), *Beyond the Market: Alternatives to Economic Rationalism*, Pluto Press, Leichardt, 1991.
6. G. Ochiltree and E. Greenblat, 'Sick Children: How Working Mothers Cope', AIFS Early Childhood Study Paper No. 2, Australian Institute of Family Studies, Melbourne, 1991.
7. P. McDonald and H. Brownlee, 'Living Day to Day: Families in the Recession', *Family Matters* 31, 1992, 8–13.
8. The Consultative Council on Obstetric and Paediatric Mortality and Morbidity, Annual Report for the Year 1992, Department of Health and Community Services, Melbourne, 1994.

7   TROUBLED THOUGHTS ON BEING A 'GOOD' MOTHER

1. A. Rich, *Of Woman Born: Motherhood as Experience and Institution*, Virago, London, 1977.
2. L. Richards, *Having Families: Marriage, Parenthood and Social Pressures in Australia*, Penguin, Ringwood, 1985.
3. J. Harper and L. Richards, *Mothers and Working Mothers*, Penguin, Ringwood, 1979.
4. C. Urwin, 'Constructing Motherhood: The Persuasion of Normal Development', in C. Steedman, C. Urwin and V. Walkerdine (eds), *Language, Gender and Childhood*, Routledge and Kegan Paul, London, 1989, 164–202.
5. Urwin, 'Constructing Motherhood'.
6. C. Hardyment, *Dream Babies: Childcare from Locke to Spock*, Jonathan Cape, London, 1983; N. Chodorow and S. Contratto, 'The Fantasy of the Perfect Mother', in N. Chodorow (ed), *Feminism and Psychoanalytic Theory*, Yale University Press, United States, 1989, 79–96.
7. P. Leach, *Baby and Child*, Michael Joseph, London, 1977, 9.
8. J. Flax, 'Lacan and Winnicott: Splitting and Regression in Psychoanalytic Theory', in *Thinking Fragments: Psychoanalysis, Feminism, and Postmodernity in the Contemporary West*, University of California Press, California, 1990, 89–134.
9. A. Oakley, *Social Support and Motherhood*, Blackwell, Oxford, 1992.
10. M. Bitman, 'Selected Findings from Juggling Time', Office of the Status of Women, Department of Prime Minister and Cabinet, Canberra, 1991.
11. Leach, *Baby and Child*.
12. Leach, *Baby and Child*; B. Spock, *The Common Sense Book of Baby and Child Care*, Duel Sloan, London, 1969.
13. Chodorow and Contratto, 'The Fantasy of the Perfect Mother'.

14 P. Chesler, *With Child: A Diary of Motherhood*, Thomas Crowell, New York, 1979.

8 THE EXPERIENCE OF MOTHERHOOD

1 S. A. Elliott, 'Commentary on "Childbirth as a Life Event"', *Journal of Reproductive and Infant Psychology* 8, 1990, 147–59.
2 Elliott, 'Commentary on "Childbirth as a Life Event"'.
3 D. C. Jack, *Silencing the Self: Women and Depression*, Harvard University Press, Cambridge, Mass., 1991.
4 H. Graham, 'Prevention and Health: Every Mother's Business'. A comment on Child Health Policies in the 1970s, in C. Harris (ed.), *The Sociology of the Family: New Directions for Britain*, Sociological Review Monograph 28, Keele, 1979; R. Pill and N. C. H. Stott, 'Concepts of Illness Causation and Responsibility: Some Preliminary Data from a Sample of Working Class Mothers', *Social Science and Medicine* 16, 1991, 43–52.
5 A. McBride, 'Mental Health Effects of Women's Multiple Roles', *American Psychologist* 45, 1990, 381–4.
6 J. S. Norbeck, 'Modification of Life Event Questionnaires For Use With Female Respondents', *Research in Nursing and Health* 7, 1984, 61–71.
7 J. Astbury, 'Making Motherhood Visible: The Experience of Motherhood Questionnaire', *Journal of Reproductive and Infant Psychology* (in press).

9 DEPRESSION: WOMEN'S VOICES

1 J. Macintosh, 'Postpartum Depression: Women's Help-seeking Behaviour and Perceptions of Cause', *Journal of Advanced Nursing* 18, 1993, 178–84.
2 P. Romito, 'Unhappiness After Childbirth', in I. Chalmers, M. Enkin and M. J. N. C. Keirse (eds), *Effective Care in Pregnancy and Childbirth*, vol. 2, Oxford University Press, Oxford, 1433–66.
3 P. N. Nott, 'Extent, Timing and Persistence of Emotional Disorders Following Childbirth', *British Journal of Psychiatry* 151, 1987, 523–7; J. L. Cox, D. Murray and G. Chapman, 'A Controlled Study of the Onset, Duration and Prevalence of Postnatal Depression', *British Journal of Psychiatry* 163, 1993, 27–31.
4 Romito, 'Unhappiness After Childbirth'; M. W. O'Hara and E. Zekoski, 'Postpartum Depression: A Comprehensive Review', in R. Kumar and I. F. Brockington (eds), *Motherhood and Mental Illness 2: Causes and Consequences*, Academic Press, London, 1988, 17–63.
5 Macintosh, 'Postpartum Depression'.

10 THE SOCIAL CONTEXT OF MOTHERHOOD

1 J. Astbury, 'Making Motherhood Visible: The Experience of Motherhood Questionnaire', *Journal of Reproductive and Infant Psychology* (in press).
2 I. G. Sarason, J. H. Johnson and J. M. Siegel, 'Assessing the Impact of Life Changes: Development of the Life Experiences Survey', *Journal of Consulting and Clinical Psychology* 46, 1978, 932–46; J. S. Norbeck, 'Modification of Life Event Questionnaires For Use With Female Respondents', *Research in Nursing and Health* 7, 1984, 61–71.
3 J. Sewell, F. Oberklaid, M. Prior, A. Sanson and M. Kyrios, 'Temperament in Australian Toddlers', *Australian Paediatric Journal* 24, 1988, 343–5.
4 I. G. Sarason, H. M. Levine, R. B. Basham and B. R. Sarason, 'Assessing Social

Support: The Social Support Questionnaire', *Journal of Personal and Social Psychology* 44, 1983, 127–39.
5 J.L. Cox, J.M. Holden and R. Sagovsky, 'Detection of Postnatal Depression: Development of the 10-item Edinburgh Postnatal Depression Scale', *British Journal of Psychiatry* 150, 1987, 782–6.
6 D. Tannen, *You Just Don't Understand: Women and Men in Conversation*, Random House, Australia, 1991.
7 Tannen, *You Just Don't Understand*.
8 Tannen, *You Just Don't Understand*.
9 J. Sewell, F. Oberklaid, M. Prior, A. Sanson and M. Kyrios, 'Temperament in Australian Toddlers', *Australian Paediatric Journal* 24, 1988, 343–5.
10 M.A. Keener, C.H. Zeanah and T.F. Anders, 'Infant Temperament, Sleep Organisation and Night Time Parental Interventions', *Pediatrics* 81, 1988, 762–71.
11 J. Bates, 'Issues in the Assessment of Difficult Temperament: A Reply to Thomas, Chess and Korn', *Merrill-Palmer Quarterly* 29, 1983, 89–97; J. Bates and K. Bayles, 'Objective and Subjective Components in Mothers' Perception of the Children From Age 6 Months to 3 Years', *Merrill-Palmer Quarterly* 30, 1984, 11–129; I. St James, I. Roberts and D. Wolke, 'Comparison of Mothers' with Trained Observers' Reports of Neonatal Behavioural Style', *Infant Behavioural Development* 7, 1984, 299–310.

11 BALANCING ACTS: WORK AND FAMILY

1 K. Gieve, *Balancing Acts: On Being a Mother*, Virago, London, 1989; S. Sharpe, *Double Identity: The Lives of Working Women*, Penguin, Harmondsworth, 1984; J. Brannen and P. Moss, *Managing Mothers: Dual Earner Households After Maternity Leave*, Unwin Hyman, London, 1991; A. Hochschild, *Double Shift: Working Parents and the Revolution at Home*, Viking Penguin, New York, 1989.
2 L. Segal, *Slow Motion: Changing Masculinities, Changing Men*, Virago, London, 1990.
3 G. Ochiltree and E. Greenblat, *Sick Children: How Working Mothers Cope*, AIFS Early Childhood Study Paper No. 2, Australian Institute of Family Studies, Melbourne, 1991.
4 M. Bitman, 'Selected Findings from Juggling Time: How Australian Families Use Time', Office of the Status of Women, Department of the Prime Minister and Cabinet, Canberra, 1992.
5 Bitman, 'Selected Findings from Juggling Time'; P. Moss and J. Brannen, 'Fathers' Employment', in C. Lewis and M. OBrien (eds), *Reassessing Fatherhood: New Observations on Fathers and the Modern Family*, Sage, London, 1987.
6 S. Arber, N. Gilbert and A. Dale, 'Paid Employment and Women's Health: A Benefit or a Source of Role Strain', *Sociology of Health and Illness* 7, 1985, 345–97.
7 G.W. Brown and T. Harris, *The Social Origins of Depression*, Tavistock Press, London, 1978.
8 P. Romito, 'Unhappiness After Childbirth', in I. Chalmers, M. Enkin and M. J.N.C. Keirse (eds), *Effective Care in Pregnancy and Childbirth*, Oxford University Press, Oxford, 1989, 1433–46; E.S. Paykel, E.M. Emms, J. Fletcher and E.S. Rassaby, 'Life Events and Social Support in Puerperal Depression', *British Journal of Psychology* 136, 1980, 339–46.

9 Hochschild, *Double Shift*; Moss and Brannen, 'Fathers' Employment'; G. Russell, *The Changing Role of Fathers*, Queensland University Press, St Lucia, 1983.
10 L. B. Tiedje and C. S. Darling-Fisher, 'Factors That Influence Fathers' Participation in Child Care', *Health Care for Women International* 14, 1993, 99–107.
11 A. Oakley, *The Sociology of Housework*, Martin Robertson, Oxford, 1974.
12 Oakley, *The Sociology of Housework*.
13 Moss and Brannen, 'Fathers' Employment'; Russell, *The Changing Role of Fathers*.
14 Hochschild, *Double Shift*; Moss and Brannen, 'Fathers' Employment'; Russell, *The Changing Role of Fathers*; Oakley, *The Sociology of Housework*.
15 E. Greenblat and G. Ochiltree, *Use and Choice of Child Care*, AIFS Early Childhood Study Paper No. 4, Australian Institute of Family Studies, Melbourne, 1993.
16 Hochschild, *Double Shift*.
17 J. Lazarre, *The Mother Knot*, McGraw Hill, New York, 1976.
18 Russell, *The Changing Role of Fathers*.

13 WHAT WOMEN DO ABOUT DEPRESSION

1 V. Welburn, *Postnatal Depression*, Fontana, Glasgow, 1980, 39.
2 J. McIntosh, 'Postpartum Depression: Women's Help-seeking Behaviour and Perceptions of Cause', *Journal of Advanced Nursing* 18, 1993, 178–84.
3 J. M. Holden, R. Sagovsky and J. L. Cox, 'Counselling in a General Practice Setting: Controlled Study of Health Visitor Intervention in Treatment of Postnatal Depression', *British Medical Journal* 298, 1989, 223–6; E. Taylor, 'Postnatal Depression: What Can A Health Visitor Do?', *Journal of Advanced Nursing* 14, 1989, 877–86; S. A. Elliot, 'Psychological Strategies in the Prevention and Treatment of Postnatal Depression', *Baillieres Clinical Obstetric Gynaecology* 3, 1989, 879–903.

APPENDIX 1 OTHER RESEARCH ISSUES

1 A. Jacoby and A. Cartwright, 'Finding Out About the Views and Experiences of Maternity Service Users', in *The Politics of Maternity Care: Services for Childbearing Women in Twentieth Century Britain*, J. Garcia, R. Kilpatrick and M. Richards(eds), Clarendon Press, Oxford, 1990, ch. 13, 238–55.
2 A. Taylor, 'Maternity Services: The Consumers View', *Journal of the Royal College of General Practitioners* 36, 1986, 157–60.
3 D. Sullivan and R. Beeman, 'Satisfaction with Maternity Care: A Matter of Communication and Choice', *Medical Care* 20, 1982, 321–30.
4 D. Locker and D. Dunt, 'Theoretical and Methodological Issues in Sociological Studies of Consumer Satisfaction with Medical Care', *Social Science and Medicine* 12, 1979, 283–92.
5 J. Green, V. Coupland and J. Kitzinger, 'Expectations, Experiences, and Psychological Outcomes of Childbirth: A Prospective Study of 825 Women', *Birth* 17, 1990, 15–23; B. Morgan, C. Bulpitt, P. Clifton and P. Lewis, 'Analgesia and Satisfaction in Childbirth' (The Queen Charlotte's 1000 Mother Survey), *Lancet* ii, 1982, 808–11.
6 S. Elliott, M. Anderson, D. Brough, J. Watson and A. Rugg, 'Relationship Between Obstetric Outcome and Psychological Measures in Pregnancy and the Postnatal Year', *Journal of Reproductive and Infant Psychology* 2, 1984, 18–22.

7 S. E. Romans-Clark, V. A. Walton, D. J. Dons et al., 'Which Women Seek Help For Their Psychiatric Problems?', *New Zealand Medical Journal* 103, 1990, 445–8; G. Brown and T. Harris, *Social Origins of Depression: A Study of Psychiatric Disorder*, Tavistock Press, London, 1978.
8 B. Barnett, K. Lockhart, D. Bernard, V. Manicavasagar and M. Dudley, 'Mood Disorders Among Mothers of Infants Admitted to a Mothercraft Hospital', *Journal of Paediatrics and Child Health* 29, 1993, 270–5.
9 J. Astbury, S. Brown, J. Lumley, R. Small, 'Birth Events, Birth Experiences and Social Factors in Depression After Birth', *Australian Journal of Public Health* 18, 1994, 176–84.
10 Brown and Harris, *Social Origins of Depression*.
11 P. A. L. Lancaster and E. L. Pedisich, *Caesarean Births in Australia, 1985–1990*, AIHW National Perinatal Statistics Unit, Sydney, 1993.

INDEX

'active say' 19, 73–80, 94–5, 126
alcohol consumption 96–7, 127
Alder and Bancroft 132, 289
Alder and Cox 132, 133, 289
Alder et al. 132, 289
amniocentesis 34, 92
anaesthesia *see* epidural; pain relief
analgesia *see* pain relief
Annual Reports of Maternal and Infant Health 1971–1980 105, 285
antenatal care
  check–ups 33–4, 35, 39–40, 96–7
  provider 17, 31–3, 35, 87
  satisfaction 19, 37–49, 58, 62–3, 94–5, 102
antenatal classes *see* childbirth education
antenatal screening 126
  see also amniocentesis; chorion villus sampling; fetal cardiotocography; glucose tolerance tests; ultrasound examination
appropriate technology *see* intervention
Arber et al. 203, 292
Armstrong et al. 4, 18, 20, 278, 280
artificial rupture of membranes (ARM) 53, 55
Astbury vii, 22, 26, 164, 190, 278, 280, 281, 291
Astbury and Bajuk 2, 278
Astbury et al. vii, 266, 278, 294
augmentation of labour 13, 53, 55, 68, 70, 92
Australian Bureau of Statistics 136, 290

Australian Institute of Health and Welfare National Perinatal Statistics Unit 54

baby
  crying problems 152–3, 178, 199, 259–60
  feeding problems 236–7
  illness 152–3, 176, 178–9, 230, 259
  sleeping problems 152–3, 236–7
'baby blues' 120
Barnett et al. 266, 294
Bartlett and Pennebaker 15, 45, 280, 282
Bastian and Lancaster 51, 282
Bates 198, 292
Bates and Bayles 199, 292
Bebbington et al. 124, 288
Beck 111, 286
Bell and Lumley 18, 280
Bennett 10, 279
Bennett et al. 41, 282
birth centre 14, 17, 31–3, 41–2, 51, 81–3, 92, 117–18, 127
birth events
  satisfaction 68–80
birthing services 31–2, 41–3, 59, 80–2, 86, 111, 116–18
birthweight 106, 131
Bitman 152, 203, 290, 292
Blazer et al. 126, 288
bottle-feeding 105–8, 133
  advice and support 107–8
Bowler 80, 284
Boyce and Todd 131, 288
Boyce et al. 26, 121, 281, 287
Bramadat and Dreidger 57, 283
Brannen and Moss 202, 292
breastfeeding 96–7, 101, 105–8, 109, 110, 113, 126–8, 131–3,

breastfeeding *(cont.)*
  178, 195–6, 233, 240
  advice and support 107–8
breech birth 65–6
British Journal of Psychiatry 3
British Medical Journal 2
Brockington et al. 120, 286
Brown, G. and Harris 124, 203, 266, 267, 287, 292, 294
Brown, S. and Lumley (1993) vii, 278; (1994) vii, 278
Brown, S. et al. vii, 278
Burnell et al. 116, 286

caesarean birth (section) 3, 4, 14, 15, 50–5, 69–70, 92, 109, 113, 126, 131, 266, 268
caring for children 139–60, 205–22, 262
  competing demands 141–2, 144, 213, 217, 219–21
  illness 243, 245–6, 248, 261–2
  see also baby, illness
  juggling time/quality time 141–2, 146–9
  mealtimes 165, 168–9, 191
  rewards 169–72, 206
  24-hour nature of 141–2, 145, 166, 205–7
Cartwright (1979) 70, 283; (1986a) 11, 12, 279, 280; (1986b) 15, 280; (1988) 11, 279
Cartwright and Smith 4, 279
Carty and Bradley 116, 286
cause 267–8
  see also depression after birth, contributing factors
Centre for the Study of Mothers' and Children's Health vii
cervical suture 92
Chalmers et al. 53, 80, 282, 284
Chesler 160, 291
child care 136, 216, 218, 231
childbirth education 62–3, 84–99, 117, 127
  attenders/non–attenders 86–9
  satisfaction 89–90
  type 88–9
Chodorow and Contratto 149, 157, 290, 291

chorion villus sampling 34
coding 22, 268–70
communication
  with family and friends 195, 250–60, 261–2
  with health professionals 194–5, 256–62
  with partner 192–5, 256–8, 261–2
complementary feeding *see* breastfeeding
confidence
  as a mother 165, 167–8, 178–9, 191, 216–17, 246–7
  with baby 95–6, 110, 113–14, 126, 129
Consultative Council on Obstetric and Paediatric Mortality and Morbidity 14, 50, 136, 137, 280, 282, 290
continuity of care 36–7, 41–9, 53, 64, 83
control *see* 'active say'
Cooper et al. (1988) 124, 288; (1993) 133, 289
coping and parenthood 191–201, 204–5, 219–20, 228, 258–60
counselling 189, 261
country of birth, mothers' 15–16, 43–9
Cox et al. (1984) 4, 278; (1987) 22, 26, 121, 122, 190, 280, 281, 286, 287, 292; (1993) 121, 122, 124, 182, 287, 288, 291
Crowell et al. 126, 288

Dalton 132, 133, 289
Day 120, 286
de facto *see* marital status
delivery *see* birth; breech birth; caesarean birth (section); forceps, birth assisted by; vaginal birth
demand feeding *see* breastfeeding
Dennerstein et al. 133, 289
Department of Health and Community Services, Victoria 14, 33
depression after birth 6, 8, 19, 20–2, 95, 110, 113, 114, 120–4, 158–9, 170, 173–89,

190–201, 210–14, 216, 222–4, 227–48, 249–62
advice 234, 239, 248, 260–2
as cause of dissatisfaction 3
contributing factors 6–8, 122–3, 125–34, 185–9, 190–201, 240–1
duration 181–6, 234–5, 239–40, 245–8
identification/diagnosis 120–1, 174–6
onset 181–6, 234–5, 239–40, 245–8
recovery 185–9, 231–2, 235, 241–2, 249–62
seeking help 250–60, 266–7
discriminant function analysis 200–1
doctor 71–2, 75, 83, 127, 233, 245, 261–2
see also general practitioner; psychiatrist; specialist obstetrician
domestic labour 146, 152–3, 176, 205–14, 235
Dragonas et al. 121, 287
Drapac and Rubinstein 101, 285

early discharge *see* length of hospital stay
Edinburgh Postnatal Depression Scale (EPDS) 13, 17, 21, 120–2, 124, 130, 175, 185–6, 190–201, 234, 241–2, 248, 266, 274
education, mothers' 17, 43–9, 76–7, 87, 127, 159, 209
see also social differences
elective caesarean *see* caesarean birth (section)
electronic fetal monitoring *see* fetal cardiotocography
Elliott (1989) 262, 293; (1990) 161, 291
Elliott et al. 68, 126, 265, 283, 288, 294
emergency caesarean *see* caesarean birth (section)
emotional support *see* support
emotional well-being 8, 95, 114, 120, 173–89, 216, 222–4
see also depression after birth

employment 136, 146, 189, 204–5, 214–21, 231–2, 262
and the experience of motherhood 214–21, 244–5
in pregnancy 127
see also unemployment
enema 51, 55, 92
epidural 3, 56, 66–7, 69–70, 90–1, 126
episiotomy 51, 53, 55, 56, 69–70, 92, 195
Erb et al. 10, 279
ethics approval 10, 13, 79
Ethnic Affairs Commission 11
exhaustion *see* fatigue
expectations about birth 96, 99
expectations about children 205–7, 228–9, 232, 243–4
experience of motherhood 2, 6, 8, 20–1, 161–72, 230–1
ambivalent feelings 170, 172, 190–1, 216–21, 238, 245
enjoyment/rewards 169–72, 206, 230, 232, 237, 244, 245
see also caring for children
Experience of Motherhood Questionnaire (EMQ) 22, 163–72, 232, 238, 245, 274–5

face-to-face interviews 16–17, 19, 23–4, 25
family income 17, 43–9, 87, 136–7, 209
see also income, women; social differences
fathers 64–6, 86, 100–1, 118, 157–8, 176–80, 189, 192–5, 198, 204–5, 207–14, 233, 235, 238–9, 256–7, 259, 261–2
at home 221–2, 242–3, 262
fatigue 168–9, 176–80, 186–9, 206, 214, 238
see also rest in hospital
fetal cardiotocography 31, 34–5, 70, 92
Fisher 131, 289
Flax 151, 290
Follow-up Study
feedback to participants 24
methodology 20–5
participation 22

Follow-up Study *(cont.)*
  representativeness 21–2
forceps, birth assisted by 3, 4, 15, 50, 51, 53, 55, 69–70, 92, 113, 126–31, 268

Garcia 37, 39, 281
gas and oxygen 66, 69–70, 90–1, 127
general anaesthetic 66, 69–70, 91
General Health Questionnaire 121
general practitioner 17, 31–3, 35, 36, 40–9, 62, 69, 87, 113, 127, 176, 250–5, 266
George and Sandler 133, 289
Gieve 202, 292
Giles et al. 49, 282
Gitlin and Pasnau 6, 279
glucose tolerance tests 34
'good' mother 139–60, 162–3, 221
Graham 162, 291
Graham and McKee 38, 281
Green et al. (1990a) 70, 79, 130, 264, 283, 284, 288, 293; (1990b) 80, 284
Greenblatt and Ochiltree 214, 293
Gregg et al. 7, 279
grief and loss 186–9, 195

Hannah et al. 130, 132, 288, 289
Harding 2, 5, 278, 279
Hardyment 149, 290
Harlow and Linet 4, 279
Harper and Richards 142, 290
Harris et al. (1989a) 131, 132, 133, 289; (1989b) 26, 121, 281, 287
health after birth 50–1, 103, 104, 108–9, 152–3, 186–9, 191, 195–8, 229–30, 236, 239–40, 259, 261–2
Health Department of Western Australia vii
Health Insurance Commission 32, 33
health-insurance status 17, 31–2, 41–9, 60–1, 87, 114–15, 116–17, 127, 136
  see also social differences
health policy 9, 80–3, 111, 116–18
  see also birthing services

Hewson and Bennett 4, 279
Hewson et al. 70, 283
Hochschild 202, 204, 213, 219, 292, 293
Holden et al. 262, 293
home birth 14, 17, 18, 51, 82, 127
home interview 22
  tape recording and transcription 23
  see also face-to-face interviews
hormones 6–8, 131–3, 186–9
  see also depression after birth, contributing factors
hospital antenatal clinic *see* public hospital clinic
hospital stay *see* length of hospital stay; postnatal care
housework *see* domestic labour
husbands *see* fathers

income
  women 136
  see also family income
induction of labour 3, 13, 52, 55, 56, 68, 70, 92
infant feeding *see* bottle-feeding; breastfeeding
information
  informal sources 97–8, 118
  see also satisfaction with information
Institute for Social Studies in Medical Care vii, 12
intervention 52–6, 68–70, 73–80, 81, 91–3
interviews *see* face-to-face interviews; home interviews
intrapartum *see* labour
involutional melancholia 6
isolation 166, 176–7, 186–9, 191, 215–16, 258–9

Jack 162, 291
Jacoby 45, 70, 282, 283
Jacoby and Cartwright 38, 264, 281, 293
James et al. 116, 286
Joffe and Grisso 4, 279

Keener et al. 198, 292
Keirse et al. 64, 283

Kozak 52, 282
Kumar and Robson 124, 287

labour 63–8
  length 67, 68, 76–80, 127, 131
  unwanted people 63–6, 74–80, 126, 129, 131
labour companion 63, 64, 65
labour management
  satisfaction 19, 56–80, 94–5, 102, 127
labour procedures *see* artificial rupture of membranes (ARM); augmentation of labour; breech birth; caesarean birth (section); enema; epidural; episiotomy; forceps, birth assisted by; induction of labour; shave; vacuum extraction (Ventouse)
labour ward 17, 51, 81–3, 127
Lancaster and Pedisich 54, 268, 282, 294
Last vii, 278
Lauren et al. 4, 279
Lazarre 221, 293
Leach 149, 153, 290
length of hospital stay 15, 102, 110–18, 126–7
  satisfaction 113
life events 195–8
Life Experiences Questionnaire (LEQ) 22, 164, 195–8, 200–1, 229, 230, 236, 240–1, 275–6
listening 262–3
  see also communication
Locker and Dunt 38, 57, 264, 281, 283, 293
logistic regression 48, 76–80, 97, 127, 130
Lord et al. 6, 278
Lumley (1985) 57, 283; (1986) 64, 283; (1993) vii, 278
Lumley and Astbury 84, 92, 284
Lumley and Brown, S. (1993a) vii, 278; (1993b) 80, 284
Lumley and Davey 100, 105, 285
Lumley et al. (1984) 13, 280; (1990) 9, 12, 33, 50, 51, 52, 53, 54, 55, 84, 110, 111, 279, 280, 281, 282, 284, 285

MacArthur et al. 50, 132, 282, 289

Macintosh 174, 189, 250, 291, 293
marital status 15–16, 43–9, 87, 106–7, 126–30, 228, 265
  see also social differences
Martin, C. (1979) 4, 279; (1990) 37, 49, 70, 281, 282, 283
Martin, J. 136, 290
material circumstances *see* social adversity
maternal age 15–16, 43–9, 87, 106, 127–30
  see also older women; social differences; young women
Maternal and Child Health nurse 118, 173, 176, 177, 181, 233–4, 246, 250–1, 253–6, 259, 260, 261–2
maternal mortality 50
maternity services *see* birthing services
McBride 162, 291
McDonald and Brownlee 137, 290
McGraw and Abplanalp 90, 284
medical case notes/records *see* women's reports and medical records
medication 189
mental health and well-being *see* emotional well-being
Michael 9, 12, 88, 279, 280, 284
midwife 17, 31–3, 61–2, 69, 71–3, 75, 83, 103–5, 127
midwives clinic 42–3
Mill 1, 278
Mill Park Maternal and Child Health Centre vii, 13
Ministerial Review of Birthing Services in Victoria 2, 9, 10, 12, 43, 51, 54–5, 59–60, 73, 80, 81, 84, 110, 116
misclassification 122
missing data 20, 76, 127
Morgan et al. 70, 264, 283, 293
Moss and Brannen 203, 204, 209, 213, 292, 293
Moss et al. 100, 116, 285, 286
mother and baby hospital 253, 259, 266–7
motherhood *see* experience of motherhood; caring for children

mother–infant relationship 170–2, 175–6
  see also caring for children, rewards
multiple births 16, 18, 74–5, 106, 119
Murray and Carothers 26, 121, 122, 281, 287

Naaktgeboren 63, 283
negative life events see life events
nitrous oxide see gas and oxygen
non-stress testing see fetal cardiotocography
Norbeck 22, 164, 190, 280, 291
Norr and Nacion 111, 286
Norr et al. 116, 286
Nott 182, 291
Nott and Cutts 121, 287
Nursing Mothers' Association 119

Oakley (1974) 208, 209, 213, 293; (1979) 31, 37, 38, 281; (1980) 1, 38, 278, 281; (1981) 23, 281; (1982) 34, 281; (1983) 57, 283; (1992) 98, 151, 285, 290
Oakley and Rajan 130, 288
obstetric complications see pregnancy and birth complications
Obstetric Physiotherapy Society 100, 101, 105, 285
obstetric procedure score 68, 69, 76–80, 81–2, 126, 201, 277
obstetric records see women's reports and medical records
obstetrician see specialist obstetrician
Ochiltree and Greenblatt 137, 203, 290, 292
O'Hara and Zekoski 125, 189, 288, 291
O'Hara et al. 124, 287
older women 106, 113, 265, 266, 268
O'Neill et al. 130, 288
operative delivery 52–6
  see also caesarean birth (section); forceps, birth assisted by; vacuum extraction (Ventouse)

oxytocin
  see augmentation of labour; induction of labour

paediatrician 267
pain 66–7, 69–70, 72, 78, 80, 90–1, 127
  see also pain relief
pain relief 55, 66–7, 69, 72, 76–80, 90–1, 105, 127
  see also epidural; gas and oxygen; general anaesthetic; pethidine
parity 16, 43–9, 59, 69–70, 71, 72, 74–80, 86, 110, 113, 115, 127–30, 265, 266, 268
  see also social differences
partners see fathers
Paykel et al. 203, 292
Perinatal Data Collection Unit, Victoria 51–2
perineal suture 51, 53–5, 92, 109
pethidine 66, 69–70, 90–1, 109, 126
Pill and Stott 162, 291
pilot testing 12–13, 19–20, 23
Pitt 132, 289
Pop et al. 121, 287
Porter and Macintyre 57, 82, 99, 118, 283, 284, 285, 286
positive life events see life events
positivistic science 5–6
Post and Ante Natal Depression Association (PaNDA) vii, 23
postal questionnaires advantages/disadvantages 16–17, 19, 56–7
post-hysterectomy depression 6
postnatal care
  lack of flexibility 100–1, 103–5, 109–10
  satisfaction 19, 95, 100–17, 126–7
postnatal depression 124–5, 175–6, 182, 227, 234, 238–9, 245, 247
  see also depression after birth
postnatal distress 120
postnatal stress 120
postpartum depression see depression after birth

Index

postpartum psychosis 120
poverty 136–7
power, statistical 18, 21–2, 81, 125–6, 130
practical support *see* support
preferences 82–3
  see also labour, unwanted people
pregnancy 31–49, 84–99
  attitude to 43, 47, 62–3, 127
  depression in 181–6
  future 126
  hospital admission 62–3, 101, 127, 131
pregnancy and birth complications 36, 41, 42, 81, 131, 265
pre-menstrual syndrome 6
preparation for childbirth *see* childbirth education
previous births *see* parity
previous psychiatric illness 186–9, 266–7
prompting 22
psychiatrist 245, 247, 250–2, 254, 266–7
psychologist 250, 255, 266
public hospital clinic 17, 31–3, 35, 36, 37, 40–9, 62, 113, 127
Pym et al. 51, 282

randomised trials 49, 53–4, 98–9, 115–16
Raskall 137, 290
Ratcliffe 6, 279
Redman et al. 88, 90, 93, 95, 97, 284
referral practices 266–7
Reid and McIlwaine 38, 281
reproduction
  and mental health and well-being 6–8
reproductive history 63, 126–7, 131
research methods 16–27, 264–70
  longitudinal 27
  qualitative 16, 25, 27, 268–70
  quantitative 16, 25, 27
  see also face-to-face interviews; home interviews; postal questionnaires; standardised questionnaires

researcher perspectives 2, 6, 7, 23–4
residence, metropolitan 15–16, 41–2, 82–3, 87, 126–8
residence, rural *see* rural women
rest in hospital 101, 103–5, 126
Rice 104, 105, 285
Rich 139, 290
Richards L. 142, 290
Richards M. 41, 282
risk 268
Romans-Clarkson et al. (1990a) 126, 288; (1990b) 266, 294
Romito 121, 125, 130, 182, 189, 203, 286, 288, 291, 292
rooming-in *see* rest in hospital; separation from baby
Roy et al. 121, 287
rural women 14, 15–16, 22, 41–2, 59, 82–3, 87, 88, 106, 126–8, 235–42, 242–8, 259
Russell 204, 209, 213, 225, 293

sample
  clinical/hospital 265–7
  population 264–7
sample size 14, 17, 18, 21–2
Sarason et al. (1978) 22, 26, 190, 280, 281, 291; (1983) 22, 190, 280, 292
satisfaction with care 3, 18–19, 26, 37–49, 56–80, 94–5, 101–5, 133–4
  assessment 56–7, 264
  timing of assessment 10, 38–9
  see also antenatal care, satisfaction; labour management, satisfaction; postnatal care, satisfaction
satisfaction with information 34–6, 39–40, 71–2, 76–80, 93–4, 102, 126–7
scan *see* ultrasound examination
Segal 202, 292
separation from baby 67, 69, 76–80, 100–1, 102, 105, 109–10, 126–7
Sewell et al. 22, 26, 190, 198, 280, 281, 291, 292
sex after birth 169, 191, 195
sex of baby 127
shared care 31–2, 41–2

Sharpe 202, 292
shave 51, 53, 55, 92
Shearer (1983) 57, 283; (1987) 57, 283; (1990a) 91, 284; (1990b) 133, 289
Shearman 9, 84, 279, 284
shopping 223–4
Silverman 98, 285
Simkin 20, 63, 280, 283
Simkin and Enkin 85, 88, 90, 97, 98, 284, 285
single women *see* marital status
Small et al. (1992) vii, 278; (1994a) vii, 278; (1994b) vii, 278
smoking 18, 96–7, 106, 127, 267
Snaith 121, 287
social adversity 130, 136–7, 186–9, 233, 261–2
 see also social differences
Social Biology Resources Centre vii, 10
social change 136–8, 202–4
social differences 17, 21, 26, 43–9, 59, 80, 82–3, 87–8, 96–7, 102, 106, 107–8, 113, 114, 125–30, 159, 265
social life 165, 166
 see also timeout
Social Support Questionnaire (SSQ) 22, 275
socio-demographic characteristics *see* education, mothers'; family income; health-insurance status; marital status; maternal age; social differences
specialist obstetrician 17, 31–3, 35, 36, 40–9, 62, 69, 79, 87, 113, 127, 195, 250–2, 254
Spock 153, 290
sport and exercise 210, 212, 223–6, 240, 243
St Clair 98, 284
St James 199, 292
Stamp and Crowther 132, 289
standardised questionnaires 25–6
 see also Edinburgh Postnatal Depression Scale (EPDS); Experience of Motherhood Questionnaire (EMQ); Life Experiences Questionnaire (LEQ); Toddler Temperament Scale (TTS)
statistical terms 271–3
Steer 80, 284
Stein A. et al. 130, 288
Stein G. 120, 286
stitches *see* perineal suture
Strasser and Davis 57, 283
stresses of parenthood 190–201
 see also coping and parenthood
study 237
 returning to 231–2, 233
Sullivan 110, 285
Sullivan and Beeman 15, 70, 264, 280, 283, 293
Sunbury Maternal and Child Health Centre vii, 13
support 186–9, 192–5, 197–8, 227, 233, 236, 240–1, 247
support group 256–8, 260, 261–2
Surtees et al. 124, 288
Survey of Recent Mothers (1989)
 methodology 9–16
 response rate 14–16
 representativeness 15–16, 18, 21, 26, 32–3, 51–2, 88, 265–7

talking *see* communication
Tamminen 132, 289
Tannen 194, 292
Taylor A. 15, 37, 102, 264, 280, 281, 285, 293
Taylor E. 262, 293
team midwifery 31, 49, 83
 see also birth centre
tear *see* perineal suture
temperament of child 186–9, 198–201, 261–2, 266
theories of knowledge 5–6
Thome 121, 287
Thorpe 121, 287
Tiedje et al. 207, 293
timeout 154–6, 165–7, 186–9, 222–6, 228, 240, 243, 261–2
 see also employment; social life
Toddler Temperament Scale (TTS) 22, 198–201, 231, 237, 244, 276–7
twins *see* multiple births

ultrasound examination   31, 34–6, 92
unemployment   137, 195
   see also employment
unplanned pregnancy   *see* pregnancy, attitude to
unwanted pregnancy   *see* pregnancy, attitude to
Urwin   145, 146, 290

vacuum extraction (Ventouse)   15, 52, 53, 54, 92, 268
vaginal birth   15, 51, 53–4, 69
Victorian Health Promotion Foundation   vii
violence   136

Wadd   105, 285
Waldenström and Nilsson   49, 282
Waldenström et al. (1987a)   116, 286; (1987b) 111, 286
Watson et al.   124, 287
Welburn   249, 293
Western Australian Ministerial Task Force to Review Obstetric, Neonatal and Gynaecological Services   12
Wieck   7, 279
Williams and Carmichael   130, 288
'woman-centred research'   5, 6
women of non-English speaking backgrounds   11–12, 14, 43–9, 88, 104–5, 106, 118, 126–30, 136–7, 265
   and translations   11–12, 15
   see also social differences
women without partners   *see* marital status

women's reports
   Follow-up Study   140, 142, 143, 144, 145, 146, 147, 148, 149, 150, 151, 152, 153–4, 155–6, 157–8, 161, 162–3, 165, 166, 167, 168, 170, 171, 172, 174, 175, 176, 177, 178–9, 179–80, 181, 182, 186, 187, 192–3, 194, 195, 196, 197, 198, 199, 200, 204–5, 206, 207, 210, 211, 212, 213, 215, 216, 217, 218, 219, 220–1, 222, 223, 224, 225, 227–48, 251, 252, 253, 254, 255, 256, 257, 258, 259, 260
   and medical records   1, 4, 13, 56–7
   reliability of   2, 3, 4, 56–7, 133–4, 198–9, 262
   survey comments   20, 26, 36, 37, 38, 39, 55, 56, 57, 60, 63, 64, 65, 66, 67, 70, 71, 72, 73, 75, 85, 89, 90, 93, 94, 101, 102, 103, 104, 107, 108, 109, 115, 116, 117, 118, 119, 122, 123
Woollett and Dosanjh-Matwala   100, 102, 105, 285
work
   paid   *see* employment
   unpaid   *see* caring for children; domestic labour
World Health Organization   52, 282

young women   15, 43–9, 113, 137
   see also social differences